D1594749

PACIFIC CREST TRAIL

From the Mexican Border to Tuolumne Meadows

Laura Randall

prior editions by Ben Schifrin, Ruby Johnson Jenkins,
Thomas Winnett, and Jeffrey P. Schaffer

 **WILDERNESS PRESS** . . . *on the trail since 1967*

PACIFIC CREST TRAIL: SOUTHERN CALIFORNIA
FROM THE MEXICAN BORDER TO TUOLUMNE MEADOWS

First edition 1973
Second edition 1977
Third edition 1982
Fourth edition 1989
Fifth edition 1995
Sixth edition 2003
Seventh edition 2020
Copyright © 1973, 1977, 1982, 1989, 1995, 2003, 2020 by Wilderness Press

Cover design: Scott McGrew
Book design: Travis Bryant
Maps: Scott McGrew
Cover photo: © Tandem Ride Photography/Shutterstock. A hiker overlooks the desert floor of Mount Laguna while
    hiking the Pacific Crest Trail.
Frontispiece photo: The PCT follows the bouldery granite and marble beds of the Whitewater River in Section C.
Opposite page: A plaque above a rest spot commemorates author and naturalist Jim Jenkins.
Interior photos: Laura Randall, unless otherwise noted on page; photos on pages 40–43 by Dan R. Lynch
Index: Potomac Indexing LLC

Library of Congress Cataloging-in-Publication Data

Names: Randall, Laura, 1967-
Title: Pacific Crest Trail : Southern California, from the Mexican border to Tuolumne Meadows / Laura Randall, Ben
    Schifrin, Ruby Johnson Jenkins, Thomas Winnett, Jeffrey P. Schaffer.
Description: Seventh edition. | Birmingham, Alabama : Wilderness Press, [2020] | Includes index.
Identifiers: LCCN 2017051196| ISBN 9780899978406 (paperback) | ISBN 9780899978413 (ebook)
Subjects: LCSH: Hiking—Pacific Crest Trail—Guidebooks. | Hiking—California, Southern—Guidebooks. | Walking—
    Pacific Crest Trail—Guidebooks. | Walking—California—Guidebooks. | Backpacking—Pacific Crest Trail—Guidebooks. |
    Backpacking—California, Southern—Guidebooks. | Pacific Crest Trail—Guidebooks. | California, Southern—Guidebooks.
Classification: LCC GV199.42.P3 R36 2018 | DDC 796.5109794—dc23
LC record available at https://lccn.loc.gov/2017051196

Published by 🐸 **WILDERNESS PRESS**
    An imprint of AdventureKEEN
    2204 First Ave. S., Suite 102
    Birmingham, AL 35233
    800-678-7006, fax 877-374-9016

Manufactured in China
Distributed by Publishers Group West

Visit wildernesspress.com for a complete listing of our books and for ordering information. Contact us at our website,
at facebook.com/wildernesspress1967, or at twitter.com/wilderness1967 with questions or comments. To find out more
about who we are and what we're doing, visit blog.wildernesspress.com.

DISCLAIMER

Although Wilderness Press and the author have made every attempt to ensure that the information in this book is accurate
at press time, they are not responsible for any loss, damage, injury, or inconvenience that may occur to anyone while using
this book. You are responsible for your own safety and health while in the wilderness. The fact that a trail is described in
this book does not mean that it will be safe for you. Be aware that trail conditions can change from day to day. Always check
local conditions, know your own limitations, and consult a map.

As any hiker knows, nature and our pathways into it are ever-changing; wildfires reshape whole forests and open up
views, floods and landslides obliterate long-established routes, roads and trails change as new routes are built and old trails are
abandoned, and businesses close. Your comments on recent developments or changes for future editions are always welcome.

While this guidebook revision has been under development for more than four years, at press time in the summer of
2020, COVID-19 is widely spread at critical levels in California, Oregon, and Washington. The Pacific Crest Trail Association is currently only recommending local, fully self-supported trips on the PCT that don't include travel to communities
along the trail. Follow local regulations and maintain physical distance between non-family members. Explore the PCT
locally or visit other beautiful trails near your home until it's safe to travel more fully. For the latest information on PCT
restrictions, visit pcta.org/covid-19.

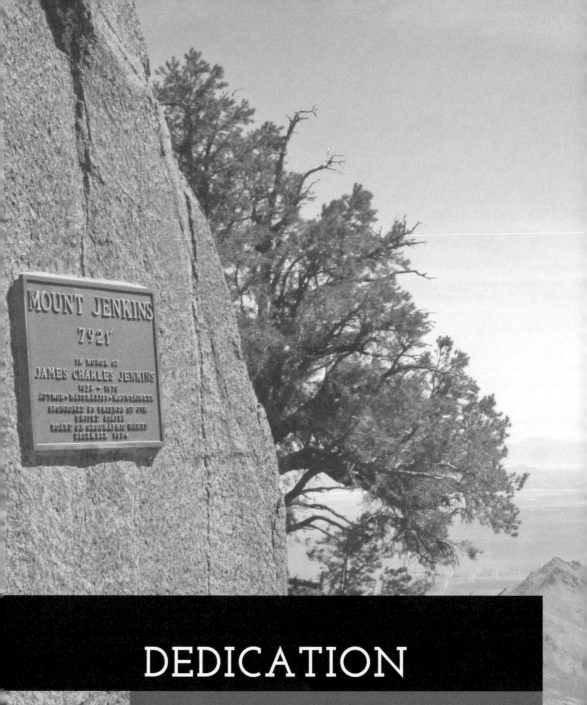

DEDICATION

To James Charles Jenkins, 1952-1979

Coauthor of the first three editions of this book

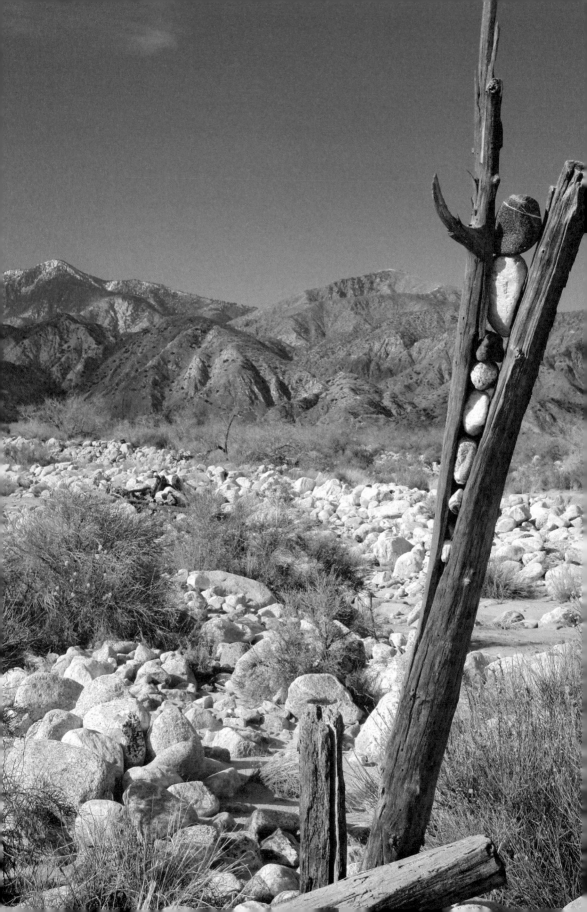

>>>CONTENTS

>>>ACKNOWLEDGMENTS

In late 2015 I was approached by the editors at Wilderness Press about updating the 2003 edition of *Pacific Crest Trail: Southern California.* I had hiked sections of the trail near my home in Los Angeles but was humbled and awed by the task being handed to me: helping a new generation of PCT hikers prepare for and understand more than 900 miles of one of the world's most famous trails. *The Pacific Crest Trail, Volume 1: California,* has been an essential resource for anyone planning a PCT trek since it was first published in 1973. The guide was last updated in 2003 by a quartet of writers with impressive backgrounds in outdoor adventure: Wilderness Press founder Thomas Winnett, who died in 2011 at the age of 89; Ben Schifrin and Jeffrey Schaffer; and Ruby Johnson Jenkins, who assumed the fieldwork for her son, James C. Jenkins, after he died in a freeway accident before completing work on the book's fourth edition.

Their dedication and obvious love for the PCT inspired me and stayed with me throughout my hikes and research. There are many, many others to thank for making the 2020 edition of this book possible: Jordan Summers, author of the 2020 editions of *Pacific Crest Trail: Northern California* and *Pacific Crest Trail: Oregon & Washington;* mapping legend Lon "Halfmile" Cooper; the entire staff of the Pacific Crest Trail Association; trail angels Jeff and Donna Saufley, Mike Herrera, Terrie and Joe Anderson, and many other unnamed folks who provided lifts, unexpected food, and kind words between Campo and Tuolumne Meadows; and Kevin Corcoran and all the volunteer Southern California Trail Gorillas, who have spent countless hours clearing, weed whacking, and doing whatever else it takes to keep the trail clear and safe for all hikers.

A special thanks must go to all those who accompanied me on long and short stretches or offered words and gestures of encouragement during the most challenging times: Ayleen Gontz, Maria Sammis, Anita Vonderheid, Amy Schad, Kit Ross, Donna Marovish, Laura Witten, Elana Verbin, and especially my family: John, Jack, and Theo Kimble for their love and support.

Finally, to the folks at Wilderness Press and AdventureKEEN, for giving me this incredible, life-changing opportunity and whose hard work, dedication, and enthusiasm were instrumental in getting this new edition on bookshelves.

—*Laura Randall*

>>>ABOUT THIS BOOK

Wilderness Press published its first book on the Pacific Crest Trail, *The Pacific Crest Trail, Volume 1: California*, in June 1973, more than 47 years ago. Since then, our PCT guidebook series has earned the reputation as the most essential resources available to anyone who is planning a PCT trek.

That first book is now covered by two books: *Pacific Crest Trail: Southern California (From the Mexican Border to Yosemite's Tuolumne Meadows)* and *Pacific Crest Trail: Northern California (From Tuolumne Meadows to the Oregon Border)*. A third book, *Pacific Crest Trail: Oregon & Washington*, first published in 1974, covers the Northwestern part of the PCT. Because only a few users of the Pacific Crest Trail are complete thru-hikers, the division of these texts makes it easier for planning the kind of shorter two- to three-week treks that most hikers do. These new editions feature all new photos and maps. Our detailed maps are based on the most current data available.

We would love to hear your comments or suggestions on how our books can be improved. Contact us at pct.wildernesspress.com, at facebook.com/wildernesspress1967, or at twitter.com/wilderness1967.

Thank you for buying and using this book. We hope it serves you well as you prepare for and set off on an incredible trip along the Pacific Crest Trail.

—Bob Sehlinger, Publisher, Wilderness Press

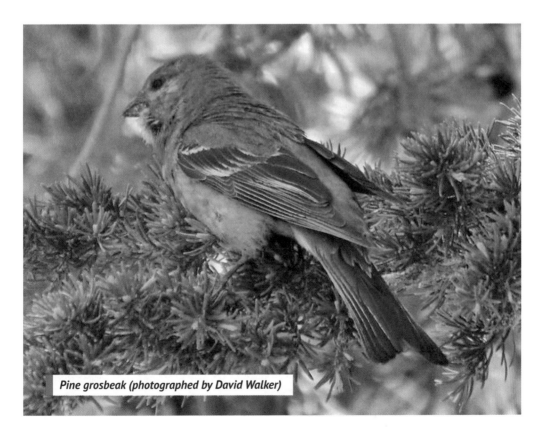

Pine grosbeak (photographed by David Walker)

>>>FOREWORD

One of the reasons I love outdoor adventures is because they are largely unscripted. Sure, you plan your precious days off and where you'll go. You meticulously pick your gear, food, and watering holes, and, hopefully, you get in and out of the wilderness without mishap. Life is good.

But the wilderness often throws you a curve, mostly because the backcountry is organized chaos. There may be a trail, even a great one like the Pacific Crest Trail, but it's often the case that Mother Nature tosses obstructions, such as downed trees, a landslide, a swollen river, a lightning storm, or even a wildfire, in your way. Seasoned veterans of the backcountry have come to expect such obstacles.

Working for the Pacific Crest Trail Association (PCTA), the nonprofit that protects, preserves, and promotes the Pacific Crest Trail, I regularly see firsthand the amazing work that dedicated volunteers do to keep the trail open and passable for hikers and horseback riders. PCTA staff and volunteers often go to the same places year after year to reopen the trail. Imagine what the trail would be like without this gargantuan effort.

All that says nothing of the risks that are still out there. Rattlesnakes, bears, and mountain lions can change things in a hurry. A simple shift in weather can bring snow at higher elevations, making that planned cowboy campout a little uncomfortable to say the least. We've all heard—or lived—stories about someone breaking an ankle or bears stealing food 15 miles from the trailhead. Suddenly, a weekend backpacking trip becomes a survival mission.

This risk comes with the territory. The more we get outside and away from our modern conveniences, the more we become comfortable facing the unknown. I love the anticipation of a

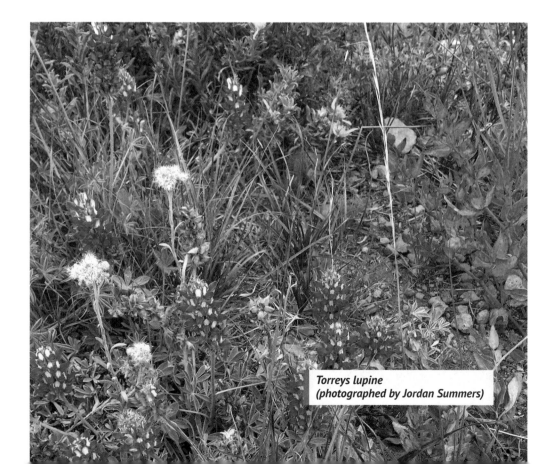

Torreys lupine
(photographed by Jordan Summers)

backcountry trip. For me, this element of wilderness travel is essential. Rising to meet challenges makes us feel alive. This guidebook will help show you the way and work out the logistics, but you never know what the day will bring. That's a good thing.

I can tell you it's always interesting. Personal contact with nature can push us to our limits and challenge our mental capacity to endure and survive. Most times it's tough but still safe and peaceful. But even experts sometimes find themselves in situations so dangerous it's foolish. The thing is, you never see it coming. You can be prepared, but each time out is a roll of the dice. I wouldn't have it any other way.

In testing ourselves outside, we live larger than is possible within the confines of our "real world" existence. Making good decisions about the weather and when to turn back is part of the challenge and the joy. Outside, I learned how to push my limits and when to back off.

It may be dangerous to, say, dodge a car flying though a downtown crosswalk, but that doesn't feed my soul. I want to do more than exist. I want to *really* feel alive. I do this on the trail, slowing down my awareness of time passing, turning minutes into hours, speeding up my heart rate, and sharpening my senses.

Contact with the natural world, wildflowers, flowing streams, wildlife, towering trees, and mountains—large, wild landscapes in general—reveals as much about who we are as it does about the natural world. Outside, we have space and time to look deep inside and reflect. We can put our worldly troubles into perspective and work through whatever it is we need to work through. We spend time in our own heads and realize how little we need to truly live large. On the trail we have time without distraction. We find enlightenment and we emerge stronger.

We build bonds with family and friends over our shared experiences and physical challenges in the wilderness. The friendships I have formed while hiking or climbing mountains are the most meaningful.

It all boils down to this: the trip you are about to take will be life changing. Whether you are going out for 26 miles or 2,650, what you will find on the Pacific Crest Trail will be nothing short of amazing. Most of the people I encounter who've hiked on the PCT—whether they've day-hiked, section-hiked, or thru-hiked—find rewards. They come away with an understanding about what's important in life. They have focus and grit. They learn determination out there. It's worth the price of admission.

The trail can teach us all of these things and more. I have never met anyone who completed a long trip on a trail or river who could not offer some kind of evidence of personal growth. Sure, we complain about the heat, the bugs, the sweat, the stench of our clothes, the dirt under our nails, and the blisters. Oh, the daily suffering! But then we launch with greater passion into the beauty and the grandeur and how small we felt out there. Have you ever seen a mountain lake so blue? A meadow so wonderfully inviting? Has a burger and a beer after a long day's walk ever tasted better? Ask any of them, even in the middle of whining about the switchbacks, and they'll tell you instantly how they would do it all again tomorrow.

This is who we are. This is how we live. We suffer, we grow, we feel alive. Then we rinse and repeat. Life is good. Definitely.

—*Mark Larabee*
PCTA Associate Director of Communications and Marketing

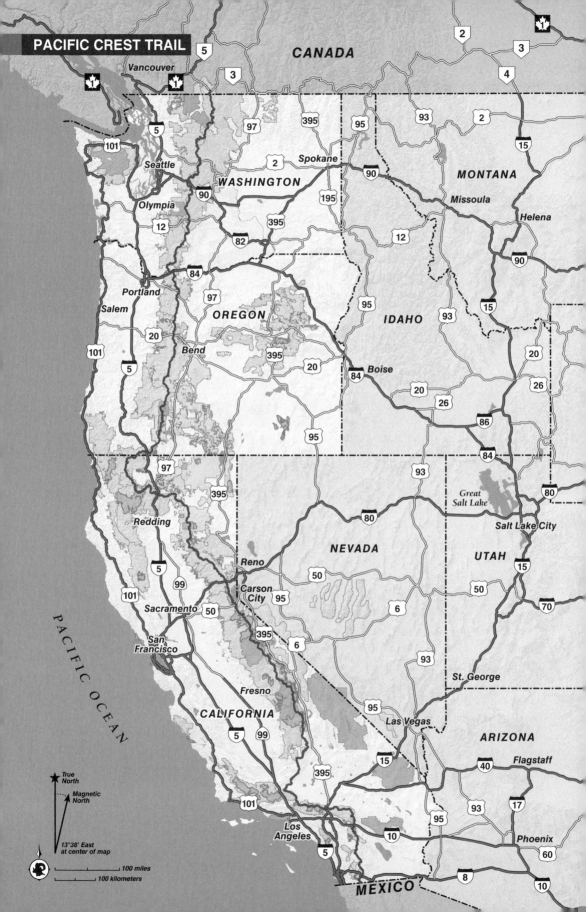

SOUTHERN CALIFORNIA

Section	Starting Mileage	Length
A: Mexican Border to Warner Springs	0.0	109.5
B: Warner Springs to San Gorgonio Pass	109.5	100.0
C: San Gorgonio Pass to I-15 near Cajon Pass	209.5	132.5
D: I-15 near Cajon Pass to Agua Dulce	342.0	112.5
E: Agua Dulce to CA 58 near Mojave	454.5	111.9
F: CA 58 near Tehachapi Pass to CA 178 at Walker Pass	566.4	85.6
G: CA 178 to John Muir Trail Junction	652.0	115.0
H: John Muir Trail Junction to Tuolumne Meadows	767.0	175.5

NORTHERN CALIFORNIA

Section	Starting Mileage	Length
I: Tuolumne Meadows to Sonora Pass	942.5	74.4
J: Sonora Pass to Lower Echo Lake	1,016.9	75.4
K: Lower Echo Lake to I-80	1,092.3	64.4
L: I-80 to CA 49	1,156.7	38.7
M: CA 49 to CA 70	1,195.4	91.5
N: CA 70 to Burney Falls	1,286.9	132.1
O: Burney Falls to Castle Crags	1,419.0	82.2
P: Castle Crags to Etna Summit	1,501.2	98.5
Q: Etna Summit to Seiad Valley	1,599.7	56.2
R: Seiad Valley to I-5 in Oregon	1,655.9	63.0

OREGON & WASHINGTON

Section	Starting Mileage	Length
A: Seiad Valley to I-5 in Oregon	1,655.9	63.0
B: I-5 near Siskiyou Pass to OR 140 near Fish Lake	1,718.9	54.5
C: OR 140 near Fish Lake to OR 138 near the Cascade Crest	1,773.4	74.4
D: OR 138 near the Cascade Crest to OR 58 near Willamette Pass	1,847.8	60.1
E: OR 58 near Willamette Pass to OR 242 at McKenzie Pass	1,907.9	75.9
F: OR 242 at McKenzie Pass to OR 35 near Barlow Pass	1,983.8	107.9
G: OR 35 near Barlow Pass to I-84 at Bridge of the Gods	2,091.7	55.5
H: Bridge of the Gods to US 12 near White Pass	2,147.2	147.7
I: US 12 near White Pass to I-90 at Snoqualmie Pass	2,294.9	98.2
J: I-90 at Snoqualmie Pass to US 2 at Stevens Pass	2,393.1	71.0
K: US 2 at Stevens Pass to WA 20 at Rainy Pass	2,464.1	127.0
L: WA 20 at Rainy Pass to BC 3 in Manning Provincial Park	2,591.1	70.3

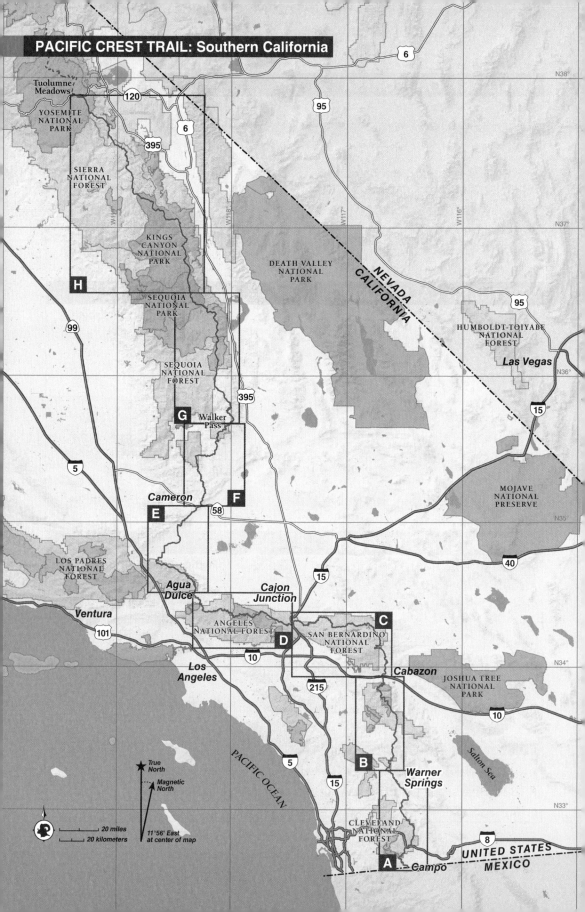

PACIFIC CREST TRAIL: Southern California

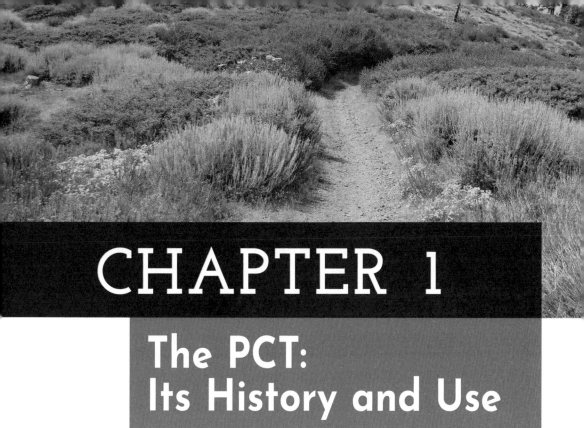

CHAPTER 1

The PCT:
Its History and Use

During the 1800s Americans traveling west toward the Pacific States were confronted with mountain barriers, such as the Cascades and the Sierra Nevada. The idea of making a recreational trek along the crest of these ranges probably never entered anyone's mind and most likely did not occur until the 1880s. However, relatively early in the 1900s, a party did make a recreational, multiday crest traverse of a part of the Sierra Nevada. From July 8 to July 25, 1913, Charles Booth, accompanied by his wife, Nora, and two friends, Howard Bliss and Elmer Roberts, made a pack trip from Tuolumne Meadows north to Lake Tahoe. Today's Pacific Crest Trail (PCT) closely follows much of their trek. (*Note:* For brevity in this book, we refer to the Pacific Crest Trail as the PCT. The official name is the Pacific Crest National Scenic Trail, abbreviated PCNST. However, that abbreviation is more cumbersome, and essentially no one uses it.)

CONCEPTION OF THE PCT

One of the earliest proposals for the creation of a Pacific Crest Trail is contained in the book *Pacific Crest Trails* by Joseph T. Hazard (Superior Publishing Co., 1946). He writes that, in 1926, Catherine Montgomery, an avid outdoorswoman and teacher at the Western Washington College of Education in Bellingham, suggested to him that there should be:

> A high winding trail down the heights of our western mountains with mile markers and shelter huts—like these pictures I'll show you of the "Long Trail of the Appalachians"—from the Canadian Border to the Mexican Boundary Line!

Above: The trail enters the Angeles National Forest above Wrightwood in Section D.

Hazard writes that, on that very night, he conveyed Montgomery's suggestion to the Mount Baker Club of Bellingham, which was enthusiastic about it. He says that soon a number of other mountain clubs and outdoors organizations in the Pacific Northwest adopted the idea and set about promoting it.

More recent research has unearthed evidence that the first written record of the idea for the PCT occurred even earlier than Montgomery's plea. In 1918 a U.S. Forest Service ranger in Oregon named Fred W. Cleator led a six-man crew in routing and posting a road from Mount Hood to Crater Lake. However, the budget was cut and so the road was left as a trail. Named the Oregon Skyline Trail, it was one of the early links of the PCT. Cleator's pencil-scrawled field diary, discovered by academic researchers in 2014, includes an August 20, 1918, entry in which he speculates "that a Skyline Trail the full length of the Cascades in Washington and Oregon, joining a similar

trail in the Sierras of California, would be a great tourist advertisement" and "fine to plan upon." In 1928 Cleator became supervisor of recreation for Region 6 (Oregon and Washington) of the U.S. Forest Service. He established and began to develop the Cascade Crest Trail, a route down the spine of Washington from Canada to the Columbia River. Later, he extended the Oregon Skyline Trail at both ends so that it, too, traversed a whole state. In 1937 Region 6 of the U.S. Forest Service developed a design for PCT markers and posted them from the Canadian border to the California border.

But the U.S. Forest Service's Region 5, which includes California, did not follow this lead. Eventually, a private citizen provided the real spark, not only for a California segment of the PCT but indeed for the PCT itself. In the early 1930s the idea of a Pacific Crest Trail entered the mind of Clinton C. Clarke of Pasadena, California, who was then chairman of the executive committee of the Mountain League

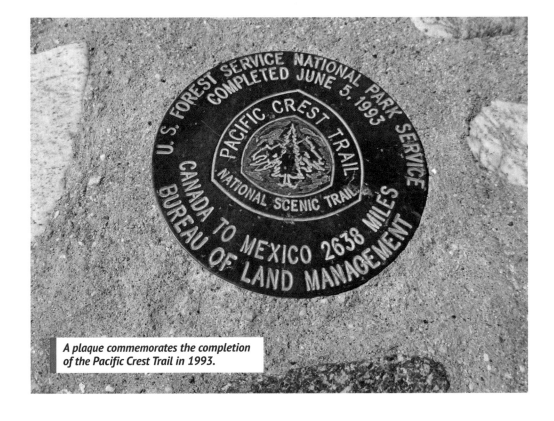

A plaque commemorates the completion of the Pacific Crest Trail in 1993.

of Los Angeles County. A graduate of Harvard who moved west and spent summers trekking the high Sierras, Clarke launched a passionate one-man letter-writing campaign, urging the heads of the U.S. Forest Service, Sierra Club, and other outdoors clubs to consider a super-trail from Mexico to Canada.

"In March, 1932," writes Clarke in *The Pacific Crest Trailway* (The Pacific Crest Trail System Conference, 1945), he "proposed to the United States Forest and National Park Services the project of a continuous wilderness trail across the United States from Canada to Mexico. . . . The plan was to build a trail along the summit divides of the mountain ranges of these states, traversing the best scenic areas and maintaining an absolute wilderness character." For years, Clarke insisted on calling his proposed wilderness corridor the John Muir Trail, but eventually relented to protests that the name belonged exclusively to the High Sierras area where Muir's legacy is so distinguished. When Harold C. Bryant, acting director of the National Park Service, wrote to Clarke in 1934 with several other name suggestions, Clarke gave in and embraced one of them, the Pacific Crest Trail.

The proposal included the formation of additional Mountain Leagues in Seattle, Portland, and San Francisco by representatives of youth organizations and hiking and mountaineering clubs, similar to the one in Los Angeles. These Mountain Leagues would then take the lead in promoting the extension of the John Muir Trail northward and southward to complete a pathway from border to border. When it became evident that more than Mountain Leagues were needed for such a major undertaking, Clarke led the formation of the Pacific Crest Trail System Conference, with representatives from the three Pacific Coast states. He served as its president for 25 years.

As early as January 1935, Clarke published a handbook/guide to the PCT, giving the route in rather sketchy terms: "The Trail goes east of Heart Lake, then south across granite fields to the junction of Piute and Evolution Creeks." This covers about 9 miles.

In the summer of 1935—and again the next three summers—groups of boys under the sponsorship of the YMCA explored the PCT route in relays, proceeding from Mexico on June 15, 1935, to Canada on August 12, 1938. This exploration was under the guidance of a YMCA secretary, Warren L. Rogers, who served as executive secretary of the Pacific Crest Trail System Conference from 1932 to 1957, when Clarke died (at age 84) and the conference dissolved. (Rogers was an enthusiastic hiker—and mountaineer—despite a bout with polio as a child that left him with a limp.) On his own, Rogers more or less kept the idea of the PCT alive until hiking and trails began receiving national attention in the 1960s. He launched a determined campaign to take possession of Clarke's papers after his death and continued to promote the trail and its joys through correspondence, camping magazines, and radio shows almost to the time of his death in 1992 at age 83.

National Trails System

In 1965 the Bureau of Outdoor Recreation, a federal agency, appointed a commission to conduct a nationwide trails study. The commission, noting that walking for pleasure was second only to driving for pleasure as the most popular recreational activity in America, recommended establishing a national system of trails of two kinds—long National Scenic Trails in the hinterlands and shorter National Recreation Trails in and near metropolitan areas. The commission recommended that Congress establish four scenic trails—the already existing Appalachian Trail, the partly existing Pacific Crest Trail, the Potomac Heritage Trail, and the Continental Divide Trail. Congress responded by passing, in 1968, the National Trails System Act, which set the framework for a system of trails and specifically made the Appalachian and Pacific Crest Trails the first two National Scenic Trails.

Today, there are 11 National Scenic Trails, totaling more than 18,000 miles, within the National Trails System. They are long-distance trails (more than 100 miles long) and are recreational in nature. Just as wonderful for a short day visit as a long-distance backpacking adventure, these trails call to all who want to explore America's natural landscapes.

The Proposed Route

Meanwhile, in California, the U.S. Forest Service in 1965 had held a series of meetings about a route for the PCT in the state. These meetings involved people from the U.S. Forest Service, the National Park Service, the State Division of Parks and Beaches, and other government bodies charged with responsibility over areas where the trail might go. These people decided that so much time had elapsed since Clarke had drawn his route that they should essentially start all over. Of course, it was pretty obvious that segments like the John Muir Trail would not be overlooked in choosing a new route through California. By the end of 1965 a proposed route had been drawn onto maps. (We don't say *mapped* because that would imply that someone had actually covered the route in the field.)

When Congress, in the 1968 law, created a citizens' advisory council for the PCT, it was the route devised in 1965 that the U.S. Forest Service presented to the council as a first draft of the final PCT. This body of citizens was to decide all the details of the final route; the U.S. Forest Service said it would adopt whatever the citizens wanted. The advisory council was also to concern itself with standards for the physical nature of the trail, markers to be erected along the trail, and the administration of the trail and its use.

In 1972 the council agreed on a route, and the U.S. Forest Service put it onto maps for internal use. Because much of the agreed-upon route was cross-country, these maps were sent to the various national forests along the route,

for them to mark a temporary route in the places where no trail existed along the final PCT. This they did—but not always after fieldwork. The result was that the maps made available to the public in June 1972 showing the final proposed route and the temporary detours did not correspond to what was on the ground in many places. A common flaw was that the U.S. Forest Service would base a segment on a preexisting U.S. Forest Service map that was incorrect, showing a trail where there was none.

Perfect or not, the final proposed route was sent to Washington for publication in the *Federal Register,* the next step toward its becoming official. A verbal description of the route was also published in the *Federal Register* on January 30, 1973. But the material in the register did not give a precise route that could be unambiguously followed; it was only a general outline, and the details in many places remained to be settled.

Private Property Glitches

As construction on PCT segments began, many hikers were optimistic that the entire trail could be completed within a decade. Perhaps it could have, if it weren't for private property located along the proposed route. While some owners readily allowed rights-of-way, many others did not, at least initially, and years of negotiations passed before some rights were finally secured. While negotiations were in progress, the U.S. Forest Service sometimes built new trail segments on both sides of a parcel of private land, expecting to extend a trail segment through it soon after. At times this approach backfired, such as in the northern Sierra Nevada in the Gibraltar environs (Section M, *Pacific Crest Trail: Northern California*). The owners of some property never gave up a right-of-way, and so a new stretch of trail on Gibraltar's south slopes was abandoned for a snowier, costlier stretch on its north slopes, completed in fall 1985. But at least the stretch was built.

The major obstacle to the trail's completion had been the mammoth Tejon Ranch, which began in Civil War days as a sheep ranch, then later became a cattle ranch, and in 1936 became a public corporation that diversified its land use and increased its acreage. This "ranch," about the size of Sequoia National Park, straddles most of the Tehachapi Mountains. An agreement between the ranch's owners and government representatives was finally reached, and in 1993 this section of the PCT was completed. However, rather than traversing the length of the Tehachapi Mountains as intended by Congress, the PCT for the most part follows miles of roads along the west side of the high desert area of Antelope Valley before ascending to the edge of ranch property in the north part of the range. This part of the trail is described in Section E.

In 2008 Tejon Ranch Company unveiled a landmark conservation and land-use agreement providing the framework for conserving up to 90% of Tejon Ranch—about 240,000 acres. In keeping with the original vision for the PCT, a significant part of the plan includes a set of easements that will protect the trail corridor and allow the PCT to be relocated from the floor of the Mojave Desert to the crest of the Tehachapi Mountains, following the route agreed upon by the U.S. Forest Service, the Pacific Crest Trail Association (PCTA), and the Tejon Ranch Company.

In May 2014, The Tejon Ranch Conservancy received the final paperwork for a 10,000-acre conservation easement from the Tejon Ranch Company, protecting habitat for the endangered California condor and other threatened, endangered, and sensitive plant and animal species and associated habitats, as well as vistas visible from a proposed new section of trail. This is the first tangible act in relocating 37 miles of the PCT from the Mojave Desert to the Tehachapi Mountains, the largest relocation project since the trail's official completion in 1993. The PCT easement still needs to be finalized, setting the route for the trail through Tejon Ranch and identifying off-trail campsites and access to critical water sources. The actual trail construction and realignment is still years away.

In 2016 an opportunity arose allowing the PCTA to acquire 245-acre Landers Meadow in Kern County, California, which was transferred into public ownership and incorporated into the Sequoia National Forest in 2018. Through member and community donations, the PCTA was able to protect this wet meadow and keep the trail uninterrupted along the route.

Finally, there is another stretch in Northern California, covered in *Pacific Crest Trail: Northern California*, where the route uses existing roads. To get the trail off a dangerous road walk, a new footbridge would need to be built across the Klamath River, an expensive and time-consuming project with little energy behind it. The lack of the bridge means that PCT travelers must tread 7.3 miles along the road. While a new bridge would cross the Klamath River just downstream of Seiad Valley, the town would remain an important resupply point for PCT hikers and horseback riders regardless.

Golden Spike Dedication

The Pacific Crest National Scenic Trail was officially dedicated on National Trails Day, June 5, 1993, a lengthy 25 years after Congress passed the National Trails System Act that had mandated it. The dedication was touted as the Golden Spike Completion Ceremony, in which a "golden" spike was driven into the trail, a reenactment of the 1869 ceremony at Promontory Point near Ogden, Utah, where the Central Pacific and Union Pacific railroad companies converged to complete the transcontinental railroad. For the PCT, there were no competing trail crews, so a PCT site close to metropolitan Southern California was chosen because it was the final easement acquired: a flat at the mouth of a small valley on the north side of Soledad Canyon (Section D, map 6). Protected under a canopy to shelter them from the unseasonably cold, windy, drizzly weather, Secretary of the Interior Bruce Babbitt and others spoke to an unsheltered audience of about 300 hearty souls (and a dozen or so others protesting various unrelated environmental issues). The trail was proclaimed to be 2,638 miles long officially, though the accuracy of this mileage is questionable because this number existed as early as 1990, before the completion of several stretches in Southern California and in the southern Sierra Nevada, and before the major relocation of the Hat Creek Rim stretch north of Lassen Volcanic National Park.

Future relocations are likely, and so the authors of the Pacific Crest Trail books, following the lead of our fellow hikers, have used the 2020 version of Lon "Halfmile" Cooper's trail mileage for all locations.

SOME WHO WALKED AND RODE

No doubt hikers in the 19th century did parts of the PCT, though that name didn't exist back then. It may be that someone walked along the crest from Mexico to Canada or vice versa many years ago. The first documented hiker to complete the entire three-state trek was Martin Papendick (1922–2000), who did so in 1952, when a tristate trail was still a dream and the PCT was decades away. It was his second attempt, and it took him 149 days to backpack from Manning Park south to Campo. The first person to receive official acknowledgment from the U.S. Forest Service for hiking the actual PCT route in one continuous journey (that is, a thru-hike)—in 1970—was Eric Ryback, who described his north-to-south trek in *The High Adventure of Eric Ryback*. This was quite a feat for anyone, much less a 130-pound 18-year-old, hiking solo in the more difficult north-to-south direction without a guidebook or detailed maps. His 1971 book focused attention on the PCT, and other people began to plan end-to-end

treks. In 2009 Ryback became a PCTA board member and designed and funded the PCT completion medal.

As mentioned earlier, in June 1972, the U.S. Forest Service maps of the PCT route became available to the public, and the race was on. The first person to hike this entire route from south to north was Richard Watson, who finished it on September 1, 1972. Barely behind him, finishing four days later, were Wayne Martin, Dave Odell, Toby Heaton, Bill Goddard, and Butch Ferrand. Very soon after them, Henry Wilds went from Mexico to Canada solo. In 1972 Jeff Smukler did the PCT with Mary Carstens, who became the first woman to make it. The next year, Gregg Eames and Ben Schifrin set out to follow the official route as closely as possible, whether by trail or cross-country. Schifrin—who would go on to coauthor early editions of the California volume of this guidebook—had to drop out with

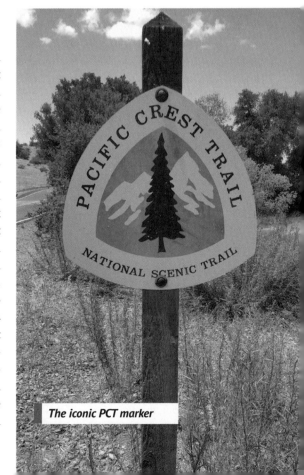

The iconic PCT marker

a broken foot at Odell Lake, Oregon (he finished the route the next year), but Eames got to Canada and is probably the first person to have walked the official route almost without deviation.

In 1975 at least 27 people completed the PCT, according to Chuck Long, who was one of them and who put together a book of various trekkers' experiences. Perhaps as many as 200–300 hikers started the trail that year, intending to do it all. In 1976 one who made it all the way was Teddi Boston, the first woman to solo the trail. Like Ryback, the 49-year-old mother of four made the trek the hard way, north to south.

Fascination with the trail steadily dropped, so that by the late 1980s, perhaps only a dozen or so thru-hikers completed the entire trail in a given year. However, as completion of the trail approached, interest in it waxed, and some notable hikes were done. As enthusiasm for the trail continued to grow, so did a thirst for chronicling the personal stories and adventures of individual hikers. Countless PCT memoirs can be found on bookstore shelves and blogs these days, providing both useful data for serious hikers and enjoyment for armchair adventurers.

However, in a trail guide, space is limited, so we will mention only a select few who set "higher" goals. In the past we recommended that the thru-hiker allow five to six months for the entire PCT. No more, thanks to ultralight backpacking first espoused by Ray and Jenny Jardine. In 1991 the couple completed the entire trail (their second thru-hike) in only three months and three weeks, and Ray subsequently wrote a how-to book (see page 11) based on the accomplishment.

A few thru-hikers not only did the PCT but also did the two other major north–south National Scenic Trails, the Continental Divide Trail (CDT) and the Appalachian Trail (AT). The first triple-crown hiker may have been Jim Podlesay, hiking the AT in 1973, the PCT in 1975, and the CDT in 1979. Back in 1975 many new stretches of the PCT had yet to be built, and in 1979 the CDT's route was still largely a matter of whatever you chose it to be. By 1980 the PCT was essentially complete, except for gaps between the Mexican border and the southern Sierra and the initial southern Washington stretch. And with the PCT mostly complete, the first person who hiked it plus the AT and CDT may have been Lawrence Budd, who did all three in the late 1980s. Starting earlier but finishing later was Steve Queen, who hiked the PCT in 1981, the AT in 1983, and the CDT in 1991. The first woman may have been Alice Gmuer, who hiked the PCT in 1987 and 1988, the AT in 1990, and the CDT in 1993. Close behind was Brice Hammack, who over eight summers completed the last of the three trails in 1994—at the very respectable age of 74.

In the 21st century, some outstanding hiker-athletes have posted speed records and other fantastic on-trail accomplishments. A PCT thru-hike can take up to six months for most hikers. In 2006 triple-crown hiker Scott Williamson made it to Canada in three months and then turned around to return to the Mexico border, which he reached in three more months. This was his second yo-yo hike (back-to-back thru-hike) on the PCT and his ninth PCT thru-hike. (His first yo-yo was completed two years before on his fourth PCT thru-hike.)

In 2013 Heather Anderson traversed the route in 60 days, 17 hours. This was her second PCT thru-hike, and as of 2020, she holds the record for women on the trail. More recently, in 2016, 26-year-old Belgian dentist Karel Sabbe completed the trail with a new fastest-known-time record of 52 days, 8 hours, and 25 minutes. (There is no official record of PCT speed records; these numbers rely on verified GPS tracks and the honor of those making the claims.)

While there have been thousands of successful thru-hikers on the PCT, few equestrians have matched this feat. Often, thru-hikers are unable to hike every foot of the trail (because of fire closures, snowpack, stream crossings, tree fall, or resupply exits), and for thru-equestrians, this feat has so far proved extremely challenging due to icy snowfields impassable for stock. Perhaps the first equestrians to do the trail were

Don and June Mulford in 1959. Barry Murray and his family rode it in two summers in the early 1970s. Much later, in 1988, Jim McCrea became the first thru-equestrian, completing the entire trail in just under five months. Retired veterinarian and former PCTA president Ben York rode the entire PCT on horseback in 1992 and again in 1996.

THE PCT IN THE 21st CENTURY

The escalation of social media and the internet had an unprecedented effect on the PCT in the last decade, creating new channels for hikers to stay connected and driving the increased popularity of the trail. Thru-hikers can now "meet" one another ahead of their starts through PCT Facebook groups, share information and ask questions on the discussion boards of Reddit, and post photos and videos from the trail on Instagram. The PCTA shares important updates and other data on its Twitter feed, @PCTAssociation, using the hashtag #PacificCrestTrail.

Cheryl Strayed's best-selling 2012 memoir *Wild* and the subsequent film of the same name, starring Reese Witherspoon, also had an impact on the PCT in the 21st century. Strayed recounted her 1,100-mile solo hike in 1995, weaving personal struggles with descriptions of stunning scenery and all the bruises, aches, and lost toenails that come with long-distance hiking. Strayed used a previous version of this guide, *The Pacific Crest Trail, Volume 1: California* (before it was split into two), to navigate the first part of the trail. *Wild* won multiple awards and inspired many people to get on the trail.

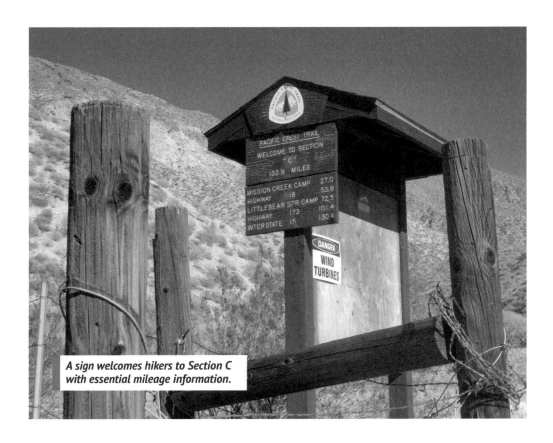

A sign welcomes hikers to Section C with essential mileage information.

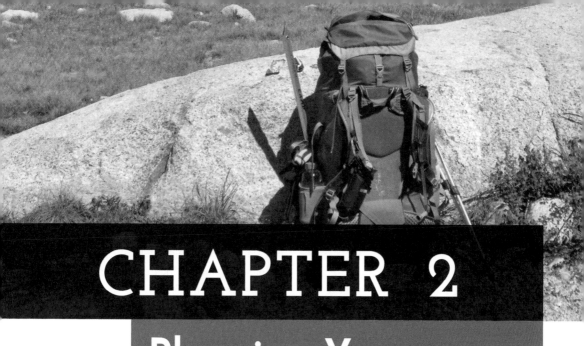

CHAPTER 2

Planning Your PCT Hike

TREKKING DAYS OR WEEKS VERSUS TREKKING MONTHS

On the basis of our limited research, we have concluded that the majority of those who buy this book will do parts of the Pacific Crest Trail (PCT) as a series of short excursions, each lasting about two weeks or less. More than 90% of all backpackers take a weekend to hike about 6 miles in from a trailhead to a known beauty spot—lake, mountain, stream—and return with memories of a wonderful trip. Others may venture out for a couple of weeks, seeing several beauty spots along the route.

For these hikers, less logistical planning is necessary than for thru-hikers, but there are still considerations. Depending on your goal, you may need to resupply once or twice. If so, identify the location—grocery store, post office, hostel—where you intend to resupply, and plan to carry sufficient food to reach the next resupply point, plus food for one extra day. Also consider what gear you will need. Will you be traveling solo, with a partner, or in a group? Going solo requires greater attention to gear weight than if you're sharing equipment with a partner or group. How long will you be gone? And what is your experience level? The answers to these questions will help you decide which items to pack. On page 10 is a checklist to help with your packing. You may want to carry more or less, but regardless of your preferences, be prepared for potentially bad weather. Without food, your backpack should weigh only about 15–20 pounds; allow an additional 2 pounds per person

Above: The average backpack, without food, weighs 15–20 pounds.
(photographed by Jordan Summers)

ITEMS TO CONSIDER FOR YOUR HIKE

day pack/backpack (plus pack cover/pack liner)	biodegradable soap
PCT permit (must carry a paper copy at all times)/wilderness permit/CA campfire permit	quick-dry towel and/or washcloth
emergency contact information	trowel
paper maps; digital maps stored on your smartphone are a bonus	toilet paper
compass	plastic zip-top bags for used toilet paper
GPS/tracking/emergency signal device	hand sanitizer
guidebook(s) (This one!)*	first aid kit and first aid notes*
emergency whistle	molefoam/blister kit
shelter (tent/tarp/mid/hammock/bivy sack)	mosquito repellent
sleeping bag	bear repellent (pepper spray)
sleeping pad or air mattress	headlamp and batteries
nylon or Tyvek ground cloth	smartphone
stuff sacks	watch
50 feet of 3-millimeter nylon cord (shelter guy outs/laundry line)	keys
hiking shoes or boots	wallet/cash/credit card/ATM card
socks (wool)	water bottle(s)/hydration bag
lightweight camp shoes or sandals	water purification system
shorts	mini lighter or matches in waterproof container
pants	stove/fuel/pot
T-shirt or short-sleeved shirt	bowl/cup
long-sleeved shirt	spoon/fork
windshirt/sweatshirt	food/beverage mixes
thermal top/bottom	salt/pepper/spices
underwear	1-gallon odor-proof zip-top freezer bags (for food and trash)
swimsuit	bear-proof food-storage container
raingear or poncho (the latter can double as a ground cloth)	small pocketknife/small multitool
down puffy (vest/hoodie/jacket)	camera and accessories
warm cap/brimmed hat	micro-tripod
lightweight gloves	compact binoculars
bandanna	trekking poles
glasses/contact lenses	ice ax
sunglasses (polarized)	microspikes/crampons
sunscreen and lip balm (with sunscreen)	fishing gear and fishing license
personal-hygiene items	duct tape for emergencies (for example, broken pack, tent pole, or shoe)
prescription medications, plus list*	

* may be stored on smartphone

per day for food. If you are out for a week, your pack initially should be under 35 pounds. One thing is certain in backpacking: when the weight goes up, the fun goes down. When day or section hiking, it is easier to pinpoint your clothing requirements for that specific time of year. However, a lot can happen between point A and point B, so it is important to research what you might encounter in each section or state that you choose to hike. Ultimately, your preparations must include, at the least, a way to return to your car or reach home at the end of your hike.

Roughly 86% of the PCT in California can be day hiked, averaging about 15 miles a day; over some sections you'll do less than 5 miles, while over others you'll do more than 25 (but less than 30). Most sections in this book include information on day hikes for each section, ranging from easy to strenuous, with information on how to reach the trailheads by car.

There are at least five advantages to day hiking. First, access is easier and less complicated. The national parks and the popular wilderness areas require wilderness permits for overnight stays, and some popular PCT stretches even have trailhead quotas for overnighters, but fewer areas require permits for day hikers. Second, day hiking does not require in-depth planning or preparation—though you should always be prepared for changing weather, carry the Ten Essentials, and know your limitations. And have a plan for emergencies—inform a trusted friend of your whereabouts and leave a list of what to do if you don't return as promised. Third, because your pack is lighter, you may enjoy the hike more because you'll expend less effort and suffer less wear and tear on your body, especially your feet. Day hikers can usually get by with running shoes or cross-training boots, which are much lighter than hiking boots and cause less wear on the trails. Fourth, you can easily carry a day's supply of water, so you won't have to worry about finding or purifying water. And finally, day hikers have less impact on the environment, as they usually use toilets near trailheads rather than

along the trail. Particularly around a popular lake, excrement can affect the water quality; for instance, excrement from humans infected with *Giardia lamblia,* discussed under "Waterborne Microscopic Organisms" (page 37), can lead to the establishment of these microorganisms in a previously untainted lake or stream.

If you prefer shorter outings, consider obtaining Wilderness Press's Day & Section Hikes series on the PCT. The series is divided by region and sold in four guides: Southern California, Northern California, Oregon, and Washington. (For books on or related to the PCT, see the "Pacific Crest Trail" section under "Recommended Reading and Source Books" [page 321]. For books on general hiking or riding, see the "Backpacking, Packing, and Mountaineering" section.)

At the other end of the spectrum of PCT trekkers are the growing number of thru-hikers (919 in 2019) who attempt to do the entire trail in one multimonth effort. Before the early 1990s there was a rather high attrition rate among these thru-hikers—typically 50%–80% didn't complete it. This need not be so. Today, there are great books and online resources available to prepare you mentally, physically, and logistically for this odyssey, as well as free smartphone apps and crowd-sourced water reports to guide you every step of the way.

Ray and Jenny Jardine were instrumental in a long-distance backpacking revolution with their 1992 how-to book *The Pacific Crest Trail Hiker's Handbook,* published by AdventureLore Press (unfortunately, out of print since the late 1990s). The Jardines' book advocated ultralight backpacking. If you have only 20 pounds on your back, you'll be able to traverse more miles per day than if you have 60. No longer do you have to take 5.5–6.5 months for a thru-hike; traveling light, you can do it in five months or less (the Jardines did it in less than four months). Ultralight gear has gained popularity since then and is championed by big and small outfitters alike. Richard A. Light's *Backpacking the Light*

Way (Menasha Ridge Press, 2015) takes a thorough look at packing lightly and efficiently without compromising safety or comfort. Geared to both beginner and advanced hikers, it is packed with tips on planning, specific gear options, helpful techniques, and winter conditions.

There are several advantages to ultralight backpacking. A lighter pack is easier on your joints and muscles, making the excursion more pleasurable. Furthermore, by traveling light, you are less likely to have an injury because 1) your body isn't overstressed; 2) you're less likely to fall; and 3) if you do, the impact isn't as great. Traveling light, you'll perspire less, which is a plus on the long dry stretches. Additionally, you'll burn fewer calories, getting by with less food and, hence, less weight. By reducing your pack's weight to less than 20% of your body weight (that is, about 25–35 pounds for most hikers), you can probably get by with lightweight

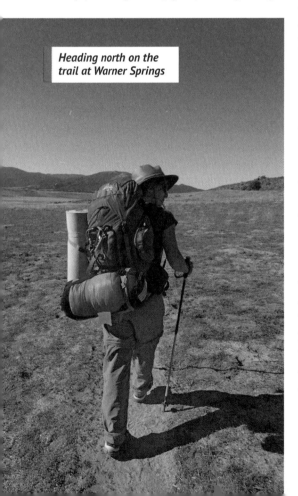

Heading north on the trail at Warner Springs

running or walking shoes, or even high-quality hiking sandals, making you less prone to the painful blisters synonymous with almost all boots. Both lighter packs and lighter footgear increase your daily mileage, providing an advantage other than comfort. You can start later and finish earlier, thereby encountering fewer storm- and-snow problems in the High Sierra early in your trek and in Washington near completion.

However, there is a drawback to ultralight backpacking. If you're caught in a blizzard or some other adverse condition, you may not have sufficient gear to survive; indeed, some ultra- lighters on long-distance trails have died. Light's book offers specifics on dealing with winter conditions, including shelter and food consider- ations and contingency planning. Also—and this applies to everyone, whether you take four or six months for a thru-hike—foremost on your mind will be keeping to your schedule, but because unexpected events or trail conditions can delay you and force you to make up for lost time, you likely won't have the time or energy to stop and smell the flowers. For this reason alone, our sug- gestion to those intent on doing the entire trail is to do it in two to five or more hiking seasons, each trip one to three months long, taking suf- ficient time to enjoy your trek. For most hikers, 15 miles per day under optimal trail and weather conditions is far more pleasurable than 25 miles per day under high-pressure conditions.

An excellent book on hiking long-distance trails is Karen Berger's *Hiking the Triple Crown: How to Hike America's Longest Trails: Appa- lachian Trail, Pacific Crest Trail, Continen- tal Divide Trail* (Mountaineers Books, 2001). Where Light's and the Jardines' books advocate ultralight backpacking, Berger offers a smorgas- bord of choices, as each successful thru-hiker has his or her own preferences. The first third of her book is a how-to on long-distance backpacking, while the remainder addresses issues specific to the AT, PCT, and CDT. A more detailed and PCT-specific volume is *The Pacific Crest Trail: A Hiker's Companion* (Countryman Press, 2014) by Berger and Daniel R. Smith; if you plan to be on the PCT for more than a month, read it.

Long-distance backpackers should consider several other books. One that many hikers feel is indispensable is *Yogi's Pacific Crest Trail Handbook* (Yogi's Books, 2019) by Jackie McDonnell, which has detailed advice on the mechanics of keeping supplied and in touch with humanity while hiking long-distance trails. Triple-crowner McDonnell offers details on things one thinks about after deciding to hike, such as resources to consult, logistics of each resupply and what supplies to expect, and services available for most PCT towns or resorts, complete with detailed maps. More than half of the pages are perforated to be sent to resupply points, along with food, maps, and so on.

Paul Bodnar's *Pocket PCT: Complete Data and Town Guide* (2016) also offers detailed accounts of supplies and services available for most PCT towns or resorts, each with a map compatible with the popular Guthooks smartphone app. The book is great for planning and, at under 5 ounces, is easy to carry.

How-to books and reference books are certainly useful in preparing for and planning a thru-hike, but so are personal accounts, and several (both in print and out-of-print) are listed under "Recommended Reading and Source Books" (page 321). Larger libraries may have copies of out-of-print books. There's nothing like firsthand accounts to give you a feel for the thru-hike and its challenges.

Given that few equestrians attempt most or all of the PCT, it is not surprising that a how-to book for them does not exist. However, PCT veterans Ben and Adeline York, who covered the entire trail on horseback twice, recommended earlier editions of the packers' bible, *Horses, Hitches, and Rocky Trails* by Joe Back (Johnson Books, 2018). You will encounter more problems than do backpackers, and so the following caution is even more important: a short horseback trip does *not* qualify you for a lengthy excursion on the PCT.

PHYSICAL FITNESS

Whether you are section hiking or thru-hiking, backpacking is exceptionally hard work. Plan to begin your conditioning long before you think you need to. There are numerous sources for conditioning routines geared specifically for hikers. *Backpacker* magazine features at least one in each issue, often including multipage, full-body routines and strategies to benefit from them. You can also find excellent conditioning advice in *The Joy of Backpacking* (also by Wilderness Press), specifically in the chapter on "Getting Fit for the Trail."

Of course, the best way to get in shape for your PCT hike is to get out and go hiking! Menasha Ridge Press publishes the 60 Hikes Within 60 Miles series for almost 30 metropolitan areas throughout the United States. Snag one of these guidebooks, get out on the trail, and get fit.

If you have any medical concerns, be sure to consult with your doctor and share your backpacking plans before you begin training.

PERMITS

If you will be traveling fewer than 500 miles on the PCT, you will need to obtain your permit from the local agency for the trailhead from which you will start. Check the website of the agency to learn about quotas and other restrictions. Permits and campsite reservations should be investigated well in advance. Increasingly, permits can be acquired on recreation .gov. This is an easy way to obtain your permit, but it is not available in all cases.

Anyone planning to hike or horseback ride 500 or more continuous miles on the PCT should obtain an interagency long-distance permit from the Pacific Crest Trail Association (PCTA). Permits are free, but there are limits to the number of permits available.

In an effort to manage the increasing numbers of long-distance hikers hitting the trail, stricter permitting regulations were implemented in 2020 for both north- and southbound hikes. All thru-hikers starting at or near the Mexican border between March 1 and May 31 need to obtain a long-distance permit from the PCTA. Through an agreement with the U.S. Forest Service, National Park Service, Bureau of Land Management, and other agencies, the PCTA usually begins accepting permit applications via its website in October for northbound hikers and in January for southbound hikers. The permit must be printed out and carried at all times. The application opening dates are subject to change, and the permits have various terms that you must follow, so be sure to visit pcta.org/discover-the-trail/permits at the start of your planning phase for the most updated information.

One such term is that travel in the southern Sierra (from Kennedy Meadows to the Sonora Pass) must be continuous with no skips or changes in direction. Thru-hikers who exit this stretch to do more than resupply or plan to reenter at a different point must obtain a new permit from the local land management agency because their PCT long-distance permit will no longer be valid for this area.

INTERNET RESEARCH AND APPS

In recent years, blogs and social media have changed the way hikers research and plan their PCT experience. Many hikers chronicle their every step with photos, anecdotes, and advice posted on personal blogs or websites created exclusively for their PCT adventures. (Trailjournals.com and postholer.com are two popular hiking sites with PCT sections.) And don't forget to join the strong PCT-based groups on social media: each year's class of thru-hikers has a Facebook group that serves as a real-time forum to ask questions, offer suggestions and updates, and post photos along the way. One intrepid hiker was even able to regain the phone he forgot at a trail angel property (places that host thru-hikers with tent sites, water, and other amenities) by communicating with fellow trekkers who had stayed behind.

The PCTA does a good job of posting current blog entries for each PCT class on its website. It also posts regular updates and photos on Facebook, Twitter, and Instagram under the moniker PCTAssociation. Favorite hashtags include #pacificcresttrail, #PCTrail, and #PCT2020 (or current year). Some hikers use the PCT's Facebook page, facebook.com/PCTAFan, to connect with others while on the trail. Another rich source of first-person accounts and advice is the PCTA's blog: pcta.org/blog.

The internet is especially helpful in looking for current trail closures and restrictions before each trip. Visit pcta.org/closures for closure information and consult local agency websites (page 25) for permit information and to find out if fire bans are in place.

Also be sure to check the essential PCT water report (pctwater.com), which provides, via hikers reporting from the trail, the most updated information on water sources. It will tell you when water tanks are empty, guzzlers are accessible, and seasonal streams are down to a trickle. Most Southern California PCTers print out a copy before heading out on the trail and keep it with them at all times.

Finally, Guthook Guides provides trail location and campsite data in a simple smartphone app that is compatible with both iPhone and Android devices.

Staying Wired

Hikers with electronics (such as smartphones, GPS, or personal location devices) can keep their batteries juiced up if they carry solar chargers or battery packs. Hikers can also use the charging blocks and cables at on- and off-trail hospitality or resupply stops, though such charging stations are sporadic. Often there is a choice of power strips, but at the least, duplex outlets are always available for hikers' use. Some trail angel properties have them, while others don't. Fast-food places and coffee shops, like the iconic McDonald's at the end of Section C, often serve as impromptu spots to charge devices for resourceful hikers. Observant hikers look for open outlets to use while eating in restaurants, doing laundry, buying groceries, drinking cool beverages, and any other temporarily sedentary activity where the lights are on. However, always be sure to ask businesses before charging and use common courtesy. Don't linger for hours at a restaurant charging your devices and taking up a table unless you've been given permission to do so. And don't expect that free power will always be available; if you really want power, consider paying for a hotel room.

Keeping your batteries charged does not imply that you'll have a signal when you most need one. Most hikers look forward to unplugging on the trail, but there are times that seeing a bar or two of service pop up in a remote area is a welcome surprise. Like many aspects of this mighty and temperamental trail, cell phone coverage on the PCT is unpredictable. Sometimes it shows up in places you least expect it, like Donohue Pass at 11,000 feet in the Ansel Adams Wilderness. On the other hand, it can be nonexistent in places where we take it for granted, like trailheads with big parking areas and nature centers. Much of Section D, for instance, where the PCT weaves over the Angeles Crest Highway and is closest to Los Angeles, has no service whatsoever. In Section E, north of CA 138 in Palmdale, hikers can expect robust service as the trail parallels the Los Angeles Aqueduct and wind farms (though howling winds can make conversation challenging).

Regardless of your carrier, you'll be disappointed with coverage along the PCT. If staying connected is vital for you, consider purchasing a second phone with another carrier or an unlocked phone with SIM cards for two carriers.

Finally, if you do use your phone on the trail, be sure to take it out of sight and earshot of others. Be courteous and don't intrude on anyone else's wilderness experience.

TRAIL ADVICE

Once you have your wilderness permit (if required) and a full pack, you are ready to start hiking. The following advice, most of it from the National Park Service and U.S. Forest Service, is provided to help make your hike safer and more enjoyable.

The wilderness permit does not serve as a registration system for hikers. Leave your itinerary, route description, and expected time of return with a responsible person back home. Also leave instructions on what to do if you don't arrive or make contact as planned. You must be specific on what the contact is to do when the deadline arrives: "Call the sheriff of the county in which I am hiking; say that I am an overdue PCT hiker, and give them my description...." Fill in all the details so your stand-in has no decisions to make. Be specific and make sure you connect as planned.

Stay on maintained trails unless you are good at using a compass and topographic maps. When off the trail, you can easily lose your sense of direction, especially in a viewless forest or in bad weather. If you become disoriented, don't panic. As soon as you think you may be off track, stop, assess your current direction, and then retrace your steps to the point where you went astray. Using a map, a compass, and this book, and keeping in mind what you have passed thus far, reorient yourself, and trust your judgment on which way to continue.

Note: About 10% of the PCT is on private land. Always obey signs and do not go off trail, camp, or follow side trails in these areas.

Solo hiking can be dangerous, particularly if you have large streams to ford. If you do set out alone, stick to frequently used trails so that you can get help if you become sick or injured.

Watch your step on trails. The mountains are no place to get a sprained ankle.

Take a wilderness first aid course. Accidents happen on the PCT, so make sure you're prepared to handle them. Your safety is your responsibility.

If you want to wear hiking boots, make sure they are well broken-in to avoid blisters. Wear two pairs of socks and carry moleskin just in case.

If you bring children along, be sure they have personal identification on them at all times. Tell them what to do if they get lost (they should stay put), and give them a whistle or other means of signaling for help. Don't leave them alone; there are mountain lions out there (see page 31).

Confusion about which trail to take at junctions frequently results in spread-out parties becoming separated. To avoid confusion and the possibility of someone getting lost, faster party members should wait for slower members at all trail junctions. If members of your party want to travel at different paces, then be sure enough of them have a marked map that shows the party's route and campsite for each night.

Be prepared for rain or snow any time of the year. Learn survival techniques, especially how to stay warm and dry in inclement weather.

Always use sun protection when hiking. Wear sunglasses and a hat, and always use a lip balm and sunscreen, both with an SPF of 30 or higher. Also note the expiration date on the tube or bottle.

Don't underestimate the power of moving water, particularly since streambeds tend to be quite slippery. One of the greatest dangers to backcountry travelers is crossing streams. Whitewater and areas above cascades and waterfalls are especially dangerous. Visit pcta.org/discover-the-trail /backcountry-basics/water/stream-crossing-safety for an in-depth discussion on how to safely navigate stream crossings.

Lightning is a hazard in the mountains. You can gauge how far away a lightning strike is by counting the seconds it takes for thunder to arrive after you see lightning flash. A 5-second delay means the strike was about a mile away. A 1-second delay means that it was about 1,000 feet away and you are too close for comfort—absolutely seek shelter. Do not continue upward into a thunderstorm. Get off ridges and peaks. Stay away from meadows and lakes, and avoid exposed lone objects such as large rocks, isolated trees, railings, cables, and

sizable objects. Find shelter in forested areas among same-size trees. Your vehicle is a safe place to wait out a storm.

It's possible to hike portions of the PCT with your dog, but it requires a great deal of planning and preparation. Dogs are allowed on the PCT in some national and state parks but not others. Visit pcta .org/discover-the-trail/backcountry-basics/dogs for everything you need to consider when thinking about bringing your dog on your PCT adventure.

Water Caches

Water caches are containers of water left on or near the trail by an informal and unorganized community of volunteers. They are especially prominent along dry stretches of the Southern California portion of the PCT. Well-known water caches are noted in the sections of this book, **but they should never be counted on, under any circumstances.**

One of the intentions of long-distance hiking on trails such as the PCT is to promote self-reliance. Hikers should be prepared to carry enough water and not depend on water caches, as they can run dry, be tampered with, and sometimes contribute to large quantities of litter on the trail. The best way to monitor the water situation on the PCT is to regularly check the crowd-sourced PCT Water Report at pctwater.com.

LEAVE NO TRACE

With thousands of hikers using the Pacific Crest Trail, there is a virtual string of people progressing down the trail, competing for drinking, camping, and bathing space—and elimination space. Welcome, Leave No Trace!

The Leave No Trace (LNT) philosophy became a movement helped along by professionals at the U.S. Forest Service and the National Outdoor Leadership School (NOLS). NOLS recorded and reported on the impact of leading students into the same areas and the effect it was having on each ecosystem they visited, specifically those that were revisited annually. Learning what worked and what did not was based on these observations. It depends a lot on locale—coastal, desert, forest, or mountain. Each ecosystem requires specific care.

There are only seven LNT principles, and they are all common sense. Most PCT hikers embrace them automatically.

The member-driven Leave No Trace Center for Outdoor Ethics teaches people how to enjoy the outdoors responsibly. These copyrighted principles have been reprinted with permission from the Leave No Trace Center for Outdoor Ethics: LNT.org.

1. **Plan ahead and prepare.** PCT hikers have no choice but to start early and plan ahead—to bring gear that can serve multiple purposes, to anticipate supply needs (food and fuel), and to handle the logistics of resupplying.

2. **Travel and camp on durable surfaces.** Just by our numbers, we stress the ecosystems we traverse. As you're hiking, stay on maintained trails, and don't cut across switchbacks, as this leads to trail erosion and wastes precious trail maintenance resources when volunteers must head out to repair damage.

Camp in existing sites, at least 200 feet away from water and the trail. Campsites too close to water sources cause water pollution. Also stay away from meadows, which are easily destroyed in one season by just a few inconsiderate acts. For an excellent sleep, try granite slabs. Never build new fire rings.

3. **Dispose of waste properly.** The old cliché is still true: if you can pack it in, you can pack it out. Litter and food scraps are not only unsightly but also an unnatural food source that attracts animals—bears and rodents in particular. Your food source is simply detrimental to their well-being. All trash, including cans, bottles, foil, tampons, disposable diapers, toilet paper, orange peels, and apple cores, must be packed out. Do not burn or bury trash or scatter organic wastes. Carry plastic bags for trash.

When it comes to human waste in the wilderness, we all need to learn to handle it properly or we'll soon literally be on top of it. Giardia spreads when waste is not disposed of away from water sources (see page 37 for information on giardia). At least 200 feet from streams, lakes, and springs is perfect. Dig a hole in the soil down to the mineral layer (sand or rock) about 6–8 inches deep and large enough for your deposit. This part is a must-do before business. Have other materials at hand—leaves, smooth rocks, wet moss, cones, or smooth sticks. If you need toilet paper, have a couple of zip-top bags in which to carry it out. Do not place a large rock over your waste. Think about this the next time before *you* move a rock to excavate beneath it. Simply cover the hole with the excavated soil.

The issue of human waste has become far more serious in the past few seasons. Campsites formerly noted for their desirability are now surrounded by a dozen paths, each leading to a stomped-out 10-foot-diameter area full of surface turds and tissue blooms. These are not only unsightly, smelly, and disgusting, but they are also an extreme health hazard. Before taking a long hike, know and practice how to safely treat human waste in the wilderness. It's your responsibility.

Chemicals found in both biodegradable and nonbiodegradable soaps and detergents pollute backcountry waters, and pollution by organic waste has caused bacteria to spread through many lakes and streams. Unfortunately, our own bodies, as carriers of bacteria, contribute to the problem. Reduce your impact by cleaning pots, washing clothes, and bathing yourself at least 100 feet away from any body of water. You can clean your pots quite well with a small piece of a scrubby sponge and some warm water. To eliminate the need for pot scrubbing, as well as the weight of pots, a stove, and fuel, you could eat cold meals; indeed, many trekkers have hiked the entire PCT this way.

4. **Leave what you find.** Along this trail, you are going to see wonderful sights. Leave each spot as you found it; do not add to or alter it. At your campsite, minimize your impact: don't clear away brush, level the ground, cut trenches, or build a fire ring. Don't destroy, deface, or carve up trees, shrubs, or any other natural or cultural features.

5. Minimize campfire impacts. Wildfires are caused by lightning strikes and human carelessness. The first cannot be prevented; the second is completely under your control. If you must build a fire, and it's legal and appropriate, use only deadwood lying on the ground, build it no larger than you actually need, and use an existing fire ring. Put it out at least half an hour before you are ready to leave, adding water to it and stirring the ashes. In the High Sierra, fires are usually banned at elevations above 9,000 feet. At a few popular backcountry lakes, camping and/or campfires are banned; these are mentioned in the text. Finally, fires are almost always banned in Southern California. And during dry summers, especially the second half of summer, campfires are often banned everywhere. Always check with the local land management agency to see if fires are allowed before you build one. For more information on wildfire safety, visit pcta.org/discover-the-trail /backcountry-basics/fire.

6. Respect wildlife. Water instabilities over the past decade have been a major stressor on wildlife in every biozone. Observing wildlife from a distance will allow you to see much more than if you approach. Wild creatures in general do not need your food. Don't hand it out, don't leave it behind, and don't surrender it. Protect it properly (see page 30), and enjoy eating it yourself.

7. Be considerate of other visitors. We each get to have our own wilderness experience, so don't, by sight or sound, deny other hikers theirs. When you meet pack stock on the trail, speak quietly and remain in plain view. Allow them to pass by stepping off the trail on the downslope side; equestrians have the right-of-way. Close all gates. They prevent stock from wandering up and down the trail.

WEATHER

If you adequately prepare for inclement weather, your backpack trip won't be all that bad even if such weather occurs. What's more, while most of the discussion below is about avoiding rain and snow, and certainly that's the goal for most hikers, don't forget that the PCT is a world-class place to ski, snowshoe, mountaineer, and enjoy snowy solitude and beauty. During fall, winter, and spring, you truly have endless opportunities for winter recreation, with hundreds of access points.

Storms

Storms come in two categories: frontal storms and thunderstorms. The farther north you are on the PCT, the more likely you are to get caught in a frontal storm moving east across the state, as the storm season is several months longer than in Southern California. In Northern California frontal storms may come in mid- or late August, but they don't get serious until sometime in September. By October you'll generally want to be out of the highlands, which likely will become snow-covered before month's end and stay that way into early next July. When you're in the Klamath Mountains, you can get snow any time of the year, though in July and August the storms are infrequent and may dump only a few inches.

In the High Sierra, from about the Lake Tahoe environs south to Sequoia and Kings Canyon National Parks, the storm season is shorter. In average years these lands are not closed by snowfall until late October or early November, but you can still have substantial snowstorms in late September and early October. Be prepared and cautious if you're starting in late September. Frontal storms are also possible in August, but the snow usually melts in several days. In Southern California frontal storms may occur in November, but the serious ones will more likely be January–March. Still, thru-hikers starting in April from the Mexican border can get snowed on anywhere en route.

Contrasting with winter-centered frontal storms, thunderstorms are centered on summer and move north up the state. If you're caught in one, you can get a real drenching from copious rain or a beating from hard-hitting hail. This can occur in the San Jacintos and the

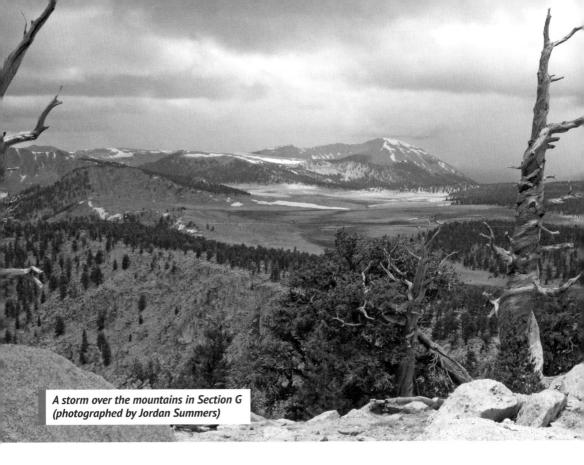

A storm over the mountains in Section G
(photographed by Jordan Summers)

San Bernardinos and in the southern and central Sierra Nevada. Especially in the high lands of Sequoia and Kings Canyon National Parks, these storms are likely, particularly in July. The cumulonimbus clouds that create these storms build in the afternoon, and the storms themselves typically occur from midafternoon into early evening—that is, from about 2 or 3 p.m. until about 7 or 8 p.m. Therefore, if you have an exposed alpine pass to cross, try to do it before midafternoon. As mentioned in "Trail Advice" earlier in this chapter, if you see the clouds looming and hear distant thunder, be prepared to seek shelter. Exposed high lands are no place to be dodging lightning strikes.

Best Times to Hike

To minimize storm encounters, hike during an optimal time. For Southern California lowlands, this can be March or April; not only are frontal storms less likely and temperatures neither too cold nor too hot, but there is also still enough groundwater for springs to be reliable, and even some seasonal streams may still be flowing. At this time of year, the higher elevations in the San Jacinto, San Bernardino, and San Gabriel Mountains will still be under snow (as may the Laguna Rim) and are best left for May or June. In July and August, they can be quite hot and, as summer progresses, flowing water becomes increasingly sparse. Temperatures become optimal by October, but the water situation is at about its worst, unless a major storm has recently moved through. However, for those who plan well, hiking Southern California in October is still feasible.

MARCH–MAY

Beyond the San Gabriels and before the High Sierra is a land of transition, essentially Sections

E and F, which traverse partly through the desert lands of Antelope Valley and the dry lands of the Tehachapi Mountains. Like Southern California lowlands, they are very hot and dry in the summer, so it's best to do them in March or April. May is pushing it, at least through the desert. Keep in mind that you may encounter snow in March at higher elevations.

JUNE–SEPTEMBER

From Section G north to the Oregon border (midway through Section R) constitutes two-thirds of the PCT in California, and most of this is relatively high lands, above 6,000 feet. In the central and northern High Sierra, terrain above 7,000 feet can remain largely snowbound through June, while in Section G, which is farther south, snow is not a likely problem in June until you reach elevations of around 10,000 feet, which are quite common in Golden Trout Wilderness. Immediately north of it is Sequoia and Kings Canyon National Parks, where much of the trail is above 11,000 feet; the snowpack is serious, even though the snow is melting fast. In years of average snowpack, Northern California snowfields can linger into late July, as is common on the approach to Sonora Pass and as far as Dicks Pass in Desolation Wilderness. Snowmelt presents another problem—swollen streams that you must ford. These can be just as life-threatening as icy passes. Therefore, don't hike there before mid-July in a year with average precipitation. August is better, but it's also the most crowded, especially in Sections G and H farther north. September usually has fair weather, and after Labor Day it lacks the crowds.

THRU-HIKING SEASON, SOUTH TO NORTH

Choosing an optimal hiking month is not an option for thru-hikers bound for the Canadian border. They must start at the Mexican border by mid-May, when there isn't too much snow at higher elevations. The hike through Antelope Valley (the western part of the Mojave Desert) can be grueling, usually too hot and always too dry. But a few weeks later, thru-hikers will be entering the High Sierra, which will be snowy. Not until early July, when hopefully they've reached I-80 at Donner Pass, will their problems be over—temporarily: snowstorms may await them in Washington in September.

Precipitation Considerations for Thru-Hikers

If you plan to thru-hike and can choose the year to do it, then pick one in which the southern half of the Sierra and all lands south of it (Sections A–H) are having a relatively dry year. (This requires some serious trust in *The Farmer's Almanac* and a huge dose of hiker optimism.) In theory, though springs will dry up earlier in Southern California, with a light Sierra snowpack you can start a month sooner, in early April rather than in early May. However, by the time you reach Oregon, perhaps in early August, the snow problems may not be that bad and the snow will continue to melt as you advance north. Another bonus of hiking in such a year is that you can finish by early or mid-September, before the frontal storms start coming in thick and fast, besieging you with one snow dusting after another.

Perhaps the worst kind of year is one with heavy precipitation both in the central and southern Sierra Nevada and in Southern California. On the plus side, springs and seasonal streams will be flowing in Southern California. On the minus side, the snowpack can slow you down in Southern California's mountains, and especially in the Sierra. Hiking slower than average, you could run out of time, for Washington's North Cascades can be snowbound and that section can be indecipherable by the time you reach it.

For the most updated information on the water situation in California, check the PCT Water Report (pctwater.com) or the PCTA's website, pcta.org. They keep track of trail conditions, including drinking-water availability, snow problems, and other issues pertinent to the PCT trekker.

Drought, Wildfires, and Flooding

Natural disasters and extreme weather conditions can cause all kinds of challenges and setbacks for thru-hikers. Preparation and awareness are essential and could save your life. Severe drought struck California between 2009 and 2016, spurring Governor Jerry Brown to declare a drought state of emergency for the entire region. This had a significant impact on the PCT and anyone who traversed it. Once-reliable natural water sources dried up, forcing hikers to carry even more water through long dry stretches. Wildfires burned longer and wider, some in areas still recovering from past fire damage. Stretches of trail were closed for months or even years to allow for recovery and trail repairs. An unprecedented string of wildfires in Oregon and Washington in late summer 2017 forced many hikers off the trail or resulted in hikes that were uncomfortably dominated by smoke and hazy views.

Conversely, the heavy rains and snowfall that hit California in the winter of 2016–17 led to dangerously high river levels; two thru-hikers drowned in separate incidents while crossing swollen rivers in the Sierra Nevada in July 2017. Others were forced to take so many detours or wait out brutal conditions that a new slogan emerged for the season: "2017—We tried."

The record rains and snowfall in the winter of 2016–17, as well as an exceptionally wet 2018–2019 season, did help pull most of the state out of its emergency drought status, but experts say its aquifers, forests, and wildlife ecosystems have a long road to recovery and may be forever altered by their desiccated states.

Regardless of the drought status, the high volume of snowmelt has an impact on the depth and velocity of creeks and rivers. Plan your stream crossing for early morning when the snowmelt is at its lowest for the day. And don't be shy about asking to buddy up with another hiker or two if you are lightweight or inexperienced.

Hypothermia

Hypothermia is the rapid and progressive mental and physical collapse that accompanies chilling of the human body's inner core. The condition is caused by exposure to cold and is intensified by wetness, wind, and exhaustion. Therefore, it's always a good idea to carry raingear. An unexpected storm could otherwise soak you to the bone. Hypothermia almost always occurs at temperatures well above freezing. Anyone who becomes fatigued in wet and windy conditions is a potential victim. If you experience a bout of uncontrolled shivering, you should seriously consider yourself a candidate for hypothermia and take appropriate countermeasures.

The best defense against hypothermia is to avoid exposure. Stay dry. When clothing is wet, it can lose as much as 90% of its insulating value, draining heat from the body. Wool and synthetic fibers such as polypropylene and Polartec retain most of their insulating value when wet, unlike cotton, down, and some synthetics. Buy breathable garments with a durable water repellent (DWR), made by various manufacturers. Be aware of the wind. Even a slight breeze carries heat away from your body and forces cold air under as well as through clothing. Wind intensifies cold by evaporating moisture from the skin's surface. Put on raingear immediately, not after you are soaked. Add a layer of clothing under your raingear before shivering occurs. Wear a hat or ski cap, preferably made of wool or polypropylene, to protect and help retain body heat.

If your party fails to take these precautionary steps, a hiker with hypothermia may develop more advanced symptoms, which include slurred speech, drowsiness, amnesia, and frequent stumbling, followed by a decrease in shivering; hallucinations; and, finally, stupor, coma, and death. The victim may strongly deny he or she is in trouble. Believe the symptoms, not the patient. This is a serious condition to prepare for if you are planning on hiking solo.

It is far more dangerous to hike alone than in a group. You may not recognize the signs of hypothermia by yourself, and if you do, you may have a harder time restoring your body heat than if you had others to help you. In the mountains it is extremely important to keep your sleeping bag and a set of clothes dry. If they get wet and threatening weather prevails, try to get out of the mountains as quickly as possible. But don't abandon your pack to make a dash for the trailhead; this risks exposing yourself to the elements even more, and losing your shelter, food, and stove can be deadly. If the weather gets too bad, set up your tent in a sheltered area, keep warm and out of the elements, and stay put until the inclement weather abates. You'll be alive and have a great story to tell, and no one at work will care if you're a day late. You should not attempt to continue hiking in inclement weather.

HIGH-ALTITUDE PROBLEMS

Altitude Sickness

Altitude sickness may occur at elevations of about 8,000 feet or more. Symptoms include fatigue, weakness, headache, loss of appetite, nausea, vomiting, and shortness of breath on exertion. Everyone is affected differently; some are not affected at all. Symptoms are usually temporary and should not affect you for more than 48 hours. Sleep may be difficult for the first night and, if you are above 10,000 feet, perhaps even for one or more additional nights. Regular periods of heavy breathing separated by periods of no breathing may awaken the sleeper with a sense of suffocation. Hyperventilation may also occur, causing lightheadedness; dizziness; and tingling of the hands, feet, and mouth. Altitude sickness results from exposure to the oxygen-deficient atmosphere of high elevations. It is aggravated by fatigue and cold. Some people are more susceptible to it than others. As the body adjusts to the lower oxygen pressure, symptoms usually disappear. Resting and drinking extra liquids are recommended. If symptoms persist, descend to lower altitudes.

High-Altitude Pulmonary Edema

Though rare, this is a serious and potentially fatal condition. Cases have been reported at altitudes of 8,500 feet, but it usually occurs considerably higher. The basic problem, as with altitude sickness, is a reduction of oxygen, and early symptoms are often unrecognized or confused with altitude sickness. However, in the case of pulmonary edema, reduced oxygen initiates diversion of blood from the body shell to the core, causing congestion of the lungs, brain, and other vital organs. Besides exhibiting symptoms similar to those of altitude sickness, the victim is restless, coughs, and eventually brings up frothy, blood-tinged sputum. The only treatment is immediate descent to at least 2,000 feet lower and, if available, administration of oxygen. You should secure medical help as soon as possible.

Blood in Urine

If you are at high elevations and exercising to the point of dehydration, you can, like serious long-distance runners, have reddish urine. You are not dying, but this is a good sign that you are overexerting yourself. Slow down.

Ultraviolet Radiation

Always use sun protection when outdoors, but it is especially important above 9,000 feet, as the dangerous ultraviolet radiation at these elevations is very intense. Wear UV-absorbing or -reflecting sunglasses and a hat to protect your eyes. You can get quite a splitting headache if your eyes get too much radiation. Prolonged exposure to ultraviolet radiation increases your risk of skin cancer, so be liberal with sunscreen, and reapply frequently, on all your exposed skin.

TRAIL REGISTERS

Trail registers give hikers an idea of who did what, relative degree of trail use, and changing trail conditions and special concerns. By signing these registers, you develop over time a camaraderie with other trekkers. Though you may never catch up to those ahead of you, by trail's end you may feel that you've come to know them. Because the locations of registers are not always obvious, a list is presented below. These locations are subject to change, though most are quite stable, especially the sites that are post offices. Unless otherwise designated, the register is located in a post office, which at some places is just a tiny room in a store or a resort.

TRAIL REGISTERS IN SOUTHERN CALIFORNIA

• Campo	• Tehachapi
• Mount Laguna	• Mojave
• Julian, Banner Store	• Onyx
• Warner Springs	• Kennedy Meadows, Kennedy Meadows Store
• Anza	• Lone Pine
• Idyllwild	• Independence
• Cabazon	• Vermilion Valley Resort, store
• Big Bear City	• Mammoth Lakes
• Wrightwood, Mountain Hardware	

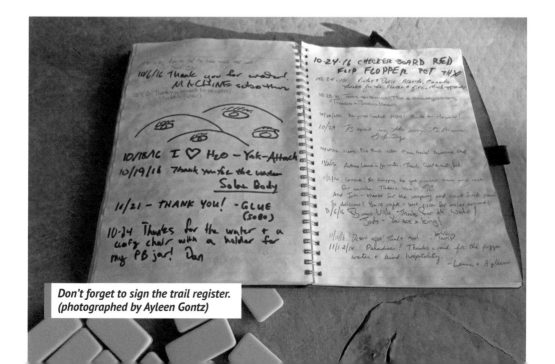

Don't forget to sign the trail register.
(photographed by Ayleen Gontz)

MAILING TIPS

If you will be on the trail long enough to bother with resupply points, you can use the table below, which lists mostly post offices but also a few private businesses. Expect to pay holding fees when mailing to private businesses, and be sure to check whether they accept UPS and FedEx only, USPS only, or all three. It's generally acceptable to mail a package to arrive about two weeks before you get there. If you mail it too early, your package may be returned to you.

Those who thru-hike the trail should consider buying *Yogi's Pacific Crest Trail Handbook* by Jackie McDonnell, as she gives up-to-date and complete post office hours, locations, and phone numbers. You should also visit pcta.org /discover-the-trail/thru-hiking-long-distance -hiking/resupply for additional sources of resupply locations. (Be aware that this kind of information has changed in the past and likely will in the future.) Finally, also check the introduction of each section for resupply information.

You can mail yourself almost any food, clothing, or equipment. Before you leave home, you should have a good idea of your consumption rate of food, clothing, and fuel for your stove. What you may not know is what you want to eat or what other items you may need in week two or three. So, when you decide what you want and need in the coming weeks, purchase those items at stores along the way and send packages forward for pickup. The buy-as-you-go approach supports local trail town economies, and the stores are nearly universally well prepared and stocked for hikers. However, if you have special dietary needs, you may want to ship your packages from home.

Address your package to:

[Your Legal Name]
PCT Hiker, ETA: MM/DD/YY
General Delivery
[Post Office, State Abbr. Zip Code]

Keep in mind that some post offices are seasonal. Hours of most are 9 a.m.–noon and 1–5 p.m. or longer. Some are open Saturday mornings. Plan your trip schedule accordingly to avoid waiting two or three days in town because an office was closed for the weekend (don't forget about the three-day weekends: Memorial Day, Fourth of July, and Labor Day).

POST OFFICES ALONG OR NEAR THE ROUTE, SOUTH TO NORTH

- Campo 91906
- Mount Laguna 91948*
- Julian 92036
- Warner Springs 92086*
- Anza 92539
- Idyllwild 92549*
- Cabazon 92230
- Big Bear City 92314*
- Wrightwood 92397*
- Acton 93510
- Lake Hughes 93532*
- Lancaster 93534
- Tehachapi 93561*
- Mojave 93501
- Onyx 93255

- Kennedy Meadows General Store*
  96740 Beach Meadows Road
  Inyokern, CA 93527
- Lone Pine 93545
- Independence 93526
- Bishop 93514
- Mono Hot Springs 93634
- Vermilion Valley Resort*
  c/o Rancheria Garage
  62311 Huntington Lake Road
  Lakeshore, CA 93634
- Mammoth Lakes 93546*
- Tuolumne Meadows 95389*
- Lee Vining 93541
  (use when Tuolumne Meadows is closed)

* = recommended for use

FEDERAL GOVERNMENT AGENCIES

The U.S. Forest Service (USFS) has overall responsibility for managing the Pacific Crest Trail (PCT). The large majority of the PCT lies on lands for which the USFS is the public steward.

The USFS partners with the Bureau of Land Management, National Park Service, and California State Parks to manage and protect the trail. While all of these land management agencies have similar regulations, each may have specific requirements. For example, some wilderness areas do not require a wilderness permit for entry, while others do. As stated earlier, the PCTA provides wilderness permits for

FEDERAL GOVERNMENT AGENCIES, SOUTH TO NORTH

• BLM–El Centro Field Office 1661 S. Fourth St. El Centro, CA 92243 760-337-4400; blm.gov/california	• BLM–Bakersfield Field Office 3801 Pegasus Drive Bakersfield, CA 93308 661-391-6000; blm.gov/california
• Cleveland National Forest* 10845 Rancho Bernardo Road San Diego, CA 92127 858-673-6180; fs.usda.gov/cleveland	• Owens Peak, Chimney Peak, Domeland (east) Wildernesses contact: BLM–Bakersfield
• Hauser Wilderness contact: Cleveland NF	• Sequoia National Forest 1839 S. Newcomb St. Porterville, CA 93257 559-784-1500; fs.usda.gov/sequoia
• Anza-Borrego Desert State Park 200 Palm Canyon Dr. Borrego Springs, CA 92004 760-767-5311; parks.ca.gov	• Kiavah, Domeland (west), South Sierra, and Golden Trout* Wildernesses Wilderness permits are recommended for overnight trips in South Sierra. Permits are required for overnight trips in the Golden Trout Wilderness. Contact the Mt. Whitney District Office, P.O. Box 8, Lone Pine, CA 93545; 760-876-6200
• BLM–Palm Springs Field Office 1201 Bird Center Drive Palm Springs, CA 92262 760-833-7100; blm.gov/california	
• Santa Rosa and San Jacinto Mountains National Monument* contact: BLM–Palm Springs	• Sequoia & Kings Canyon National Parks* 47050 Generals Highway Three Rivers, CA 93271 559-565-3341; nps.gov/seki
• San Bernardino National Forest 602 S. Tippecanoe Ave. San Bernardino, CA 92408 909-382-2600; fs.usda.gov/sbnf	• Inyo National Forest 351 Pacu Lane, Ste. 200 Bishop, CA 93514 760-873-2400; fs.usda.gov/inyo
• San Gorgonio Wilderness contact: San Bernardino NF and BLM–Palm Springs	• John Muir Wilderness* contact: Inyo NF
• Angeles National Forest 701 N. Santa Anita Ave. Arcadia, CA 91006 626-574-1613; fs.usda.gov/angeles	• Sierra National Forest 1600 Tollhouse Road Clovis, CA 93611 559-297-0706; fs.usda.gov/sierra
• Sheep Mountain Wilderness* contact: Angeles NF	• Ansel Adams Wilderness* contact: Mammoth Lakes Welcome Center 2510 Main St. Mammoth Lakes, CA 93546 888-466-2666, 760-924-5500

* = wilderness areas and national parks that require a wilderness permit for an overnight stay

trips of 500 miles or more on the PCT; however, hikers who plan to do less than 500 miles may need to apply directly to a federal government agency for a permit. You may also want to inquire about trailhead parking fees or check for temporary road or trail closures. (Also visit pcta .org/discover-the-trail/closures for information about closures on the trail.) The appropriate Bureau of Land Management, National Forest, and National Park offices are listed on page 25.

If you need a wilderness permit, obtaining it online is often the most painless way to do so. In many wilderness areas, including those with quotas, permits are available through the National Recreation Reservation Service (NRRS) at recreation.gov. In most cases, reserved permits can be printed at home or picked up at a USFS ranger station within 14 days prior to date of entry. In some instances, hikers are required to pick up the permit in person. If you're in doubt, call the issuing authority for clarification. If you are seeking permits for single sections covering any wilderness, recreation.gov is the most efficient source for obtaining your permits.

Remember that each permitting authority may have different procedures. For example, in the Desolation Wilderness, each campsite is identified and its quota is posted on a map to use when reserving. Once your application is accepted and dates are approved, you can print your permit at home. In nearby Mokelumne Wilderness, the campsite quota system is the same, but permits must be picked up at the ranger station. Always check with each agency.

You must have a California Fire Permit to use a stove, lantern, or have a campfire on most of the PCT in California. The permit is your agreement to follow the campfire restrictions and regulations in effect. Beyond being your agreement to follow safe practices, the permit is a tool to educate you on how to use fire safely and appropriately. Get yours after watching a video and, yes, taking a test at ready forwildfire.org/permits/campfire-permit.

This permit does not actually give you permission to have a campfire! Campfires are not allowed or appropriate along much of the PCT. Campfires are generally not allowed in Southern California or during dry, hot summers. They're also generally not allowed on private land, which accounts for about 10% of the trail.

ORGANIZATIONS RELEVANT TO THE PACIFIC CREST TRAIL

The previously mentioned books should answer most of your questions about hiking or riding the PCT. But if questions linger, they may be answered by contacting one or more of the following organizations.

Pacific Crest Trail Association (PCTA)

The PCTA is part of the legacy (the PCT itself is the other part) of many advocates and volunteers, including Warren Rogers. As a young man, Rogers worked with Clinton C. Clarke, known as the father of the trail. Clarke put the trail on the map beginning in the 1930s, forming the Pacific Crest Trail System Conference and advocating for the idea of the trail with a reluctant USFS. World War II contributed to the slow demise of his beloved conference. He died in 1958.

Rogers eventually picked up the baton in 1971, forming the Pacific Crest Club to be a "worldwide fellowship of persons interested in the PCT," as his son, Don, put it. Then, in 1977, he founded the Pacific Crest Trail Conference, which addressed the needs of both the trail and its users. In 1987, when Rogers was no longer able to run these organizations, the club was merged with the conference, and for several years volunteer Larry Cash of Eugene, Oregon, was its chief officer. The conference campaigned against trailside clear-cutting, against mountain bikes, for additional water sources along the drier stretches, and for volunteer trail maintenance. In 1992 the organization changed its name to the Pacific Crest Trail Association (1331 Garden Highway, Sacramento, CA 95833; 916-285-1846; pcta.org).

Over the years, the PCTA has become increasingly active in coordinating volunteer trail maintenance and leading efforts to promote safe and responsible use of the trail. The association has a formal partnership with the USFS, National Park Service, Bureau of Land Management, and California State Parks through a Memorandum of Understanding. In 2018 PCTA volunteers spent 118,524 hours maintaining the trail, promoting the PCTA, and helping to raise awareness. That same year, the organization raised more than $4 million in private donations.

In addition to issuing long-distance permits and keeping members up-to-date on all things trail-related via its website and social media (its Twitter handle is @PCTAssociation), the PCTA publishes a monthly e-newsletter, "Trail Dirt," and a quarterly print magazine, *The Pacific Crest Trail Communicator*. While addressing general issues and timely matters, it provides informative and inspirational accounts by those who have hiked or ridden horses on much or all of the PCT. The association's website contains an active blog and more than 100 pages of content, including trip-planning aids, current trail and snowpack conditions, trip calculators, permit applications, and links to other useful sites.

While it's impossible to keep track of exactly how many people use the trail every year, the PCTA provides estimates on use via the number of annual long-distance permits it issues. The group maintains a 2,600-Miler List on its website and sends hikers who notify it of completion a medal or certificate. In 2018 the organization issued a record 7,313 permits to section and thru-hikers and horseback riders, who came from all 50 states and 41 countries and territories.

Finally, the PCTA lobbies Congress to support trail maintenance and for adequate funding for the USFS and other federal land management agencies. Private donors provide the bulk of its funding, which supports volunteer programs, public engagement, and advocacy. The organization is also raising money to help acquire the nearly 10% of the PCT that remains on private land, working with willing sellers to ensure that future generations of users have a protected corridor. In 2019, in a historic leap toward achieving this goal, the PCTA announced that along Northern California's Trinity Divide in the Klamath and Shasta-Trinity National Forests, 17 miles of the PCT that was previously on private property—as well as 10,300 acres of land surrounding the trail—are now in public ownership and permanently protected. The organization also consults with and advises government agencies on future reroutes to make the trail safer, more practical, or more scenic.

American Long Distance Hikers Association–West

In 1993 Ray Jardine founded the Western States Chapter. After a couple of years, Ray left his organization, and a few of its members took it over and reorganized it. Its mission is to promote fellowship and communication among long-distance hikers and anyone who supports long-distance hiking. As the association's name implies, it is aimed at long-distance backpackers (that is, not day hikers and equestrians). It addresses relevant backpacking matters on long trails or treks, not only in the Western United States but also overseas, and members hail from around the country, not just from the West. If you're a long-distance hiker, there are at least two reasons to join the association: First, "The Distance Hiker's Gazette" contains good descriptions of various trails and routes, plus backpacking advice. Second, you can find camaraderie among distance hikers at the ALDHA-West Gathering, held each fall. To join the organization, visit aldhawest.org.

Equestrian Organizations

The vast majority of PCT users are hikers, but there is fair use from equestrians on certain stretches. Occasionally an equestrian party will attempt to do the whole trail. This is more difficult than hiking, as horses don't wear crampons and don't cross logs over deep, raging streams. Consequently, it's virtually impossible to do the whole trek in one long season without making serious diversions, such as skipping the High Sierra entirely or doing it later, after the snow has melted and streams are safe.

If you want to ride the entire trail without any diversions or leapfrogging, then do it over two or more summers, making sure you do the High Sierra between mid-July and mid-September (and Washington during August—before that, there is too much snow, and after that, too much chance of snowstorms). For help on planning your trip through California, contact the Backcountry Horsemen of California; for Oregon and Washington, start with the Back Country Horsemen of America (see below for more on both). The PCTA also offers invaluable planning information on its website at pcta .org/discover-the-trail/equestrian-center.

BACKCOUNTRY HORSEMEN OF CALIFORNIA

This organization (which is open to men and women) was created in 1981. BCHC is dedicated to conserving backcountry wilderness and protecting stock users' enjoyment of wilderness

trails. Among other things, the organization offers clinics on how to pack with a horse and/ or mule in the mountains. Besides teaching the fundamentals of packing, it stresses low-impact use, courtesy, and common sense. It is a partner with Leave No Trace, a member-driven movement to protect the outdoors by teaching people to enjoy it responsibly (see page 16). BCHC is a member organization of the Back Country Horsemen of America. Find more information at bchcalifornia.org.

BACK COUNTRY HORSEMEN OF AMERICA

Like the organization profiled above, BCHA is open to both men and women, but it does not include all of the United States; it covers only 11 Western states plus several others of the contiguous 48 states. If you plan to continue riding north beyond California, into Oregon or Washington, you might start with this organization. It publishes a quarterly newsletter (available via its website, bcha.org). Plus, Back Country Horsemen of Montana publishes a book—very relevant for California equestrians—*Back Country Horsemen's Guidebook* (see "Recommended Reading and Source Books: Backpacking, Packing, and Mountaineering," page 322).

ANIMAL AND PLANT CONCERNS

If you hike the entire California PCT, you'll see dozens of bird species. You'll also pass by dozens of mammal species but will see very few, except for deer, marmots, pikas, and squirrels, particularly the nearly ubiquitous California ground squirrel. However, the animals are around; just camp near a spring in Southern California, and you'll hear quite a flurry of activity during the night. Without a tent, you may hear or feel toads and mice traversing around or over you, and a scorpion or two may get under or, worse, into your sleeping bag. What follows is a brief synopsis of animal and plant problems you might face on the PCT.

Black Bears

With the possible exception of cougars, most animals will be scared of you and will not be a threat as long as you respect the animal's space. The wilderness of California is the black bears' home; we can only visit. The threat they pose is that they are very intelligent and always searching for large quantities of food to build their nutrition stores.

Black bears, which can be a variety of colors and hues, are almost as far-ranging as cougars and are present along the entire PCT. Conflicts between bears and humans usually occur because bears want your food. It's easy pickings, after all. And if a bear can nab your food, it will nab someone else's too. So, the bear becomes known as a nuisance bear. This is not the bear's fault. Human food needs to be properly stored by humans (more on that below).

Despite weighing up to 500 pounds, black bears can run up to 35 miles an hour. One day shy of Monument 78, we watched as a fully filled-out, lustrously black-coated adult bear moved itself quickly from the canyon creek up 2,000 vertical feet on the opposite mountainside.

Most bears actually fear people and will leave when they see you. You are more likely to see the back end of a bear than to meet one face-to-face. If a bear woofs, snaps its jaws, slaps the ground or brush, or bluff charges, you are too close. Back away! Don't take any pictures! Seriously, don't.

Take precautions to avoid this kind of bear–human interaction. Control your food, toiletries, and trash—anything with a smell that may

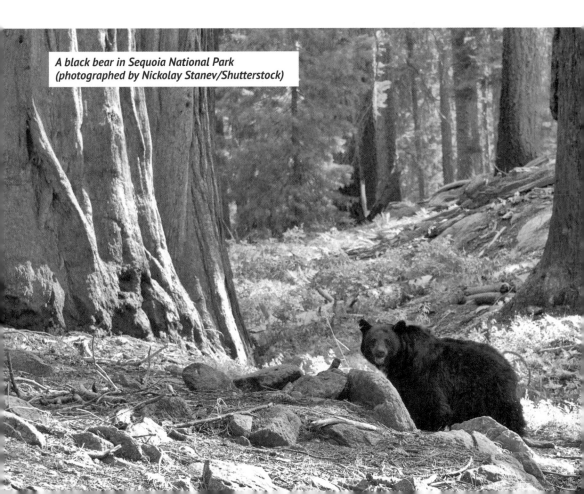

A black bear in Sequoia National Park (photographed by Nickolay Stanev/Shutterstock)

be an attractant. Locate your camp kitchen away from your sleeping area, and keep the area free of food spills. It's also best if your backpack doesn't smell of trout and your candy supply is stored away from your tent.

Don't leave food out or unattended—not even for a few minutes. Secure your food for the protection of yourself and the bear. Use a bear-proof canister to carry and store your food when backpacking. These work and can be rented at most U.S. Forest Service visitor centers.

If a bear is eating your food or shredding your pack in search of your snacks, don't throw rocks at its head or face, and don't attempt to retrieve your food items until the bear has left the area. You can yell, wave your arms, and bang pots, but you've lost. In the bear's mind, it is now his food. Let him have it. Now you can walk away with a great story. If you try to reclaim the food from the bear, you won't.

In the unlikely event that you do encounter a black bear on the trail, don't run. Make eye contact without staring. Pick up small children to keep them from running. Back away slowly. Speak calmly but firmly to the bear to identify yourself as a human and not a prey animal; never scream.

If a bear approaches within about 75 feet, make yourself appear larger by spreading your arms, waving hiking sticks or branches, or holding your jacket open. Do not block the bear's escape route.

Attacks are rare, but if a bear is after you and not your food, throw rocks and make every attempt to frighten it away or fight it off aggressively with anything at hand (now is the time to use your bear spray). Don't bother to run; they're very fast.

Waking up in the dark of night to have one sniffing your head certainly gets your adrenaline rushing. However, although bears are carnivores by nature, in California they are mostly herbivores by habit; only about 10% of their diet is animal matter, and that is mostly insects. Humans are not part of their diet. For example,

in Yosemite National Park's history, not even one visitor has been killed by any of these usually gentle creatures (unlike grizzlies, which once ranged over much of California but went extinct there in the 1920s).

SAFEGUARDING YOUR FOOD

Today's national park regulations now require all section and thru-hikers in all of Yosemite and Lassen Volcanic National Parks and parts of Sequoia and Kings Canyon National Parks to carry bear canisters, which are available for rent at most main visitor centers and permit offices. Food-storage boxes are also available for use by long-distance hikers on the PCT and John Muir Trail (JMT). Their locations are highlighted in Sections G and H in this guide; a detailed list of their locations on parts of the JMT and PCT, along with other helpful info, can also be found at nps.gov/seki/planyourvisit/bear_box.htm and sierrawild.gov/bears/food-storage-map.

As a last resort, and only where bear canisters are not required, you may consider suspending your food in trees using the counterbalancing technique. (For step-by-step instructions on this method, consult nps.gov/seki/planyourvisit/bearhang.htm.) However, black bears are incredibly good tree climbers and very intelligent, so suspending your food in trees is generally not secure. In fact, it is so insecure that it is not really a deterrent, preventative, or protection as much as it is a mere delaying tactic. We recommend storing your food in an approved canister even in areas where they are not required. For more information on safeguarding your food, visit pcta.org/discover-the-trail/backcountry-basics/food/bear-canister-protecting-your-food.

BEAR TIPS

The U.S. Forest Service offers tips on how to avoid negative encounters with bears.

- **Never give food to a bear.**
- **Carry and use a food-storage container** designed to prevent access by bears.

• Be sure that your food, toiletries, and trash are stored and that your canister is closed properly at all times—bears are active 24 hours a day. Ensure that all your food, toiletries, and trash fit in the canister. To do this, remove all your food and toiletries from their original packaging to reduce bulk.

• Pack your canister before leaving the permit office to be sure that all items fit inside.

• If you do see a bear, do not approach it.

Bear canisters are available for purchase at most outdoors outfitters. They are also available for rent in permit offices and visitor centers throughout the national parks. They can be returned to the same location or mailed back to the U.S. Forest Service for a small fee (obtain a return label at the time of rental).

Cougars

These large cats, also called pumas or mountain lions (but they also live in lowlands), weigh up to about 200 pounds for males (about half that for females) and are about 7 feet long from nose to tail. The adults are tan-coated and have black-tipped ears and tail. Cubs are usually cuter and covered with dark-brown spots. There seem to be two views about how threatening they are to humans. One is that they are merely curious, and that is why they track you. The other is that they are hungry, so they stalk you. In California, attacks on humans by cougars are rare. Certainly, if it wanted to, a cougar could easily kill you while you're asleep, tent or no tent. So far this has not happened, and the five verified attacks that occurred in California in the last decade were all nonfatal attacks, not on or near the PCT. However, a 2018 cougar attack, which occurred west of Snoqualmie Pass in Washington, and appeared to be a case of a hungry animal stalking a cyclist who acted like prey, was fatal. Another fatal attack occurred that year in Oregon's Mount Hood National Forest.

Before the mid-1990s cougars were hunted throughout the state, which kept their numbers down and gave them a fear of humans. With hunting now banned, their numbers have increased and they may lose this fear.

Cougars are important to the natural community, and this is their home. They are seldom seen but have been known to attack humans without warning, so hikers need to be alert. Avoid hiking alone at dawn or dusk, and closely supervise children. Cougars are drawn to children and dogs because their size and motions mimic those of prey. If the trail tread is soft, look for their tracks: paw prints about 3 inches across, like those left by a large dog, but without claw marks, because cats walk with retractable claws.

Cougars inhabit every corner of California and range over a 100-square-mile home territory. They are present wherever deer are abundant.

For hikers, here is amended advice offered by the National Park Service: Foremost, avoid hiking alone; there is safety in numbers. If you hike alone, you may be safer with a backpack than with a day pack because with the latter, more of your body, especially your neck, is exposed. Second, if you bring children, watch them closely; they are easy prey. Never approach a cougar. If you hear or see one, stay calm and don't scream. If you stumble upon an animal's corpse—whether fresh or rotting—depart the area immediately. This is probably a cougar's well-guarded meal.

If confronted by a cougar, do anything to make yourself appear larger: raise your outspread arms, wave hiking sticks or tree limbs, and gather other hikers next to you (pick up children). Act threatening, but allow the animal a path to escape. Absolutely avoid bending over or turning your back on mountain lions. Cougars will interpret these actions as those of their prey. Maintain eye contact and do not run. Prey such as deer run, so don't act like prey and excite its killing instinct. Stay calm, not fearful (this is not easy). Hold your ground, or back away slowly. To flee is to die. If the cougar behaves aggressively, wave your arms, shout, and throw sticks and/or stones at its body. Convince the cougar that you may be dangerous. If you are attacked, try to remain standing, as it will try to bite the neck or head. Use any instrument at hand to repel the cat. Always try to fight back. In 2007 an Auburn, California, woman successfully defended herself using a tree branch and ballpoint pen to fight off the cougar that was attacking her husband. The couple survived.

Rattlesnakes

Few animals are more unjustly maligned in legend and in life than the western rattlesnake, and no other animal, with the possible exception of the American black bear, causes more concern among walkers and riders along the California PCT. Indeed, most thru-hikers will have several encounters with these common reptiles by the time they reach the High Sierra. Even so, PCT hikers are much more likely to be taken down by dehydration or a bout of giardia than by a rattlesnake.

Frequenting warmer climes generally below the red fir belt (although they have been seen much higher), rattlers are most often encountered basking on a warm rock, trail, or pavement, resting from their task of keeping the rodent population in check. Like other reptiles, rattlesnakes are unable to control their internal body temperature (they are cold-blooded), and therefore venture from their underground burrows only when conditions are suitable. Just as rattlers won't usually be seen in freezing weather, it is also no surprise that they are rarely seen in the heat of day, when ground temperatures may easily exceed 150°F—enough to cook a snake (or blister human feet, as many will learn). One will usually see rattlers toward evening, when the air is cool but the earth still holds enough heat to stir them from their lethargy for a night of hunting. They naturally frequent those areas where rodents feed—under brush, in rock piles, and beside streams.

It is their nocturnal hunting equipment that has inspired most of the legends and fears concerning rattlesnakes. In their wedge-shaped heads, rattlers have heat-sensitive pits, resembling nostrils, that can sense nearby changes in temperature as subtle as 1°F. Rattlers use these pits to locate prey at night, as they do not have well-developed night vision. More important perhaps is their sensitivity to vibrations, which can alert a rattler to footfalls more than 50 feet away. With such acute sensibilities, useful for detecting a meal or danger, a rattler will usually begin to hurry away long before a hiker spots it. Furthermore, if you do catch one of these reptiles unawares, these

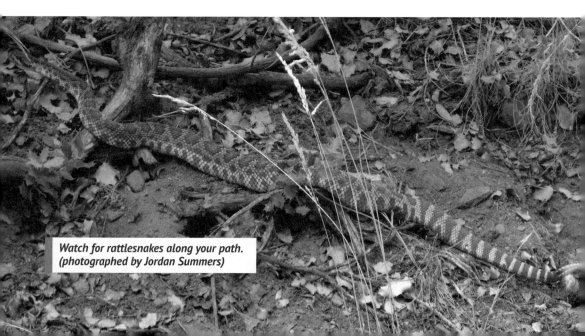

Watch for rattlesnakes along your path. (photographed by Jordan Summers)

gentlemen among venomous snakes will usually warn you away with buzzing tail rattles if you get too close for comfort.

The easiest way to avoid a snakebite is to avoid snakes. More than 75% of rattler bites are inflicted on people who are handling a snake, and more than 80% of all bites are on the hand. The lessons: Don't catch snakes, and look before you put your hands under rocks or logs, or into tall grass. Snakes will usually graciously depart as you approach, if you make enough noise—a good reason to carry a walking stick.

If bitten, get help immediately. The only truly useful treatment for a rattlesnake bite is intravenous antivenin, which can be administered in most emergency departments in California. The sooner it is given, the better, even if you must hike a distance for help. If you are solo, hike out immediately and call 911 as soon as you have service or hit the SOS on a satellite emergency notification device. If you are part of a group and are distant from possible medical attention, have the victim lie down, while another hiker goes for help. Keep the victim calm, and keep the puncture site below the heart. Because antiquated first-aid measures such as cold packs, tourniquets, and incision and suction devices are dangerous, they should never be used. There is no substitute for rapid evacuation to a hospital.

Finally, some special mention should be made of one of the West's most feared vipers, the uncommon Mojave Green rattlesnake. This desert denizen may be encountered along the Southern California PCT. Thankfully it, like other rattlers, is not aggressive. Its real danger is the lack of early symptoms of envenomation in its victims. These are delayed for the first 6–12 hours after a strike. This quiescent period may be followed by severe neurologic symptoms and shock, too late for treatment. Hence, all victims of a rattler bite should seek immediate medical attention. No special treatment is needed for a Mojave rattler bite—one type of antivenin treats all North American pit viper cases.

Mosquitoes

"Truth bids me to say that mosquitoes swarmed in myriads, with not one-tenth the fear but with twice the ferocity of a southern Secessionist." So wrote William H. Brewer about his evening in Yosemite National Park's upper Lyell Canyon on July 1, 1863. This statement is still very true for most of the High Sierra, for Lassen Volcanic National Park, and for the Klamath Mountains. Still, trekkers may encounter mosquitoes even in Southern California and wherever there is a water source suitable for their breeding. They can be quite abundant along the Sacramento River, which you encounter at a low elevation in Northern California's Castle Crags State Park. Mosquitoes occur near water from sea level up to around 11,000 feet—that is, near treeline. All mosquitoes can transmit various diseases, such as West Nile virus. For those not normally bothered by the buzzing and biting, this should be reason enough to use some protection in the evening.

By late July mosquito populations wane in the high mountains, as snow melts and meadows dry out (although they can still be abundant lower down, where water is available). Until then, you'll probably want to carry a tent with mosquito netting just to get a good night's sleep. This is especially true in June. From midmorning until late afternoon, when you are likely to be on the trail, wind usually keeps their numbers down. Of course, you can postpone your hike until August, but this is not an option for thru-hikers. Mosquitoes are pollinators, which explains why they are near their maximum numbers when wildflowers are so profuse. Without them, perhaps mountain wildflower gardens would be less glorious.

Ticks

Ticks, the slow-moving relatives of spiders, are another potential carrier of disease. They are usually found in brushy areas below 6,000 feet in Southern California and below 4,000 feet in Northern California and seem most prevalent in late winter and spring. They neither jump nor fly but transfer from grass or brush to animals or you. You hardly see them and often do not feel their bite. This eight-legged creature can be as tiny as the dot of an *I* (larvae) or up to 0.25 inch (adult).

Bites by these blood-sucking arachnids cause two general problems for hikers and equestrians: 1) how to get them off and treat the wound, and 2) rare infections. Lyme disease has raised concern about infections from tick bites.

Ticks burrow their heads into the skin of the groin, armpits, hairline, or other body areas, especially where there is a constriction created by snug clothing, such as the waistband. The trick is to remove them, whole, without further injury. The most effective method is also the simplest—grasp the tick with tweezers as close to its attachment point as possible and pull gently upward and outward but firmly until it lets go. Try not to crush it, as doing so releases its fluid into the bite. After removing the tick, take precautions to prevent infection: Wash the wound with soap and water, apply a small amount of antibiotic ointment, and try to keep it clean. No further treatment is necessary.

Tick-borne infections are the feared hazard of tick bites and are sometimes difficult to diagnose, even by doctors, so prompt hospital attention is recommended for anyone who has symptoms that suggest such an infection.

Lyme disease is characterized by a migrating rash, fever, flulike symptoms, and worsening joint pain. It is easily treated with antibiotics in its early stages.

Spotted fever is marked by high fever, headache, and a red, spotty rash that becomes purple over time. This very serious illness should be promptly treated by antibiotics. It is quite rare throughout the Pacific West. Spotless forms of the fever are also occasionally contracted. Though difficult to diagnose, the victim's history of a prolonged tick bite will help steer the doctor toward the correct diagnosis.

Tick paralysis is a rarer condition of progressive severe weakness. It is usually completely reversed by removal of the tick. It rarely affects adults and is almost never seen outside of the Pacific Northwest.

Ticks need a few hours of attachment before they can transmit any disease they may harbor, so the quicker you remove them the better. Check your clothing and skin carefully for ticks a couple of times daily, and especially after hiking through brush at low elevations. Wear long-sleeved clothing, with cuffs tucked under socks or into boots. Insect repellent is also of some use for ticks—apply it liberally and often to skin and clothing.

Other Invertebrates

Flies can be a problem at lower elevations. Small black flies typically become numerous in warm weather—from about June through early October. One favored habitat is among shady canyon live oaks, which can be locally common in Southern California. The flies are attracted to sweat from your face and body, but if you clean up, they generally cease to bother you. Occasionally, at low to mid elevations, you'll meet large, biting flies (usually deer flies), but they don't attack in numbers. Furthermore, when one is preoccupied with biting into your skin, it is easy to swat.

Another problem is the **yellow jacket,** a wasp that occasionally builds a ground nest under or beside a trail; if you trample on it, the yellow jackets will swarm you. You are very unlikely to meet them, though your chances increase if you ride a horse, for it tramples the ground far more than a hiker does. Their stings are multiple and painful, but not dangerous unless you happen to be allergic to bee stings.

(More people in the United States die from bee stings than from rattlesnake bites.)

One of the best arguments for avoiding squirrels, which frequent popular campsites looking for food, is that they may be rabid or their **fleas** may carry the plague. Avoid fleas by avoiding rodents and their nests. Often rodents will opportunistically winter in a shelter that isn't visited until spring, when hikers will find the animals' nest, dust, and feces covering the surrounding floor. Hantavirus has been reported in California, and it is caused, in every case in North America, by human contact with rodent excrement. Avoid areas where you find abandoned rodent nests.

Finally, there are **scorpions,** which are not strictly desert creatures. You may find them in Southern California up to about 7,000 feet and in Northern California up to about 5,000 feet. These creatures, active at night, can give you a painful sting, although the species found along the PCT is not life-threatening.

Poison Oak

In some locations along the PCT, optimal conditions allow the waist-high shrub to assume the proportions of a small tree or a thick, climbing vine. Certainly, many PCT travelers would agree that, with the possible exception of flies or mosquitoes, poison oak is the most consistent nuisance along the trail in California. The allergic rash it causes in most people leads to several days of insane itching and irritation. It may, however, completely incapacitate a luckless few.

Poison oak dermatitis is best managed by avoidance, and avoidance is best accomplished by recognition of the plant, in all phases of its life cycle: In spring and summer, it puts forth shiny green leaves, each divided into three oval, lobed leaflets, which, even on the same plant, exhibit an unusual variety of sizes. Toward fall, the leaves and stems turn reddish, and the small whitish flowers become smooth berries. In winter and early spring, when its leaves are gone, identification is most difficult: look for dusty-gray bark on stems, with smooth green, red-tipped new growth and possibly some white-green berries left over from the previous season.

Avoid touching any part of the plant in any season—all parts contain urushiol, an oil in the sap, that will, in a few days, cause an allergic reaction where it has penetrated the skin. If you do brush against the shrub, immediately wash the area with soap and water. Water helps to deactivate the toxin, and soap helps to extract the oil from skin. If you can't wash the area right away, try to avoid rubbing, which will spread the oil around. Better yet, avoid exposure entirely by wearing long-sleeved shirts and pants tucked into boot tops. But beware: Urushiol on clothing can be transferred to the skin even hours later. If you must wear shorts, try applying a commercial barrier cream, which helps keep the oil from reaching the skin. Above all, avoid smoke from burning poison oak, and never eat any of the plant—fatal internal reactions have occurred.

If you do develop the itchy, red, blistering, weeping rash of poison oak dermatitis, console yourself with the knowledge that it will be gone in a week or so. In the meantime, try not to

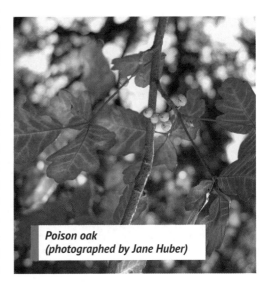

Poison oak
(photographed by Jane Huber)

scratch it—infection is the biggest hazard. Use calamine lotion, topical hydrocortisone cream, and oral Benadryl for itch relief. Severe allergic reactions, characterized by trouble breathing, dizziness, or swelling around the eyes or mouth, should be treated as soon as possible by a doctor.

Poodle-Dog Bush

Poodle-dog bush, or *Eriodictyon parryi,* is a pretty purple-flowered plant native to California that often proliferates in areas ravaged by wildfires. The plant is covered in sticky hairs, which can dislodge easily and be passed on to hikers who touch it or brush up against it.

Swelling, rash, and itching often appear 12 hours to two days after contact. Volunteers have worked hard in recent years to clear it from the trail, but it continues to rear its nasty head, especially in burn areas. It can be found in nearly all habitat types that have recently burned, including conifer forests, chaparral, oak woodland, and riparian areas. It is most rampant in recent years in burn areas of Sections C and D of the Southern California PCT, most notably between Three Points in the Angeles National Forest and Soledad Canyon Road near Acton. The U.S. Forest Service recommends wearing long sleeves and pants in these areas and avoiding the plant at all costs.

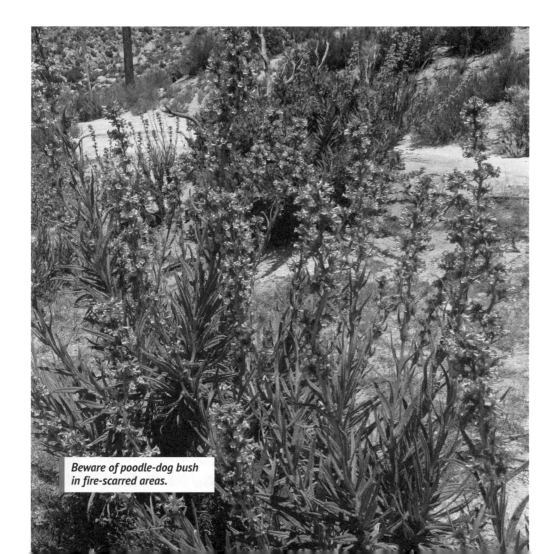

Beware of poodle-dog bush in fire-scarred areas.

Waterborne Microscopic Organisms

Many of the PCT's springs, streams, and lakes have clear water, but what you can't see might make you ill. The microscopic organisms are perhaps more threatening than any black bear you'll meet on the trail. One microscopic organism is *Giardia lamblia,* which causes giardiasis. Although the condition can be incapacitating, it is not usually life-threatening. After ingestion by humans, giardia organisms normally attach themselves to the small intestine, and disease symptoms usually include diarrhea, increased foul-smelling gas, loss of appetite, abdominal cramps, and bloating. Weight loss may occur from nausea and loss of appetite. These discomforts may last up to six weeks. Most people are unaware that they have been infected and return home before the onset of symptoms. If not treated, the symptoms may disappear on their own, only to recur intermittently over a period of many months. Other diseases have similar symptoms, but if you drank untreated water, you should suspect giardiasis and so inform your doctor. If properly diagnosed, the disease is curable with prescribed medication.

There are several ways to treat found water to make it relatively safe to drink. The treatment most certain to destroy giardia is to bring the water to a boil (no need to boil for minutes; once it comes to a boil, the little assassins are gone). Chemical disinfectants such as tablets or drops may not be as reliable: although they work well against most waterborne bacteria and viruses that cause disease, they are not effective against a certain intestinal parasite, **cryptosporidium,** which can occur at water holes fouled by cattle. The most convenient safeguard is to use a portable water purifier. While relatively expensive and somewhat bulky, an ultraviolet-light water purifier or hollow-fiber technology in a straw or gravity filter gives you safe water in a minute or two—and there's no chemical taste and no waiting for chemicals to act or for boiled water to cool.

Valley Fever

Also known as *Coccidiodes,* this lung infection can be picked up through exposure to a fungus that lives in the soil in the Southwestern United States, notably California and Arizona. The Pacific Crest Trail likely passes through areas where this fungus exists. Its spores can get into the air with dust when it is windy or when dirt is disturbed. Symptoms include fever, exhaustion, cough, and chest pain. While most victims fully recover from Valley fever, there have been rare severe or fatal cases in which it has infected the brain, joints, and other organs. The Centers for Disease Control and Prevention recommends talking to a doctor about the condition if you have its symptoms. More information is available at the California Department of Health: cdph.ca.gov.

CHAPTER 3

PCT Natural History

GEOLOGY   *by Dan R. Lynch*

It is difficult to fully appreciate the Pacific Crest Trail's sights without a basic understanding of the earth, its rocks, and the forces strong enough to build mountains. Here, we will cover some of the fundamentals of geology and a brief history of how the Pacific Coast's mountain ranges came to be. Then, when you're resting after a difficult portion of your hike, you'll be able to look back on your route and admire it for the natural forces that produced such a picturesque landscape.

Rock Types Along the Pacific Crest Trail

The Pacific Crest Trail (PCT) follows the ridges and peaks of the Sierra Nevada and the Pacific Coast Ranges, but some of the regions connecting these mountains include low-lying deserts, valleys, and gorges. This diverse topography will lead you through an equally diverse assortment of rock types from all three categories of rocks—igneous, metamorphic, and sedimentary. These terms refer to how the rocks formed and are crucial to understanding geology.

IGNEOUS ROCKS

Many of the PCT's most rugged landscapes and highest peaks, including Mount Whitney and Mount Hood, are composed of igneous rocks. **Igneous rocks** are formed directly from the cooling of

Above: Quartzite is common along the trail.

fluid molten rock originating from deep within the earth, where temperatures can reach thousands of degrees. Molten rock still deeply buried is called **magma,** and if undisturbed, it will cool and harden very slowly to form **intrusive igneous rocks,** such as granite. But movement within our planet can force magma upward toward Earth's surface. During an **eruption,** when magma breaks through Earth's **crust,** or the outer, most rigid layer of the planet, magma becomes **lava** and can flow across the landscape, where it cools very quickly in the atmosphere. **Extrusive igneous rocks,** such as basalt, are the results of cooled, hardened lava. Aside from how quickly they cool, a primary difference between magma and lava is the amount of gas trapped within the molten rock. All molten rock contains various gases, and within the earth, magma's gases have nowhere to go. When magma erupts as lava, however, those trapped gases can rise and escape, creating bubbles in the resultant rock and, if the gases escape very quickly, even causing powerful explosions when erupting.

Igneous rocks are defined and distinguished from each other by their mineral compositions and structural variations, particularly their grain sizes. All rocks are composed of different mixtures of minerals; the mixtures in igneous rocks are determined by the varying properties of the magma or lava that formed them. **Minerals** can therefore be thought of as the building blocks of rocks; minerals are not rocks, but all rocks contain minerals. Minerals are solid materials composed of specific chemical compounds that crystallize, or harden in a particular repeating shape that reflects their molecular structure. This can be a fairly complex subject, but put more simply, a **crystal** is the natural shape a chemical takes on when it hardens. Table salt, for example, is a mineral called halite, which is composed of the chemical compound sodium chloride and

crystallizes in the shape of a cube (look at table salt through a magnifying glass to see for yourself). Quartz, the most common mineral, is a constituent of many rocks, as are minerals from the feldspar, mica, olivine, pyroxene, and amphibole groups, all of which form different crystal shapes.

As hot, thick, fluid magma or lava begins to cool, the minerals within it begin to crystallize. The longer the molten rock takes to cool, the larger the crystals are. In granite, for example, which cools for many years within the earth, the various minerals within it can crystallize to large, visible sizes. But in rhyolite—a rock with essentially the same mineral composition as granite but which instead cools rapidly on the earth's surface—the minerals have a much shorter time to crystallize, remaining small and nearly invisible without magnification. In both, each individual grain is a mineral crystal, no matter its size. This is called **grain size,** which helps identify rocks.

In the Cascade Range, you may encounter rocks that appear to be both coarse- and fine-grained. These rocks, which show large, angular grains suspended in a very fine-grained body of rock, are described as **porphyritic,** meaning that they have a mixture of textures. These rocks are the result of a body of magma that was beginning to cool within the earth, allowing some minerals to crystallize to visible sizes, but was then suddenly erupted, causing the rest of the rock to cool much more quickly around the large grains.

Intrusive igneous rocks form much of the backbone of the PCT; granite is particularly common along the trail, but others can also be found in the mountains. Extrusive igneous rocks are also very prevalent along your journey. While definitively identifying each type of rock is beyond the scope of this book, learning some of their key traits will help point you in the right direction.

PRIMARY IGNEOUS ROCKS ALONG THE PCT

Granite (*intrusive*)	Coarse-grained, hard; mottled coloration but predominantly white, gray, tan, or pink. It is composed primarily of quartz and feldspars, with some micas, amphiboles, and other minerals. As one of the most common igneous rocks, you will find it in many places; Yosemite and the rest of the Sierra Nevada Range are composed primarily of granite and granitelike rocks.	
Rhyolite (*extrusive*)	Fine-grained, hard; usually even coloration in shades of tan, gray, or pink, but may have faint bands. It has essentially the same composition as granite but cooled on the earth's surface and thus has very fine grains and some rounded gas bubbles. It is common throughout the Cascade Range; it is one of the rocks produced by volcanoes.	
Diorite (*intrusive*)	Coarse-grained; mottled coloration but predominantly white or gray. While visually similar to granite, it has far less quartz but more feldspars, amphiboles, and pyroxene minerals, making it less variable in color. It can be found throughout most of the PCT's ranges.	
Gabbro (*intrusive*)	Coarse-grained; mottled, dark gray to black or greenish-black. It mostly contains feldspars, olivine, pyroxenes, and iron-rich minerals, but very little quartz. It is less plentiful than other igneous rocks in the region but will still turn up in the Cascade and Sierra Nevada Ranges.	
Basalt (*extrusive*)	Fine-grained; very dark coloration, usually dark gray to black, but may also have brown surfaces. It has mostly the same composition as gabbro but cooled quickly on the earth's surface, particularly in large flows; it often contains rounded gas bubbles. The Columbia River Gorge is part of one of the largest basalt formations; basalt forms the valley's black walls.	
Andesite (*extrusive*)	Typically porphyritic with lighter colored larger grains embedded in a finer, darker mass. Andesite forms when oceanic crust melts and is mixed with continental magma; it is essentially a blend of basalt and rhyolite. Very common throughout the entire Cascade Range and forms much of the mountains and volcanoes there.	

A body of intrusive igneous rock still underground is called a **pluton;** rocks that formed deep underground are known as **plutonic rocks.** Sometimes magma is forced upward into cracks within older rocks, forming a near-vertical wall of rock within a different type of rock; this is called a **dike.** Bodies of extrusive igneous rocks are called **flows,** as their lava flowed away from its source. A **volcano** is a vent in the earth's crust from which lava erupts; the Cascade Range is well known for its large, cone-shaped volcanoes, known as **stratovolcanoes.** All these igneous bodies, and many more, are present along the PCT.

SEDIMENTARY ROCKS

All rocks, no matter how hard or high, eventually succumb to the effects of weather. Wind, rain, chemical exposure, and especially ice are all destructive forces that wear down and degrade rocks, reducing their once solid masses into mere grains of sand and silt. These particles, or **sediments,** end up being washed into rivers, lakes, and seas, where they settle into **beds,** or flat layers. But for the remains of many weathered rocks, these beds are just the first step in becoming a new type of rock.

Sedimentary rocks are those formed when sediments—particularly the remnants of older rocks, but also organic remains—are compacted and cemented to form a new rock body. As the weight of water and newer sediments press down on bedded sediments, the grains compress and lock together. In many cases, the addition of dissolved minerals, particularly calcite, can crystallize between grains of sediment and act as a glue to further adhere them. The resultant rocks are often flat, broad, and layered.

These rocks are identified by and often named for the type of sediment that comprises them. Sandstone, for example, is formed from compacted, solidified sand. Others, like shale, have more specific identifying traits, such as dense layering. But in general, whatever their composition, most sedimentary rocks (with the

exception of chert) tend to be fairly soft and susceptible to weathering, their particles often only loosely adhered together. As a result, some sedimentary rocks may have harder and softer layers that weather at different rates, creating sculpted rock formations with dramatic layers, arches, and caves, such as the Vasquez Rocks along the trail north of Los Angeles.

Sedimentary rocks can offer us insight as to the climate and conditions at the time of their formation, including what kind of body of water in which the rock formed. The type of sediment is, of course, a key clue, but equally important is how those sediments are organized within the rock. For example, in shale, the size of the sediments is extremely fine—tiny particles of mud and clay—and such tiny, lightweight particles sink and settle very slowly. Therefore, for large beds to build up, the body of water—usually deep—must remain calm for long periods of time. Layer after layer of sediments were undisturbed, which resulted in shale, a very fine-grained rock with many soft but well-preserved layers. When the same kinds of sediments settle in more turbulent waters, the fine layering does not occur, and the resultant rock—mudstone—is more of a mass with fewer features.

Not all sedimentary rocks are formed from rock and clay particles, however. Limestone, an extremely prevalent rock in the western United States, is formed entirely of ancient sea life. Coral reefs, both in ancient times as well as today, are home to corals, mollusks, and many other types of marine plants and animals that produce shells and skeletons made of calcium carbonate. As those organisms die and settle, the reefs build upon themselves through successive growth. The buried calcium carbonate skeletons begin to create a solid mass, and the sediments adhere together in the form of the mineral calcite. The result is limestone, a soft rock consisting primarily of calcite and frequently containing visible fossils. Similarly, chert is a sedimentary rock that forms from the compaction of thick

PRIMARY SEDIMENTARY ROCKS ALONG THE PCT

Sandstone	Composed of sand-size particles that settled in ancient lakes and seas. Usually gray or yellow to brown but can contain bands. The sand grains within sandstone are typically quartz held together by calcite and clays; grains can often be separated by hand. Common along the PCT in both desert and coastal areas.	
Limestone	Composed of very fine particles derived from ancient coral reefs and thus made almost entirely of calcite. Usually light to dark gray or brown; may occasionally show faint layering. Fairly soft and easily scratched with a knife; often has a chalky feel and a slightly glittery appearance on a fresh break. Common everywhere but especially in drier areas, such as Southern California.	
Chert (*black chert is known as flint*)	Composed of extremely fine particles invisible to the eye. May be almost any color; usually gray to black, tan to brown, or reddish. Derived from seafloor sediments rich in diatoms, this silica-rich rock is extremely hard—a knife will not scratch it. When worn, especially in riverbeds, it can appear smooth and almost polished; freshly broken pieces will have very sharp edges. Common all along the PCT.	
Conglomerate	Composed of coarse pebbles embedded in a much finer grained mass; usually very mottled and variable coloration. Conglomerate formed in active bodies of water, particularly riverbeds, where larger rounded pebbles were buried in finer sediments, such as sand. When cemented and hardened, the result appears as though many river rocks were glued together. Most common in areas closer to the Pacific Coast.	

beds of silt rich in skeletons of diatoms, tiny aquatic organisms that make shells of silica, or quartz. Many of the low-lying or desert regions of the PCT and surrounding areas are home to sedimentary rocks, but they can be prevalent in mountainous areas as well. As plutons and other igneous rock formations were forced upward due to movement within the earth, they were often forced up through sedimentary rocks. As a result, sedimentary rocks that formed long ago at the bottom of seas and lakes can now be found high on mountainsides or comprising foothills.

You'll see a few natural features throughout the PCT that are a result of weathering and are closely related to sedimentary rocks. **Talus** slopes, also known as scree, are the fragments and boulders that have fallen from mountains and cliffs and collected at their bases, forming steeply slanted hills comprised of loose rocks. **Alluvial** fans are fan-shaped accumulations of rocks, sand, and mud that originate from the mouth of a river or canyon. These are common where rivers meet flatter, broader planes and the flow slows and spreads outward, creating the fan shape. In desert areas, rivers that create alluvial fans are typically the result of flash floods, which later dry up to reveal the alluvial fan as a land feature.

METAMORPHIC ROCKS

On the earth's surface, the weather is the primary force that changes rocks, but within the earth things are very different. Beginning less than 0.5 mile down into the earth's crust, the temperature begins to increase dramatically, and at greater depths it becomes hot enough to soften or melt rock. And the deeper within the earth you go, the greater the pressure becomes as well, as the weight of the world bears down from above. It is in these extreme conditions that rocks undergo their most dramatic changes, being softened and compressed and becoming entirely new types of rocks in the process. The resulting rocks are called **metamorphic rocks** and are sometimes so completely changed by heat and pressure that it can seem impossible to tell what rock they originally were.

The movement that occurs within our planet can force rocks downward beneath the earth's crust. Although an extremely slow process (discussed in detail later), this movement is how rocks like limestone—consisting of ancient seafloor sediments from the earth's surface—can achieve such deep burial that they can be affected by the earth's interior heat. Igneous rocks, sedimentary rocks, and other metamorphic rocks can be **metamorphosed,** or changed, into metamorphic rock types. And depending on the varying amounts of heat and pressure, rocks can undergo varying amounts

PRIMARY METAMORPHIC ROCKS ALONG THE PCT

Schist (*foliated*)	Schist results from a fairly strong heating and compaction of many different kinds of rocks; the original rock determines the type of schist that results. Many schists are a result of metamorphosed sedimentary rocks and can show many fine layers, ample glittering micas, and pockets of hard gemstones, such as garnets. Schists are common throughout the PCT.	
Gneiss (*foliated*)	Gneiss (pronounced "nice") is the result of advanced metamorphism and can be derived from many types of rock. Gneisses tend to have broad layering and loosely organized bands of minerals, often with many glittering layers of micas. Gneisses are named for their parent rock; granitic gneiss, for example, began as granite and can appear to share many traits with granite. Gneisses are common throughout the PCT.	
Quartzite (*non-foliated*)	Quartzite began as sandstone; it can form when quartz-rich solutions harden between sandstone's quartz grains, or when heating and compression solidify the grains in sandstone. Quartzite is an extremely quartz-rich rock that is very hard. Usually light-colored; white, gray, tan, or pink. It has a rough texture, often with sharp edges, and a slightly flaky appearance when freshly broken. Water-worn pebbles can appear translucent and nearly polished. It is common all along the trail, especially in rivers.	

or different kinds of metamorphosis, all with potentially different resultant rocks.

Heat and pressure can plasticize, or soften, rocks, which can have a variety of effects: consolidation and hardening of the rock, reorganization of a rock's minerals into tightly packed layers (called **foliation**; any metamorphic rocks that exhibit layering are described as being foliated), or recrystallization of a rock's minerals into entirely new minerals, to name a few. Shale, for example, is a soft, layered sedimentary rock that, when metamorphosed, turns into slate, a much harder and more densely layered rock that still somewhat resembles the original shale. Sturdier rocks, like granite, require more extreme conditions to metamorphose but can be changed as well.

Metamorphosis occurs on a gradient, and with increasing heat and pressure, a rock can continue changing. The shale-to-slate transformation, for example, is a low-grade metamorphism and can continue, with the slate eventually becoming phyllite, then schist, then gneiss—all increasingly harder, more foliated, more crystallized, higher-grade metamorphic rocks—if the heat and pressure continue to build. Along the way, the rock's minerals can recombine to form new minerals. Schist, for example, is an intermediate-grade metamorphic rock that can contain garnets, which are gems typically not present in the original rock.

There are many kinds of metamorphism, most of which are associated with movement in the earth's crust or the rising of hot plutons. As a result, metamorphic rocks are particularly common in mountainous areas—especially the Klamath Range—and in foothills that have often been pushed and transformed to make way for the growing mountains. Along the trail, you'll likely encounter metamorphic rocks in the form of hard, dark, layered rocks that frequently appear to glitter with countless mineral flakes. Cliffs and other rock faces may also reveal metamorphic layers that bend or wrap around each other—these are called folds, and they illustrate the immense power that has affected these rocks.

Tectonic Plates

Many of the rocks you'll encounter along the PCT exist as a direct result of movements within our planet. Earth is not a solid, unchanging mass; it is dynamic and always evolving. This is due in large part to its layered structure. Earth has distinct zones of varying temperature and composition as they progress downward toward the planet's solid metal core. Earth's crust, the outermost layer upon which all life resides, is the top of the lithosphere, a rigid, rocky layer that is broken up into enormous segments called **tectonic plates.** These plates are like ill-fitting puzzle pieces; some plate boundaries rest on top of or beneath the edges of other plates. Generally, each continent and major ocean sits atop its own plate, and the boundaries or joints at which these plates meet are called **faults,** which can be the sites of major geological events.

Beneath the lithosphere is the asthenosphere, a molten layer upon which the tectonic plates sit. The asthenosphere consists of hot, soft rock and is in constant motion due to convection. Currents of rock rise, fall, and flow very slowly, taking the tectonic plates above them along for the ride. As the rigid tectonic plates of the lithosphere move, some collide, some spread apart, and others slide past each other. All these types of movements have played a role in the formation of the Pacific Coast region and the modern-day PCT.

CONVERGENT MOVEMENT

This type of tectonic plate movement sees plates converging, or coming together, and is frequently associated with building mountains. Many times, mountains are a result of one plate being forced beneath another, causing the upper plate to rise and develop a mountain range. Along the Pacific Coast, however, the process was a little more complex, resulting not only in mountains but volcanoes as well. This process was particularly important in the development of the Cascade Range; this will be discussed in detail later.

DIVERGENT MOVEMENT

This type of movement occurs when two tectonic plates spread apart, leaving a gap between them. This typically occurs on ocean floors where two oceanic plates are separating. Divergent movement is particularly prominent in the Atlantic Ocean but occurs in the Pacific as well. When two oceanic plates separate, the space between them fills in with rising molten rock. This tectonic spreading can be a driving factor for convergent plate collisions on the other sides of the plates.

TRANSFORM MOVEMENT

Transform movement is the general term for when tectonic plates slide past each other, often grinding against each other in such a way as to cause earthquakes, as occurs along the San Andreas Fault in California. But smaller mountain ranges can also form when the two plates don't slide along each other cleanly. Angular pressure between the plates can push material upward between them; this is how Southern California's Transverse Ranges were formed.

Formation of the Pacific Crest Trail

With a basic understanding of rock types and tectonic plates, we can now begin to piece together the story of how the PCT's mountain ranges formed.

The PCT begins near Campo in Southern California, at the Mexico border, in the foothills of the Peninsular Ranges. The **Peninsular Ranges** are a series of mountain ranges that run north–south along the Baja Peninsula of Mexico and into Southern California; the Laguna, Santa Rosa, and San Jacinto Ranges are the Peninsular Ranges that PCT hikers will pass through. All the Peninsular Ranges formed around the same time as the Sierra Nevada Range and from similar geological events stemming from the movement of an ancient tectonic plate, called the Farallon Plate.

Today, the Farallon Plate is mostly gone, almost completely subducted beneath North America, but around 200 million years ago, it was a major oceanic plate spreading eastward, toward the Pacific Coast, bringing islands along with it. As the islands docked with North America, collecting on the edges of the continent and building out the western coasts, the Farallon Plate began to dive below the North American Plate, heating up as it got deeper. As the plate melted, the resultant soft, hot rock began to rise toward the surface as plutons, or massive blobs of intrusive igneous rocks, particularly granite. In simplest terms, as the Farallon Plate continuously sank and melted, the hot rock produced rose and displaced the rock above it; as a result, the plutons were continuously pushed upward. As the Farallon Plate moved eastward, the overlying older rock moved westward and the younger granite plutons were exposed, composing the Peninsular Ranges as we know them today. The Peninsular Ranges' north-south-trending direction mainly follows the plate boundary, or fault, where the Farallon Plate was subducted, and where the Pacific Plate currently meets the North American Plate.

Just north of the Peninsular Ranges are the **Transverse Ranges,** named such because their east–west orientation is transverse to the north–south nature of the coast. The Transverse Ranges, which include the San Bernardino, San Gabriel, and Tehachapi Ranges, extend from the Pacific Coast to the Mojave Desert and generally follow the San Andreas Fault. The San Andreas Fault is an extremely active fault system on the boundary of the Pacific and North American Plates in Southern California, notorious for the frequent and destructive earthquakes it causes. While technically a transform fault, the Pacific and North American Plates are not sliding past each other smoothly. Instead, they grind together as they pass, pressing into each other and generating incredible forces that not only shake the land but also push rocks upward. As the rocks were forced higher and higher, the Transverse Ranges were born.

California's most significant portion of the PCT runs along the **Sierra Nevada Range,** famous for dramatic sites like Yosemite National Park, Lake Tahoe, and Mount Whitney. This iconic mountain range also has a particularly interesting geological history. While the range's oldest rocks originate from the Cambrian period, around 541 million years ago, the soaring, snowy peaks we see today weren't present until around 70 million years ago.

Much like the Peninsular Ranges, the subduction of the Farallon Plate caused the formation of intrusive plutons that rose and began to collect near the earth's surface in modern-day eastern California. As the multitude of plutonic rocks formed, they came to act as a singular massive body of rock known as the **Sierra Nevada Batholith** (a batholith is a large mass of intrusive rock, usually granite, that measures more than 100 square kilometers in size), which was not originally exposed on the earth's surface.

How it rose to form the Sierra Nevada Range is still actively debated; traditionally, it was thought to have been uplifted as a result of tectonic activity farther east. In a geologic region known as the Basin and Range Province (underlying much of Nevada, Arizona, and eastern California today), intense volcanic heat below the easternmost portion of the batholith is thought to have thinned it, making it lighter weight than the western portion. This may have caused the

batholith to tilt and rotate westward as the eastern end rose to become the peaks of the range. This theory, which stems from the tilted shape of the range, has been proposed for decades and is one that many may already be familiar with. Modern research, however, has suggested that perhaps there wasn't much uplift at all, but rather a collapse of the surrounding rock. As tectonic forces in the region lessened, surrounding areas may have subsided—especially the Basin and Range Province to the east—exposing the batholith and leaving it elevated. New research is still being conducted, but evidence for this theory is strong.

In either proposed method of formation, modern research suggests that the Sierra Nevada Range has towered over the eastern portion of the state for at least 70 million years. The range as we see it today has since been shaped by weathering, with notable help from the past glaciers (thick masses of ice indicative of ice ages). The glaciers scoured through valleys and down the range's slopes, creating many of the lakes found there today.

As you pass from the Sierra Nevada Range to the **Klamath Range** in Northern California and southern Oregon, you also pass into dramatically different geology. As the Farallon Plate was subducted beneath the North American Plate, large islands and microcontinents (similar to New Zealand today) atop the Farallon Plate were pulled toward North America. As they collided with the West Coast, they accreted, or became part of the North American continent. The Klamath Mountains represent the accumulation of several of these accreted islands, forced upward as further plate collisions occurred. Later volcanic activity injected the Klamath Range with intrusive rocks from below, heating and heavily metamorphosing many of the range's bodies of rock, resulting in some of the stranger kinds of rocks along the PCT.

As you leave the Klamath Range and continue northward, you'll enter the longest section

GEOLOGIC TIME SCALE

Throughout the book, we'll refer to various geological periods during which parts of the PCT were formed. This scale shows how these periods relate to each other and how many years ago they began.

ERA	PERIOD	BEGAN (in millions of years)
Cenozoic		
	Quaternary	2.58
	Neogene	23.03
	Paleogene	66.0
Mesozoic		
	Cretaceous	145.0
	Jurassic	201.3
	Triassic	251.9
Paleozoic		
	Permian	298.9
	Carboniferous	358.9
	Devonian	419.2
	Silurian	443.8
	Ordovician	485.4
	Cambrian	541.0

The Precambrian eon has not been included here. These dates are derived from the latest sources available in 2020, but, as in the past, they are bound to be slightly revised in the future. The oldest known rocks are about 4.3 billion years old; Earth's crust solidified about 4.6 billion years ago.

of the PCT: the **Cascade Range.** These iconic mountains, stretching from Northern California into Canada, are famous for their active volcanoes and rugged valleys formed during the subduction of the Juan de Fuca Plate beneath the North American Plate. The Juan de Fuca Plate, thought to be a remnant of the Farallon Plate, is a small plate off the coast of Oregon and Washington that is still actively subducting beneath North America. As it does, it descends eastward to where portions of it begin to melt, many miles from the plate boundary. As a result, when the rising magma formed by this melting is forced to the surface, it erupts inland. Due to the makeup of the magma, it produces lots of pulverized rock and ash when it erupts; subsequent eruptions can create a buildup of rock and ash around the vent, giving rise to a stratovolcano, or layered, cone-shaped volcano. Throughout the past 37 million years or so, many Cascade volcanoes have erupted for a short time and then stopped when their magma supply moved to a new spot, where a new volcano began. Peak after peak began to rise and accumulate in this way, building much of the modern range. But this is just the most recent chapter in a long history of Pacific Coast eruptions along the Cascade Range. Much earlier, the adherence of a microcontinent that already contained a chain of volcanoes laid much of the groundwork for today's Cascades.

Along your way through the Cascades, you'll have to cross the **Columbia River** along the Washington–Oregon border, where you'll notice a marked change in geology. The black-walled river valley is part of the **Columbia Plateau,** a landform composed almost entirely of basalt formed during a series of eruptions between 17 million to 6 million years ago. In one of the largest continuous lava formations in the world, the Columbia Plateau formed during a flood basalt, in which basalt lava flowed over huge, broad expanses, creating a relatively flat landscape. This unique section of your hike is in stark contrast to most of the PCT's geology, taking you to one of the lowest elevation portions of the entire route: the Bridge of the Gods, which you'll take to cross the river.

In many areas along the PCT, particularly the Sierra Nevada and Cascade Ranges, glaciers have played a large role in shaping the mountains as they appear today. Glaciers are massive formations of ice that appear at the poles and in high elevations during the glacial periods of ice ages. As they accumulate more ice, or as warming temperatures melt their ice, they grow or recede, flowing like a very slow river. But the immense weight of the ice can crush and break up rocks, the fragments of which become incorporated within the glaciers and add to its abrasive quality. As a result, mountain glaciers can carve large valleys. The point at which a glacier begins to accumulate, high in the mountains, is called a **cirque,** and it is usually bowl-shaped. As glaciers melt, cirques often collect glacial meltwater, creating small but pristine mountain lakes called **tarns.** Tarns often have a natural dam, called a **moraine,** that keeps them filled—moraines are piles or ridges of rock created by glaciers as the pulverized rock within the ice is deposited. **Lateral moraines** form along the sides of a glacier, parallel to its flow direction, from gravel left behind as a glacier begins to melt. Conversely, **terminal or end moraines** form at the front of a glacier as gravel and sand are dumped when a glacier begins to melt and recede. Keep an eye out for these features as you make your way along the trail.

From the shadow of Mount Whitney to the Columbia River banks, the PCT follows some of the most dramatic geology on the West Coast, and you'd be remiss to let it pass you by without taking notice of the millions of years of history just beneath your feet.

BIOLOGY

Just as there is a great variety of minerals, rocks, landscapes, and climates along the PCT, so too is there a great variety of plants and animals. Even if you don't know much about basic ecology, you can't help noticing that the natural scene along the PCT changes with elevation. The most obvious changes are in the trees, simply because they are the largest organisms. Furthermore, they don't move around or migrate in their lifetimes, as do animals. When you pay close attention, you notice that not only the trees but also the shrubs and wildflowers change with elevation. Then you begin to find latitudinal differences in the animal populations. In other words, there are different life zones.

Life Zones

In 1894 C. Hart Merriam divided North America into seven broad ecosystems, which he called life zones. These zones were originally based primarily on temperature, though today they are based on the distribution of plants and animals. The zones correspond roughly with latitude, from the Tropical Zone, which stretches from Florida across Mexico, to the Arctic Zone, which includes the polar regions. Between these two are found, south to north, the Lower Sonoran, Upper Sonoran, Transition, Canadian, and Hudsonian Zones. All but the Tropical Zone are encountered along the California PCT.

Just as temperature decreases as you move toward the earth's poles, so too does it decrease as you climb upward—between 3°F and 5.5°F for every 1,000 feet of elevation gain. Thus, if you were to climb from broad San Gorgonio Pass 10,000 feet up to the summit of San Gorgonio Peak, you would pass through all the same zones that you would if you walked from Southern California north all the way to Alaska. It turns out that 1,000 feet of elevation is roughly equivalent to 170 miles of latitude. Although the California PCT is about 1,600 miles long, the net northward gain in latitude is only about 650 miles—you have to hike 2.5 route-miles to get 1 mile north. This 650-mile change in latitude should bring about the same temperature change as climbing 3,800 feet up a mountain. On the PCT, you enter Oregon at a 6,000-foot elevation, finding yourself in a dense, Canadian Zone pine-and-fir forest. Doing your arithmetic, you would expect to find an equally dense fir forest at the Mexican border 3,800 feet higher—at a 9,800-foot elevation. Unfortunately, no such elevation exists along the border to test this prediction. However, if we head 85 miles north from the border to the Mount San Jacinto environs, and subtract 500 feet in elevation to compensate for this new latitude, what do we find at the 9,300-foot elevation? You guessed it, a Canadian Zone pine-and-fir forest. Ah, but nature is not quite that simple, for the two forests are unmistakably different.

Plant Geography

Every plant (and every animal) has its own range, habitat, and niche. Some species have a very restricted range; others, a very widespread one. The sequoia, for example, occurs only in about 75 groves at mid-elevations in the western Sierra Nevada. It flourishes in a habitat of tall conifers growing on shaded, gentle, well-drained slopes. Its niche—its role in the community—consists of its complex interaction with its environment and every other species in its environment. Dozens of insects use the sequoia's needles and cones, and additional organisms thrive in its surrounding soil. The woolly sunflower, on the other hand, has

a tremendous range: from California north to British Columbia and east to the Rocky Mountains. It can be found in brushy habitats from near sea level up to 10,000 feet.

Evidently, some species can adapt to environments and competitors better than others. Nevertheless, each is restricted by a complex interplay of climatic, physiographic (topographic), edaphic (soil), and biotic (living organism) influences.

Climatic Influences

Of all climatic influences, temperature and precipitation are probably the most important. Although the mean temperature tends to increase toward the equator, this pattern is camouflaged in California by the dominating effect of the state's highly varied topography. As was mentioned earlier, the temperature decreases between 3°F and 5.5°F for every 1,000-foot gain in elevation. The vegetational changes reflect this cooling trend. For example, the vegetation along San Gorgonio Pass in Southern California is adapted to its desert environment. Annuals are very ephemeral; after heavy rains, they quickly grow, blossom, and die. Perennials are succulent or woody, have deep roots, and have small hard or waxy leaves—or no leaves at all. Only the lush cottonwoods and other associated species along the dry streambeds hint at a source of water.

As you climb north up the slopes of San Gorgonio Mountain, not only does the temperature drop, but the annual precipitation also increases. On the gravelly desert floor below, only sparse, drought-adapted vegetation survives the searing summer temperatures and the miserly 10 inches of precipitation. A doubled precipitation on the mountainside allows growth of chaparral, here a thick stand of ocean spray, birchleaf mountain mahogany, Gregg's ceanothus, and great-berried manzanita. By 7,000 feet the precipitation has increased to 40 inches, and the moisture-loving conifers—first

Jeffrey pine, then lodgepole pine and white fir—predominate. As the temperature steadily decreases with elevation, evaporation of soil water and transpiration of moisture from plant needles and leaves are both reduced. Furthermore, up here the precipitation may be in the form of snow, which is preserved for months by the shade of the forest and even when it melts is retained by the highly absorbent humus (decayed organic matter) of the forest soil. Consequently, an inch of precipitation on the higher slopes is far more effective than an inch on the exposed, gravelly desert floor. Similar vegetation changes can be found wherever you make dramatic ascents or descents. In Northern California significant elevation and vegetation changes occur as you descend to and then ascend from CA 70 at Belden, I-5 at Castle Crags State Park, and CA 96 at Seiad Valley.

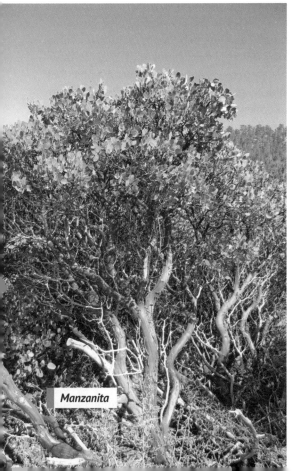

Manzanita

Physiographic Influences

As we have seen, elevation largely governs temperature and precipitation. For a given elevation, the mean maximum temperature in Northern California is about 10°F less than that of the San Bernardino area. Annual precipitation, however, is considerably more; it ranges from about 20 inches in the Sacramento Valley to 80 inches along the higher slopes, where the snowpack may last well into summer. When you climb out of a canyon in the Feather River country, you start among live oak, poison oak, and California laurel and ascend through successive stands of Douglas-fir and black oak; incense cedar and ponderosa pine; white fir and sugar pine; and finally red fir, lodgepole, and western white pine.

The country near the Oregon border is one of lower elevations and greater precipitation, which produces a wetter but milder climate that is reflected in the distribution of plant species. Seiad Valley is hemmed in by forests of Douglas-fir, tanbark oak, madrone, and canyon live oak. When you reach Cook and Green Pass (4,750'), you reach a forest of white fir and noble fir. To the east, at higher elevations, you encounter weeping spruce.

A low minimum temperature, like a high maximum one, can determine where a plant species lives, as freezing temperatures can kill poorly adapted plants by causing ice crystals to form in their cells. At high elevations, the gnarled trunks of the whitebark, limber, and foxtail pines give stark testimony to their battle against the elements. The wind-cropped, short-needled foliage is sparse at best, for the growing season lasts but two months and a killing frost is possible in every month. Samples of this subalpine forest are found on the upper slopes of the higher peaks in the San Jacinto, San Bernardino, and San Gabriel Mountains and along much of the John Muir Trail. Along or near the High Sierra crest and on the highest Southern California summits, all vestiges of forest surrender to rocky, barren slopes pioneered only by the most stalwart perennials, such as alpine willow and alpine buttercup.

Other physiographic influences are the location, steepness, orientation, and shape of slopes. North-facing slopes are cooler and tend to be wetter than south-facing slopes. Hence on north-facing slopes, you'll encounter red fir forests that, at the ridgeline, abruptly give way to a dense cover of manzanita and ceanothus on south-facing slopes. Extremely steep slopes may never develop a deep soil or support a coniferous forest, and of course cliffs will be devoid of vegetation other than crustose lichens, secluded mosses, scattered annuals, and a few drought-resistant shrubs and trees.

Edaphic Influences

Along the northern part of your trek, at the headwaters of the Trinity River and just below Seiad Valley, you'll encounter outcrops of serpentine, California's official state rock. (Technically, the rock is serpentinite, and it is composed almost entirely of the mineral serpentine, but even geologists call it serpentine.) This rock weathers to form a soil poor in some vital plant nutrients but rich in certain undesirable heavy metals. Nevertheless, there are numerous species, such as leather oak, that are specifically or generally associated with serpentine-derived soils. There is a species of *Streptanthus* (mustard family) found only on this soil, even though it could grow better on other soils. Experiments demonstrate that it cannot withstand the competition of other plants growing on these soils. It therefore struggles, yet propagates, within its protected environment. Another example is at Marble Mountain, also in Northern California, which has a local assemblage of plants that have adapted to the mountain's limey soil.

Soil can change over time and, with it, the vegetation. An illuminating example is found in formerly glaciated Sierran lands, where young soils today are thin and poor in both nutrients and humus. However, with passing millennia they will evolve into more mature soils and eventually could, given enough time, support sequoias up in the red fir zone. These trees likely grew mostly in that zone, but glaciers removed the soils, so the trees that manage to survive today do so in the lower, unglaciated lands, that is, mostly down with the white firs and sugar pines. Once glaciation ceases in the Sierra Nevada, which could be a few million years away, the sequoias could recolonize the lands they lost some 2 or more million years ago.

Biotic Influences

In an arid environment, plants competing for water may develop special adaptations besides their water-retaining mechanisms. The creosote bush, for example, in an effort to preserve its limited supply of water, secretes toxins that prevent nearby seeds from germinating. The result is an economical spacing of bushes along the desert floor.

Competition is manifold everywhere. On a descending trek past a string of alpine lakes, you might see several stages of plant succession. The highest lake may be pristine, bordered only by tufts of sedges between the lichen-crusted rocks. A lower lake may exhibit an invasion of grasses, sedges, and pondweeds thriving on the sediments deposited at its inlet. Corn lilies and Lemmon's willows border its edge. Farther down, a wet meadow may be the remnant of a former shallow lake. Water birch and lodgepole pine then make their debut. Finally, you reach the last lake bed, recognized only by the flatness of the forest floor and a few boulders of a recessional moraine (glacial deposit) that dammed the lake. In this location, a thick stand of white fir has overshadowed and eliminated much of the underlying lodgepole. Be aware, however, that lake–meadow–forest succession is very slow, the lakes being filled with sediments at an average rate of about 1 foot per 1,000 years. At this rate, it will take about 20,000–30,000 years to fill in most of the lakes, and more than 100,000 years to fill in Tenaya Lake, between Tuolumne Meadows and Yosemite Valley. However, barring significant man-induced atmospheric warming, California's climate should cool in a few thousand years, and another round of glaciation should commence.

When a species becomes too extensive, the lack of diversity makes it more vulnerable to attack. One of the hazards of a single-species stand is the inherent instability of the system. The large, pure stand of lodgepole pine near Tuolumne Meadows has for years been under siege by a moth known as the lodgepole needle miner. Within a well-mixed forest, however, lodgepoles are scattered and the needle miner is not much of a problem.

Species need not always compete, though. Sometimes two species cooperate for the mutual benefit, if not the actual existence, of both. That is true of the Joshua tree and its associated yucca moth, which are discussed in the Antelope Valley portion of Section E. Another most important association goes unseen: nearly all the plants you'll encounter have roots that form a symbiotic relationship with fungi. These mycorrhizal fungi greatly increase the efficiency of the roots' water and nutrient uptake, and the roots provide the fungi with some of the plants' photosynthesized simple sugars.

Unquestionably, the greatest biotic agent is people. (They are also the greatest geomorphic agent, directly or indirectly causing more erosion—and therefore more habitat degradation—than any natural process.) For example, people have supplanted native species with introduced species. Most of California's native bunchgrass is gone (as are the animals that grazed upon it), replaced by thousands of acres of one-crop fields and suburban sprawl. Forests near some mining towns have been virtually eliminated. Others have been subjected to ravenous scars inflicted by human-caused fires and by clear-cutting. The Los Angeles

basin's smog production has already begun to take its toll on mountain conifers, and Sierra forests may experience a similar fate. Widescale use of pesticides has not eliminated the pests, but it has greatly reduced their natural predators. Through forestry, agriculture, and urban practices, people have attempted to simplify nature, and by upsetting its checks and balances have made many ecosystems unstable. Along the PCT, you'll see areas virtually unaffected by people as well as areas greatly affected by them. When you notice the difference, you'll have something to ponder as you stride along the quiet trail.

The Role of Fire

Fires were once thought to be detrimental to the overall well-being of the ecosystem, and early foresters attempted to prevent or subdue all fires. This policy led to the accumulation of thick litter, dense brush, and overmature trees—all prime fuel when a fire inevitably sparked. Human-caused fires can be prevented, but how does one prevent a lightning fire, so common in the Sierra?

The answer is that fires should not be prevented but only regulated. Left unchecked, natural fires burn stands of mixed conifers about once every 10 years. At this frequency, brush and litter do not accumulate enough to result in complete devastation; only the ground cover is burned, while the trees remain intact. Hence, through small burns, the forest is protected from flaming catastrophes.

Some pines are adapted to fire. Indeed, the relatively uncommon knobcone pine, growing in scattered localities particularly in the Klamath Mountains of Northern California, requires fire to survive: the short-lived tree must be consumed by fire for its seeds to be released. The lodgepole pine will also release its seeds after a fire, although a fire is not necessary. Particularly adapted to fires, if not dependent on them, are plants of Southern California's chaparral community, which is discussed in the introduction of Section B. But fire is important in the Sierra and other high ranges too. For example, seeds of the genus *Ceanothus* are quick to germinate in burned-over ground, and some plants of this genus are among the primary foods of deer. Hence, periodic burns will help a deer population thrive, but without them, shrubs become too woody and unproductive for a deer herd. Similarly, gooseberries and other berry plants that sprout after fires help support several different bird populations.

Without fires, a plant community evolves toward a climax, or end stage of plant succession. Red fir is the main climax species in higher forests in California's mountains. A pure stand of any species, as mentioned earlier, invites epidemic attacks and is therefore unstable. But even climax vegetation does not last forever. Typically the climax vegetation is a dense forest, and eventually the trees mature, die, and topple over. Logs and litter accumulate to such a degree that when a fire starts, the abundant fuel causes a crown fire, not a

ground fire, and the forest burns down. Over time, succession results in an even-age stand of trees, and the cycle repeats itself. In the past, ecologists believed that stable climax vegetation was the rule, but we now know that unstable, changing vegetation is more common, even where man is not involved.

Fire also unlocks nutrients that are stored in living matter, topsoil, and rocks. Vital compounds are released in the form of ash when a fire burns plants and forest litter. Fires can also heat granitic rocks enough to cause them to break up and release their minerals. Even in a coniferous forest, the weathering of granitic rock is often due primarily to periodic fires. This may be true even in the high desert. For example, a large fire ravaged many of the granitic slopes in Anza-Borrego Desert State Park, and a postfire inspection revealed that the fire was intense enough to cause thin sheets of granite to exfoliate, or sheet off, from granitic boulders.

Natural, periodic fires, then, are beneficial for a forest ecosystem and should be thought of as an integral process in the plant community.

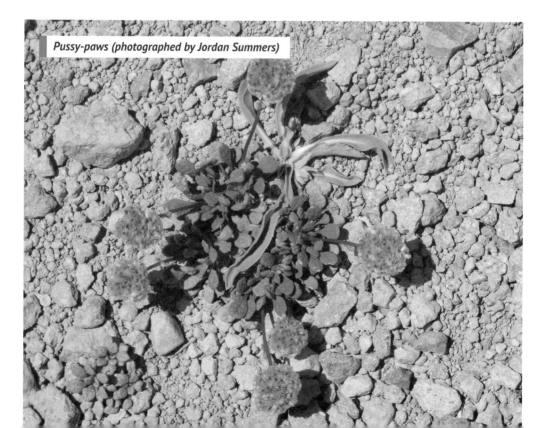

Pussy-paws (photographed by Jordan Summers)

They have, after all, been around as long as terrestrial life has, and for millions of years have been common in California plant communities.

More than ever in our lifetime, we are faced with a forest emergency unlike we've ever seen. Since 2010, it is estimated that California forests have lost more than 100 million trees to drought, disease, pests, wind, and fire. Hikers will see this impact often on the trail, though it won't always be noted in the route description because change happens so rapidly. The borders of a forest can morph quickly into the devastation caused by pine beetles or into areas of blown-down trees. More important are the possible hazards presented to hikers, whether on the trail or in a camp; burned trees have weakened roots and therefore don't stand up well in high winds. Widow-makers are plentiful wherever you spot standing tree carcasses.

A few notes of caution:

- Take extra care with any open flame; have water on hand to completely extinguish the fire and its coals.

- Use existing fire rings, and never set a fire near dry leaves, forest duff, grasses, bushes, and branches.

- Be cautious in drainages around burn areas; flash floods are more common and destructive after a fire. Do not camp in drainages.

- Use a stove with a shut-off valve and a contained fuel source that cannot spill.

- Travel through burn areas quickly. Do not camp below hazard trees, especially on windy days.

Plant Communities and Their Animal Associates

Plant communities are quite complex, and the general life-zone system doesn't account for California's diverse climates and landscapes. Consequently, we'll elaborate on the biological scenario by looking at California's plant communities. Philip Munz, one of California's leading native-plant authorities in his day, used the term *plant community* "for each regional element of the vegetation that is characterized by the presence of certain dominant species." Using this criterion, we devised our own list of California plant communities, which differs somewhat from the list proposed by Munz. We found that for the PCT, the division between Red Fir Forest and Lodgepole Pine Forest was an artificial one. True, you can find large, pure stands of either tree, but very often they are found together, and each has extremely similar associated plant and animal species. For the same reason, we grouped Douglas-Fir Forest with Mixed Evergreen Forest. Finally, we added two new communities that were not recognized by Munz, though they are recognized by other biologists: Mountain Chaparral and Mountain Meadow, each being significantly different from its lowland counterpart. Certainly, there is overlapping of species between adjacent communities, and any classification system can be quite arbitrary. Regardless of how you devise a California plant community table, you'll discover that along the PCT you'll encounter more than half of the state's total number of communities—only the Coast Range and Eastern Desert communities are not seen.

As mentioned earlier, each species has its own range, which can be very restricted or very widespread. Birds typically have a wide—usually seasonal—range, and therefore may be found in many plant communities. In the following list we've included only the plants and animals that have restricted ranges; that is, they generally breed in a range of 31,000 miles (50,000 kilometers) or less. Of the thousands of plant species we reviewed, we found that most of them failed to serve as indicator species, as they either inhabited too many plant communities or grew in too small a geographic area. Terrestrial vertebrates pose a similar classification problem. For example, in the majority of the PCT plant communities, you can find the dark-eyed junco, robin, raven, mule deer, coyote, badger, and Pacific tree frog, so we didn't include them.

The following list of plant communities will be useless if you can't recognize the plants and animals you see along the trail. Our trail descriptions mention plant communities, such as "you hike through a ponderosa pine forest." This would clue you into that plant community, and by referring to it, you could get an idea of what other plants and animals you'll see there. But then you'll need a guidebook or two to identify the various plants and animals. We have a few suggestions. If you can spare the luxury of carrying 12 extra ounces in your pack, obtain a copy of *Sierra Nevada Natural History* (University of California Press, 2004) by Tracy I. Storer, Robert L. Usinger, and David Lukas, which identifies more than 270 plant and 480 animal species and contains more than 500 color photographs. Not only does it provide identifying

characteristics of plant and animal species, but it also describes their habits and gives other interesting facts. The title is misleading, for it is generally applicable to about three-fourths of the California PCT route: Mount Laguna; the San Jacinto, San Bernardino, and San Gabriel Mountains; and from the Sierra Nevada north almost continuously to the Oregon border. Elizabeth Wenk's *Wildflowers of the John Muir Trail and High Sierra* (Wilderness Press, 2015) highlights wildflowers and shrubs between the Mount Whitney region and south Yosemite. Finally, Laird Blackwell's *Wildflowers of California* (University of California Press, 2012) covers 600 species in 10 geographical regions. This certainly beats carrying the 4-pound authoritative reference, *The Jepson Manual* (University of California Press), though this comprehensive guide to California plants is also available in electronic format.

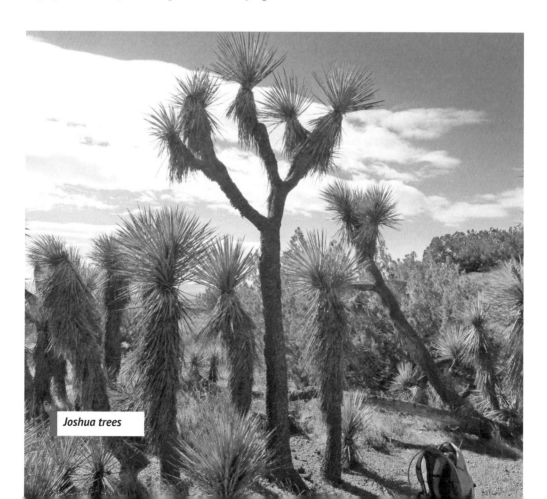

Joshua trees

PLANT COMMUNITIES OF SOUTHERN CALIFORNIA'S PACIFIC CREST TRAIL

CREOSOTE BUSH SCRUB

Shrubs: Creosote bush, bladderpod, brittle bush, burroweed, catclaw, indigo bush, mesquite

Cacti: Bigelow's cholla, silver cholla, calico cactus, beavertail cactus, Banning prickly pear, desert barrel cactus

Wildflowers: Desert mariposa, prickly poppy, peppergrass, desert primrose, spotted langloisia, desert aster, Mojave buckwheat

Mammals: Kit fox, black-tailed jackrabbit, antelope ground squirrel, Mojave ground squirrel, desert kangaroo rat, Merriam's kangaroo rat, cactus mouse, little pocket mouse

Birds: Roadrunner, Gambel's quail, Le Conte's thrasher, cactus wren, phainopepla, Say's phoebe, black-throated sparrow, Costa's hummingbird

Reptiles: Spotted leaf-nosed snake, coachwhip, western blind snake, Mojave rattlesnake, western diamondback rattlesnake, chuckwalla, desert iguana, collared lizard, zebra-tailed lizard, long-tailed brush lizard, desert tortoise

Amphibian: Red-spotted toad

Where seen along PCT: Base of Granite Mountains, southern San Felipe Valley, San Gorgonio Pass, lower Whitewater Canyon, Cajon Canyon, L.A. Aqueduct in Antelope Valley, lower Tehachapi Mountains

SHAD SCALE SCRUB

Shrubs: Shad scale, blackbush, hop sage, winter fat, bud sagebrush, spiny menodora, cheese bush

Mammals: Kit fox, black-tailed jackrabbit, antelope ground squirrel, desert woodrat, desert kangaroo rat, Merriam's kangaroo rat

Bird: Black-throated sparrow

Reptiles: Gopher snake, Mojave rattlesnake, zebra-tailed lizard

Where seen along PCT: L.A. Aqueduct in Antelope Valley

SAGEBRUSH SCRUB

Shrubs: Basin sagebrush, blackbush, rabbit brush, antelope brush (bitterbrush), purple sage, Mojave yucca

Mammals: Kit fox, white-tailed hare, pigmy rabbit, least chipmunk, Merriam's kangaroo rat, Great Basin pocket mouse

Birds: Green-tailed towhee, black-chinned sparrow, sage sparrow, Brewer's sparrow

Reptiles: Side-blotched lizard, desert horned lizard, leopard lizard

Where seen along PCT: Doble Road, Soledad Canyon, southern Antelope Valley, terrain near Pinyon Mountain

VALLEY GRASSLAND

Grasses, native: Bunchgrass, needlegrass, three-awn grass

Grasses, introduced: Bromegrass, fescue, wild oats, foxtail

Wildflowers: California poppy, common muilla, California golden violet, Douglas meadow-foam, Douglas locoweed, whitewhorl lupine, Kellogg's tarweed, red-stem filaree, roundleaf storksbill

Mammals: Kit fox, Heermann's kangaroo rat, California meadow mouse

Birds: Horned lark, western meadowlark, burrowing owl, Brewer's blackbird, savannah sparrow

Reptile: Racer

Amphibians: Western spadefoot toad, tiger salamander

Where seen along PCT: Buena Vista Creek area, Big Tree Trail near Sierra Pelona Ridge, Dowd Canyon, Seiad Valley (man-made grassland)

PLANT COMMUNITIES OF SOUTHERN CALIFORNIA'S PACIFIC CREST TRAIL *(cont.)*

CHAPARRAL

Trees: Bigcone Douglas-fir, gray (digger) pine, interior live oak

Shrubs: Chamise, scrub oak, birchleaf mountain mahogany, chaparral whitethorn, Gregg's ceanothus, bigpod ceanothus, hoaryleaf ceanothus, bigberry manzanita, Eastwood's manzanita, Mexican manzanita, Parry manzanita, pinkbracted manzanita, toyon, ocean spray, hollyleaf cherry, California coffeeberry, redberry, coyote brush (chaparral broom), poison oak

Wildflowers: California poppy, fire poppy, Parish's tauschia, charming centaury, Cleveland's monkey flower, Fremont's monkey flower, scarlet bugler, Martin's paintbrush, foothill penstemon, Coulter's lupine, buckwheat spp.

Mammals: Gray fox, brush rabbit, Merriam's chipmunk, dusky-footed woodrat, nimble kangaroo rat, California mouse, California pocket mouse

Birds: Turkey vulture, California quail, scrub jay, California thrasher, green-tailed towhee, brown towhee, rufous-sided towhee, orange-crowned warbler, Lazuli bunting, blue-gray gnatcatcher, wrentit, bushtit

Reptiles: Striped racer, western rattlesnake, western fence lizard, southern alligator lizard, coast horned lizard

Where seen along PCT: Mexican border, Hauser Mountain, Fred Canyon, Monument Peak, Chariot Canyon, Agua Caliente Creek, Combs Peak, Table Mountain, upper Penrod Canyon, middle Whitewater Canyon, Crab Flats Road, west slopes above Silverwood Lake, west of Pinyon Flats, Fountainhead Spring, North Fork Saddle, Soledad Canyon, Leona Divide, Spunky Canyon, Sawmill and Liebre Mountains, Lamont Canyon to north of Kennedy Meadows

JOSHUA TREE WOODLAND

Trees: Joshua tree (treelike stature but really a yucca), California juniper, singleleaf pinyon pine

Shrubs: Mojave yucca, Utah juniper, boxthorn, bladder sage, saltbush

Wildflowers: Wild buckwheat, rock echeveria, rock five-finger, heartleaf jewelflower, coiled loco-weed, pigmy-leaved lupine, Parish's monkey flower, mousetail, Mojave pennyroyal, two-colored phacelia, tetradymia

Mammals: Kit fox, antelope ground squirrel, desert woodrat, Merriam's kangaroo rat, white-eared pocket mouse

Birds: Pinyon jay, loggerhead shrike, Scott's oriole, Bendire's thrasher

Reptiles: Mojave rattlesnake, California lyre snake, desert night lizard, desert spiny lizard, desert tortoise

Amphibian: Red-spotted toad

Where seen along PCT: Middle Whitewater Canyon, Nelson Ridge, Antelope Valley, western Mojave Desert, Walker Pass

PINYON–JUNIPER WOODLAND

Trees: Singleleaf pinyon pine, California juniper

Shrubs: Utah juniper, scrub oak, Mojave yucca, basin sagebrush, blackbush, boxthorn, curl-leaf mountain mahogany, antelope brush, ephedra

Wildflowers: Rock buckwheat, Wright's buckwheat, golden forget-me-not, adonis lupine, yellow paintbrush, Hall's phacelia

Mammals: Black-tailed jackrabbit, California ground squirrel, Merriam's chipmunk, southern pocket gopher, pinyon mouse

Birds: Pinyon jay, rock wren, poorwill, California thrasher, gray vireo, black-throated gray warbler, ladder-backed woodpecker

Reptiles: Speckled rattlesnake, Mojave rattlesnake, leopard lizard, sagebrush lizard, western fence lizard, desert spiny lizard, coast horned lizard, Gilbert's skink

Amphibian: Red-spotted toad

Where seen along PCT: Just south of Burnt Rancheria Campground, Onyx Summit, Camp Oakes, Van Dusen Canyon, West Fork Mojave River, CA 58 to Kennedy Meadows

PLANT COMMUNITIES OF SOUTHERN CALIFORNIA'S PACIFIC CREST TRAIL *(cont.)*

NORTHERN JUNIPER WOODLAND

Trees: Western juniper, singleleaf pinyon pine, Jeffrey pine

Shrubs: Basin sagebrush, antelope brush, rabbit brush, curl-leaf mountain mahogany

Wildflowers: Sagebrush buttercup, ballhead ipomopsis, three-leaved locoweed, Humboldt milk-weed, western puccoon, sagebrush Mariposa tulip

Mammals: Least chipmunk, Great Basin kangaroo rat, sagebrush vole

Birds: Sage grouse, pinyon jay, sage thrasher, northern shrike, gray flycatcher, sage sparrow

Reptiles: Striped whipsnake, sagebrush lizard, short-horned lizard

Amphibian: Great Basin spadefoot toad

Where seen along PCT: Kennedy Meadows, Little Pete and Big Pete Meadows, upper Noble Canyon, much of the volcanic landscape between CA 108 and CA 50, Hat Creek Rim, Buckhorn Mountain

SOUTHERN OAK WOODLAND

Trees: Coast live oak, Engelmann oak, interior live oak, California juniper, Coulter pine, digger pine, bigcone Douglas-fir, California black walnut

Shrubs: Sugar bush, lemonade berry, gooseberry, bigberry manzanita, fremontia, squaw bush, poison oak

Wildflowers: Elegant clarkia, slender eriogonum, wild oats, California Indian pink, golden star, wild mountain sunflower, Kellogg's tarweed, Douglas locoweed, Douglas violet

Mammals: Gray fox, raccoon, western gray squirrel, dusky-footed woodrat, brush mouse, California mouse

Birds: California quail, acorn woodpecker, scrub jay, mourning dove, Lawrence's goldfinch, common bushtit, black-headed grosbeak, plain titmouse, Nuttall's woodpecker, western wood-pewee, band-tailed pigeon, red-shouldered hawk

Reptiles: California mountain kingsnake, Gilbert's skink, western fence lizard, southern alligator lizard

Amphibians: California newt, California slender salamander, arboreal salamander

Where seen along PCT: Lake Morena County Park, Cottonwood Valley, Flathead Flats, Barrel Spring, Cañada Verde, Warner Springs, Tunnel Spring, Vincent Gap, Three Points, upper Tie Canyon, Mount Gleason, Big Oak Spring, San Francisquito Canyon

PONDEROSA PINE FOREST

Trees: Ponderosa pine, sugar pine, Jeffrey pine, incense cedar, white fir, Douglas-fir, black oak, mountain dogwood, grand fir

Shrubs: Deer brush, greenleaf manzanita, Mariposa manzanita, mountain misery, western azalea, Scouler's willow, spicebush

Wildflowers: Elegant brodiaea, spotted coralroot, draperia, rigid hedge nettle, Indian hemp, slender iris, leopard lily, grand lotus, dwarf lousewort, Sierra onion, Yosemite rock cress, shy Mariposa tulip

Mammals: Black bear, mountain lion, mountain beaver, porcupine, western gray squirrel, golden-mantled ground squirrel, yellow-pine chipmunk, mountain pocket gopher

Birds: Steller's jay, hairy woodpecker, white-headed woodpecker, western tanager, band-tailed pigeon, pigmy nuthatch, western bluebird, flammulated owl

Reptiles: Rubber boa, California mountain kingsnake, western rattlesnake, western fence lizard

Amphibians: Foothill yellow-legged frog, ensatina

Where seen along PCT: Laguna Mountains, upper West Fork Palm Canyon, Apache Spring, upper Whitewater Canyon, much of the Big Bear Lake area, most of the San Gabriel Mountains, Piute Mountain, Haypress Creek, Chimney Rock, Burney Falls, lower Rock Creek, Castle Crags, lower slopes of Lower Devils Peak

PLANT COMMUNITIES OF SOUTHERN CALIFORNIA'S PACIFIC CREST TRAIL *(cont.)*

MOUNTAIN CHAPARRAL

Trees: Jeffrey pine, sugar pine, western juniper

Shrubs: Huckleberry oak, snow bush, tobacco brush, greenleaf manzanita, bush chinquapin

Wildflowers: Showy penstemon, dwarf monkey flower, hound's-tongue hawkweed, pussy-paw, mountain jewelflower, golden brodiaea

Mammals: Bushy-tailed woodrat, brush mouse

Birds: Mountain quail, dusky flycatcher, fox sparrow, green-tailed towhee

Reptiles: Western rattlesnake, sagebrush lizard

Where seen along PCT: Near Tahquitz Peak, near Strawberry Cienaga, in small areas from north of Walker Pass to Cow Canyon, above Blaney Hot Springs, slopes north of Benson Lake, upper North Fork American River canyon, Sierra Buttes, Bucks Summit, slopes west of Three Lakes, lower Emigrant Trail, upper Hat Creek Valley, Pigeon Hill, above Seven Lakes Basin, slopes south of Kangaroo Lake, South Russian Creek canyon, upper Right Hand Fork canyon, south slopes of Lower Devils Peak and Middle Devils Peak, between Lily Pad Lake and Cook and Green Pass, Mount Ashland Ski Road (FS 20)

MOUNTAIN MEADOW

Shrubs: Arroyo willow, yellow willow, mountain alder

Wildflowers: California corn lily, wandering daisy, elephant's-head, tufted gentian, Douglas knotweed, monkshood, swamp onion, Lemmon's paintbrush, meadow arnica, mountain carpet clover, California coneflower, Gray's lovage, Kellogg's lupine, meadow monkey flower, tall phacelia, Jeffrey's shooting star, Bigelow's sneezeweed

Mammals: Belding's ground squirrel, California meadow mouse, long-tailed meadow mouse, deer mouse, ornate shrew

Birds: Northern harrier, Lincoln's sparrow, white-crowned sparrow, Brewer's blackbird

Amphibians: Mountain yellow-legged frog, Yosemite toad

Where seen along PCT: Little Tahquitz Valley, Vidette Meadow, Grouse Meadows, Evolution Valley, Tully Hole, Tuolumne Meadows, Grace Meadow, upper Truckee River canyon, Benwood Meadow, Haypress Meadows, Corral Meadow, Badger Flat, Shelly Meadows, Donomore Meadows, Sheep Camp Spring area, Grouse Gap

RED FIR–LODGEPOLE PINE FOREST

Trees: Red fir, Shasta red fir, noble fir, lodgepole pine, western white pine, Jeffrey pine, aspen, mountain hemlock, weeping spruce

Shrubs: Pine-mat manzanita, bush chinquapin, snow bush, red heather, Labrador tea, mountain spirea, caudate willow, MacKenzie's willow, Scouler's willow, black elderberry, thimbleberry

Wildflowers: Snow plant, pinedrops, nodding microseris, broadleaf lupine, western spring beauty

Mammals: Black bear, red fox, mountain beaver, porcupine, yellow-bellied marmot, golden-mantled ground squirrel, lodgepole chipmunk, mountain pocket gopher

Birds: Blue grouse, great gray owl, mountain chickadee, red-breasted nuthatch, dusky flycatcher, olive-sided flycatcher, Williamson's sapsucker, three-toed woodpecker, ruby-crowned kinglet, Cassin's finch

Where seen along PCT: Upper Little Tahquitz Valley, upper San Bernardino Mountains, Mount Baden–Powell, Kern Plateau, lower portions of John Muir Trail, much of northern Yosemite, most of the stretch from Yosemite to central Lassen Volcanic National Park, Bartle Gap, Grizzly Peak, most of the trail from Seven Lakes Basin to Mount Ashland

PLANT COMMUNITIES OF SOUTHERN CALIFORNIA'S PACIFIC CREST TRAIL *(cont.)*

SUBALPINE FOREST

Trees: Whitebark pine, foxtail pine, limber pine, lodgepole pine, mountain hemlock

Shrubs: Sierra willow, Eastwood's willow, white heather, bush cinquefoil

Wildflowers: Eschscholtz's buttercup, Coville's columbine, mountain monkey flower, Suksdorf's monkey flower, Sierra penstemon, Sierra primrose, mountain sorrel, cut-leaved daisy, silky raillardella, rock fringe

Mammals: Red fox, yellow-bellied marmot, pika, Douglas squirrel (chickaree), alpine chipmunk, heather vole, water shrew

Birds: Clark's nutcracker, mountain bluebird, mountain chickadee, Williamson's sapsucker

Amphibian: Mount Lyell salamander

Where seen along PCT: Mount Baden–Powell summit, much of the Sierra Nevada (above 10,000 feet in the southern part, above 8,000 feet in the northern part), higher elevations in Marble Mountain Wilderness

ALPINE FELL-FIELD

Shrubs: Alpine willow, snow willow

Wildflowers: Alpine gold, Sierra pilot, alpine paintbrush, alpine sandwort, ruby sandwort, dwarf lewisia, dwarf ivesia, Muir's ivesia, Brewer's draba, feeble saxifrage, Sierra primrose

Mammals: Pika, alpine chipmunk

Birds: Rosy finch, mountain bluebird, rock wren

Where seen along PCT: At and just below Forester, Glen, Pinchot, Mather, Selden, Silver, and Donohue Passes; high traverse along Leavitt Peak ridge

A Final Word

Plant communities aren't the final word in plant and animal classification, as each community could be further subdivided. For example, Edmund Jaeger divides the desert environment into even more compartments than Munz does, including Desert Sand Dunes, Desert Wash, Saltwater Lake (Salton Sea), Desert Canal, Colorado River Bottom, Desert Urban, and Desert Rural. Farther north, in a glaciated basin near Yosemite's Tioga Pass, Lionel Klikoff has identified eight vegetational patterns within the subalpine forest plant community, each distribution pattern the result of a different set of microenvironmental influences. Once you start looking and thinking about organisms and their environments, you'll begin to see that they are more than random groups of species. There is continual interaction between similar organisms, between different organisms, and between organisms and their environment. They are there because they fit into the dynamic ecosystem; they currently are adapted to it; they belong.

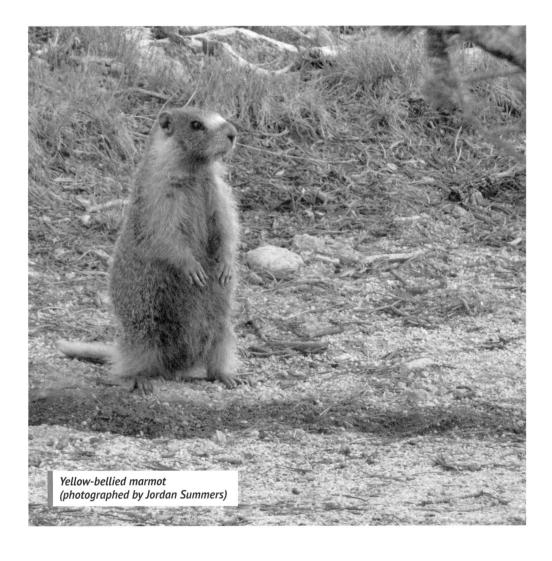

*Yellow-bellied marmot
(photographed by Jordan Summers)*

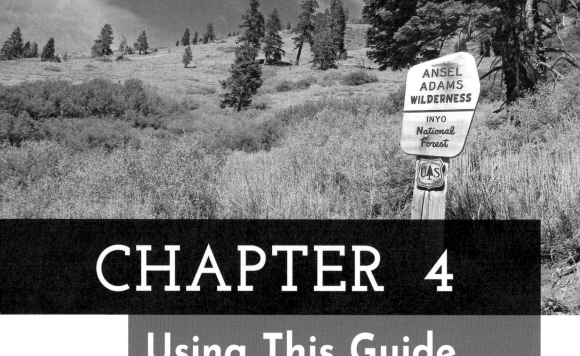

CHAPTER 4
Using This Guide

OUR ROUTE DESCRIPTION

Pacific Crest Trail: Southern California is composed of the route description and area maps of the Pacific Crest Trail (PCT). In eight section chapters, this guide covers the California PCT from the Mexican border north to Tuolumne Meadows in Yosemite National Park. The route description is divided into sections because most PCT hikers will be hiking only a part of the trail, not all of it. In this book's companion volume, *Pacific Crest Trail: Northern California* by Jordan Summers, the PCT description picks up from Tuolumne Meadows and ends at the Oregon border (Sections I–R).

Each section starts at or near a highway and/or supply center (town, resort, or park) and ends at another similar point. The one exception is the end of Section G and start of Section H, which occurs where the PCT joins the John Muir Trail near Crabtree Meadow. From this point most PCT hikers will go east to climb Mount Whitney and perhaps descend to Lone Pine to resupply. We also chose this break point because many hikers skip Southern California and start their PCT hike on the John Muir Trail—this guide's Section H. This section is the only one that is too long for *most* hikers to do without resupplying. All the other sections are short enough to make comfortable backpacking trips ranging from 3 to 10 days, and most of these have resupply points along or close to the actual route, thereby allowing you to carry a little less food.

At the beginning of each section is an introduction that mentions:

Above: The PCT enters the Ansel Adams Wilderness just beyond Agnew Meadows and climbs past rock outcrops, alpine meadows, and backcountry lakes.

- The attractions and natural features of that section

- The declination setting for your compass

- The 7.5-minute topographic maps that cover that section, arranged south to north

- A mileage table of points on the route

- A campsite table with GPS coordinates and other pertinent information

- Weather and best times to go

- Supply points on or near the route

- Water availability or scarcity

- Wilderness permits (if required)

- Special concerns (such as rattlesnakes, snow, and difficult-to-ford rivers and creeks)

Attractions and natural features will help you decide what part of the trail you want to hike.

The **declination setting** for your compass is important if you want to get a true reading. The declinations in this guide vary from 11°04'E near the Mexican border to 12°16'E near Tuolumne Meadows. They were calculated in 2020 and are accurate within 30 minutes of arc, but note that declination changes over time. Visit ngdc.noaa.gov/geomag-web for the most current information before your hike.

If your compass does not correct for declination, you'll have to add the appropriate declination to get the true bearing. For example, if your compass indicates that a prominent hill lies along a bearing of 75° and the section you're hiking has a declination of 12°E, then you should add 12°, getting 87° (due east) as the true bearing of that hill. If you can identify that hill on a map, then you can find where you are on the PCT by adding 180°, getting 267° (due west) in this example. Be aware that this procedure is correct only for true-bearing (true field-sighting) compasses, which list degrees from 0° to 360° in a counterclockwise direction. Most hikers, however, use the generally less expensive reverse-bearing

compasses, which are harder to use. (Indeed, an entire book has been written on using them for map-orienteering purposes.) Reverse-bearing, or backsight, compasses list degrees in a clockwise direction. With these compasses, you subtract. **No one should ever attempt a major section of the PCT without a thorough understanding of his or her compass and of map interpretation.**

Maps of the Pacific Crest Trail can be ordered from REI at rei.com, where you can find various waterproof maps covering the PCT and the wilderness, parks, and forests it crosses. At the USGS Store (store.usgs.gov), you can order waterproof strip maps featuring the PCT. And National Geographic sells its waterproof topographic maps, which were created in partnership with Halfmile and the Pacific Crest Trail Association, online at natgeomaps.com.

The **Points on the Trail table** for each section lists the location, mileage, elevation, and GPS coordinates in degrees, minutes, and seconds (DMS) of major points in that section. If you average 22 miles a day—the on-route rate you'll need to do to complete the tristate PCT in four months—you can determine where to camp and estimate when you'll arrive at certain supply points. Specific information on camping is listed in a **Campsites and Bivy Sites table.**

On page xi, we've included a mileage table for the entire PCT. Any two adjacent points represent the start and end of a section. (We have also listed mileages for the 10 sections covered in *Pacific Crest Trail: Northern California* and the 12 sections covered in *Pacific Crest Trail: Oregon & Washington.*) The table also lists how long each section is. Then you can pick one of appropriate length, turn to that section's introduction, and see if it sounds appealing. Of course, you need not start at the beginning of any section, as a number of roads cross the PCT in most sections. (Section H is an exception, having only a few access points.)

Supply points on or near the route are mentioned, as is what you might expect to find at each. You will realize, for example, that you can't get new clothes at Cajon Pass but can at Wrightwood, about 11 miles farther northwest. Many supply points are just a post office and/or small store with minimal food supplies. By *minimal* we mean a few odds and ends that typically cater to passing motorists, for example, beer and potato chips (which nevertheless are devoured by many a trail-weary trekker).

Water is self-explanatory, as are **weather** and **permits.**

Finally, each section's introduction may mention **special concerns** you could encounter along the route, such as desert thirst, snow avalanches, and early-season fords. If you are hiking all of the California PCT, you will be going through some of its sections at very inopportune times and will face many of these problems. Backpackers hiking a short stretch can pick the best time to hike it, thereby minimizing their problems.

When you start reading the text of a section, you will notice that a pair of numbers follows the more important trail points. For example, at CA 120 in Tuolumne Meadows (end of Section H) this pair is (942.5–8,596'), which means that this point is at mile 942.5 and an elevation of 8,596 feet. Our example is at a junction by Tuolumne Meadows Lodge. By noting these figures, you can determine the distance you'll need to hike from point A to point B, and you can get a good idea of how much elevation change is involved.

The route description tells something about the country you are walking through—the geology, the biology (plants and animals), the geography, and sometimes a bit of history. Longer highlights of interest are noted.

In the descriptions, an **alternate route** is a trail segment that the author thinks is worth considering given certain circumstances. Along this guide's alternate routes, there are occasional second mileage figures, which represent the distance along the alternate route to that point. A **side trip,** unlike an alternate route, returns to the main trail.

Note: If alternate routes and side trips vary considerably from the PCT, especially in wilderness areas that require their own backcountry permits, your PCT long-distance permit may not comply with local regulations.

FOLLOWING THE TRAIL

The route of the PCT is mostly along trail tread, but occasionally it lies along a stretch of road. Except where the trail tread may momentarily die out, there is no cross-country trekking, although early-season hikers may go miles on snow, when accurate route finding becomes imperative. Quite naturally, you want to stay on the route. For that purpose, we recommend relying on the route description and maps in this book. To be sure, there are various markers along the route—PCT emblems and signs, metal diamonds and discs nailed to tree trunks, plastic ribbons tied to branches, blazes, and ducks. (A blaze is a place on a tree trunk where bark has been removed in the shape of a lowercase letter *i*. Typically a blaze is about 4–6 inches long. A duck is a stack of two or three rocks placed on a large boulder, log, sand, or gravel. It may be more elaborate, such as a pile of several small rocks whose placement is obviously unnatural.)

Our route descriptions depend on these markers as little as possible because they are so ephemeral. Furthermore, the blazes or ducks you follow, not having any words or numbers, may or may not mark the trail you want to be on.

One way to find a junction is to count mileage from the previous junction. If you know the length of your stride, that will help. We have used yards for short distances because 1 yard approximates the length of one long stride. Alternatively, you can develop a sense of your ground speed. Then, if it is 2 miles to the next junction and your speed is 3 miles an hour, you should be there in 2/3 hour, or 40 minutes. Be suspicious if you reach an unmarked junction sooner or later than you expect. We sometimes go to great lengths to describe the terrain so that you can be alerted to upcoming junctions. Without these clues, you could easily miss the junction in early season, when snow still obscures many parts of the trail.

THE MAPS

Each section contains topographic maps complete with shaded relief, contour elevation, and both UTM and latitude/longitude grids. All individual section maps are at a scale of 1:63,360, or 1 inch equals 1 mile, and include a north indicator. Refer to the legend below for the different stylings between the PCT and other trails, as well as the many symbols featured on the maps.

Map Legend

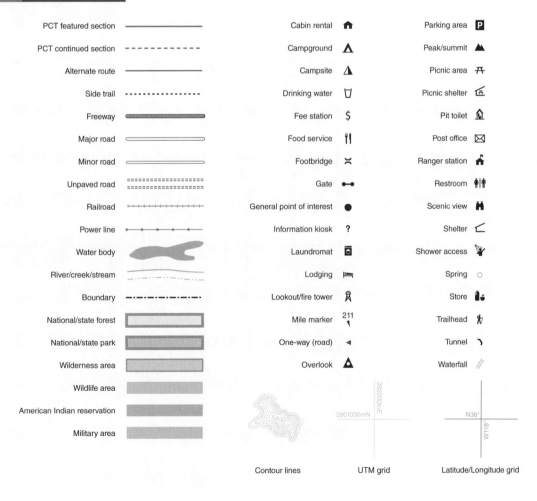

PCT featured section	————————
PCT continued section	– – – – – – –
Alternate route	————————
Side trail	················
Freeway	━━━━━━━
Major road	═══════
Minor road	═══════
Unpaved road	▭▭▭▭▭▭
Railroad	┼┼┼┼┼┼┼
Power line	•—•—•—•
Water body	
River/creek/stream	
Boundary	–·–·–·–·–
National/state forest	
National/state park	
Wilderness area	
Wildlife area	
American Indian reservation	
Military area	

Cabin rental	♠
Campground	⌂
Campsite	⚠
Drinking water	⛆
Fee station	$
Food service	⑂
Footbridge	⤫
Gate	•—•
General point of interest	●
Information kiosk	?
Laundromat	▣
Lodging	⊨
Lookout/fire tower	⍟
Mile marker	211 ↘
One-way (road)	◄
Overlook	▲

Parking area	Ⓟ
Peak/summit	▲
Picnic area	⚘
Picnic shelter	⌂
Pit toilet	⚲
Post office	✉
Ranger station	♠
Restroom	⚹
Scenic view	🔭
Shelter	⊏
Shower access	⚿
Spring	○
Store	🛍
Trailhead	🚶
Tunnel	⌐
Waterfall	//

Contour lines	UTM grid	Latitude/Longitude grid

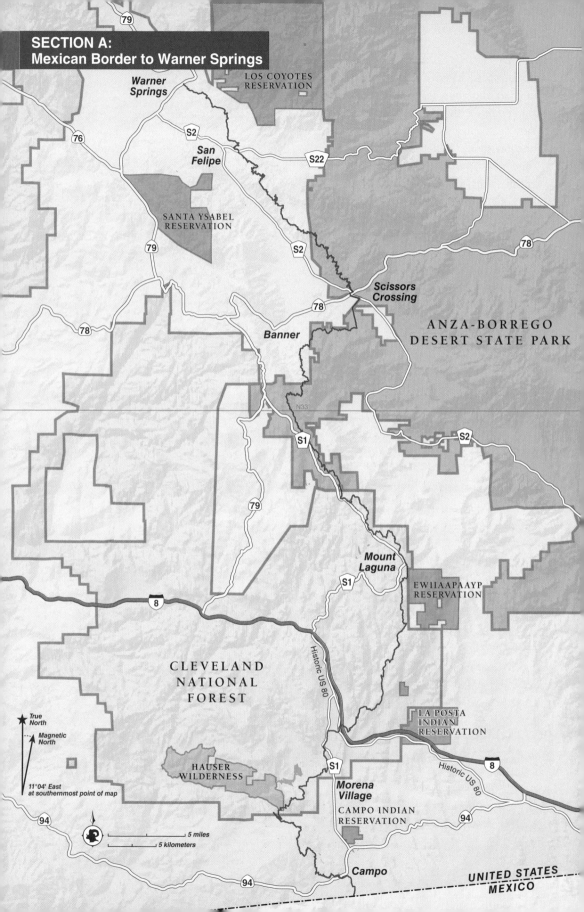

79

76

79

78

S2

S22

S2

S2

78

Warner
Springs

LOS COYOTES
RESERVATION

San
Felipe

SANTA YSABEL
RESERVATION

Scissors
Crossing

78

Banner

N33

ANZA-BORREGO
DESERT STATE PARK

S1

S2

79

Mount
Laguna

S1

EWIIAAPAAYP
RESERVATION

8

CLEVELAND
NATIONAL
FOREST

Historic US 80

LA POSTA
INDIAN
RESERVATION

★ True
North

⋯ Magnetic
North

↓ 11°04' East
at southernmost point of map

HAUSER
WILDERNESS

S1

Morena
Village

CAMPO INDIAN
RESERVATION

Historic US 80

8

94

5 miles

5 kilometers

94

94

Campo

UNITED STATES
MEXICO

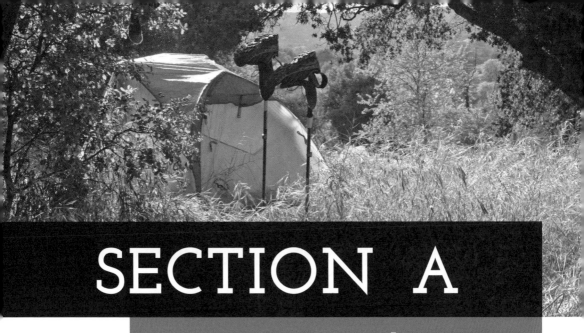

SECTION A

Mexican Border to Warner Springs

THIS SOUTHERNMOST SECTION of the Pacific Crest Trail (PCT) is among the most varied of all. It traces a fine line between scorching desert and dense, rolling brushlands, occasionally in fine midmountain forest. Although you encounter cacti and sand often, and late-spring and summer temperatures frequently rise above 100° F, the PCT in this section does not traverse true desert, but rather keeps just west of the searing Colorado Desert—which you often glimpse—passing through a transitional area influenced by moist Pacific Ocean air. At the time when most long-distance hikers will be traversing the southernmost part of the PCT, in April and May, they are quite likely to encounter late-season snowstorms as they climb into the Laguna Mountains.

The Lagunas are a fault-block range of granitic rock closely related to the Sierra Nevada geologically. Here, walkers might forget sun and thirst

Above: A tent site at Lake Morena County Park

while walking beneath shady oaks and pines also similar to those found in the Sierra. But the next day, as they swoop down to San Felipe Valley, the stifling heat returns as the route enters Anza-Borrego Desert State Park and the Colorado Desert. The furnace breath of this arid land above the Salton Sea follows you from the San Felipe Hills to Warner Springs.

DECLINATION 11°04'E

USGS MAPS

Campo	Monument Peak	Tubb Canyon
Potrero	Cuyamaca Peak	Ranchita
Morena Reservoir	Julian	Hot Springs Mountain
Cameron Corners	Earthquake Valley	Warner Springs
Mount Laguna		

POINTS ON THE TRAIL, SOUTH TO NORTH

	Mile	Elevation in feet	Latitude/Longitude
Mexican border, Southern terminus monument	0.0	2,918	N32° 35' 23.040" W116° 28' 01.140"
Campo	1.4	2,586	N32° 36' 30.240" W116° 28' 27.780"
Seasonal Hauser Creek (camping)	15.4	2,317	N32° 39' 41.100" W116° 32' 43.800"
Lake Morena County Park (camping, water, food)	20.0	3,074	N32° 40' 57.180" W116° 31' 00.120"
Fred Canyon Road to Cibbets Flat Campground	32.6	4,409	N32° 46' 17.880" W116° 26' 20.640"
Long Canyon	36.9	5,195	N32° 48' 43.680" W116° 25' 16.500"
Lower Morris Meadow (piped water)	38.8	5,889	N32° 49' 42.060" W116° 25' 04.080"
Trail junction to Burnt Rancheria Campground and Mount Laguna	41.5	5,955	N32° 51' 30.000" W116° 24' 56.340"
Desert View Picnic Area (water)	42.6	5,956	N32° 52' 09.570" W116° 24' 51.260"
Laguna Campground access trail near Sunrise Highway	47.5	5,422	N32° 53' 45.480" W116° 26' 54.540"
Pioneer Mail Picnic Area	52.6	5,274	N32° 55' 28.000" W116° 28' 52.000"
Kwaaymii Point parking lot	53.4	5,472	N32° 56' 05.040" W116° 28' 57.240"
Upper Chariot Canyon jeep road	63.7	3,857	N33° 00' 48.120" W116° 31' 37.920"
Rodriguez Spur Truck Trail (well and camping)	68.4	3,653	N33° 03' 03.720" W116° 31' 25.440"
County Highway S2 (paved road)	76.4	2,255	N33° 05' 35.960" W116° 27' 45.360"
CA 78 to Julian	77.3	2,261	N33° 05' 56.930" W116° 28' 10.200"
Montezuma Valley Road, near Ranchita	101.2	3,453	N33° 13' 00.540" W116° 35' 16.620"
San Ysidro Creek	105.0	3,354	N33° 14' 53.160" W116° 36' 00.000"
Spur trail to Eagle Rock	106.2	3,524	N33° 15' 17.160" W116° 36' 41.700"
CA 79, Warner Springs	109.5	3,045	N33° 16' 24.420" W116° 38' 41.940"

CAMPSITES AND BIVY SITES

Mile	Elevation in feet	Latitude/ Longitude	Number of tents	Feature	Notes
4.6	2,378	N32° 36' 26.220" W116° 30' 04.800"	Small	Meadow	
15.4	2,317	N32° 39' 41.100" W116° 32' 43.800"	Large	Seasonal Hauser Creek nearby	East of trail
20.0	3,074	N32° 40' 57.180" W116° 31' 00.120"	Dozens	Lake Morena County Park with designated PCT tent sites and showers	Check in at ranger office 0.3 mile west of trail on Lake Morena Drive
26.0	3,183	N32° 43' 42.900" W116° 28' 57.900"	Dozens	Boulder Oaks Campground	Pit toilet, tables
32.6	4,155	N32° 46' 39.720" W116° 26' 43.500"	Dozens	Cibbets Flat	0.8 mile west of trail, pit toilets, tables, seasonal stream
36.1	5,292	N32° 48' 06.060" W116° 25' 15.780"	<5	Long Canyon Creek	Just off trail amid dead trees
37.1	5,247	N32° 48' 46.800" W116° 25' 10.920"	<5	Long Canyon	Just off trail
41.5	5,936	N32° 51' 30.900" W116° 24' 59.700"	109	Burnt Rancheria	West of trail, usually opens in mid-April; large campground with bathrooms and showers
47.5	5,510	N32° 53' 20.700" W116° 27' 01.560"	104	Laguna Campground	0.8 mile west of trail
63.7	3,864	N33° 00' 48.120" W116° 31' 37.920"	>5	South of dirt Chariot Canyon Road	Near dry creekbed
68.4	3,653	N33° 03' 03.720" W116° 31' 25.440"	5	Rodriguez Spur	Wind-prone open area with a nearby water tank (often dry by late spring)
79.4	2,974	N33° 06' 36.420" W116° 28' 30.480"	>2	Dry creekbed	North of trail
80.4	3,066	N33° 06' 49.620" W116° 28' 52.140"	2		2 sites near each other by wash
81.6	3,074	N33° 07' 12.840" W116° 29' 04.020"	5		Below trail
85.4	3,289	N33° 08' 17.940" W116° 30' 10.980"	>5		Flat area next to trail, past burn area
86.0	3,363	N33° 08' 25.800" W116° 30' 27.060"	2	View	At a ridge saddle
86.6	3,237	N33° 08' 42.840" W116° 30' 28.140"	>10	Dry creekbed	Adequate but waterless
88.2	3,596	N33° 08' 52.140" W116° 31' 04.500"	>5	View	At a ridgecrest
91.2	3,550	N33° 10' 01.200" W116° 32' 36.540"	>5	Some shade	100 feet north of the third gate
94.4	4,296	N33° 10' 51.000" W116° 33' 29.460"	>5	View	Small campsite on a ridge surrounded by brush
101.1	3,482	N33° 12' 55.860" W116° 35' 17.160"	Large	Barrel Spring	300 feet west of trail, under a canopy of canyon live oaks

Note: Remote camping is not allowed in Laguna Mountain Recreation Area (miles 41.0–52.6).

SECTION A

WEATHER TO GO

South-to-north thru-hikers typically begin their journeys in April and early May, as biting winter winds and snow flurries in the Lagunas are usually gone, but extreme heat hasn't yet developed in the San Felipe Hills. By late May, this section's lower reaches can be uncomfortably hot. Section hikers may prefer hiking here in the fall, when it's less crowded and temperatures are typically moderate.

SUPPLIES

Last-minute supplies may be bought in Campo, 1.4 miles along the walk. It has a small store, laundromat, post office, railroad museum, and ranch-supply store. Cameron Corners, 1 mile north of Campo on CA 94, has a taco stand, a convenience store, and an all-day café. Sophisticated camping items still needed must be bought in San Diego before starting out.

Inbound airline passengers may reach the PCT's southern terminus via the following links: Take bus route 992 from the San Diego Airport to American Plaza in downtown San Diego (sdmts .com). Next, take the Orange or Green Line trolley to the El Cajon Transit Center. The Southeastern Rural Route bus #894 departs the center four times a day, Monday–Friday, and arrives in Campo about 2 hours later (sdmts.com). It does not run on weekends or holidays. For contact information on trail angels in the San Diego area, check the PCTA website (pcta.org/discover-the-trail /backcountry-basics/pct-transportation).

Morena Village, with a small store and café, lies 0.3 mile off-route at Lake Morena County Park, 20 miles into the journey. Mount Laguna, a tiny mountain community with a store, a post office, restaurants, an outdoors outfitter, and a lodge, is the next opportunity, about 43 miles into the hike. Mount Laguna Post Office has no morning service, except on Saturday.

The tourist-oriented, apple-growing, former mining town of Julian, with stores, restaurants, lodging, and a post office, lies 12.5 miles west of the PCT where it strikes CA 78 in San Felipe Valley. Julian is a welcome respite when you're sporting your first set of desert-induced blisters.

Borrego Springs is a desert resort community with complete supplies, motels, a laundromat, and the Anza-Borrego Desert State Park headquarters, with camping and a natural history museum. You can reach it from two points along the PCT. From Scissors Crossing, about 77.3 miles into your journey, find Borrego Springs by hitchhiking about 5 miles east on CA 78 to County Highway S3, then heading north about 10 miles. From County Highway S22 where the PCT strikes it, just north of Barrel Spring, at about the 101-mile point of this section, hitchhike 15 miles east on S22.

Warner Springs, at the end of this section, is the last supply point. This little resort community is clustered around a rejuvenating hot spring on the Aguanga Fault. Warner Springs Ranch Resort (31652 CA 79, Warner Springs, CA 92086; 760-792-4200; warnerspringsranchresort.com) boasts a casual bar and grill and simple bungalows. Golf and horseback riding round out the experience. Warner Springs has a post office; also, no visit here is complete without a stop at the volunteer-run community resource center (30950 CA 79, Warner Springs, CA 92086; 760-782-0670; wscrcenter.org), which provides a store and a communal room with tables, couches, computers, and books, as well as potable water outside. Check the website or call for hours and to ensure the center is still open.

WATER

Groundwater in the dry mountains of Southern California dries up rapidly after winter snows melt. Especially late May through summer, hikers should not count on any water away from civilization—in Section A, this could require some waterless camps and, most likely, some long detours for water. Plan to carry at least 8 quarts of water per person, per day, more if dry camping is expected.

In dry years, the Southern California PCT's meager accompaniment of streams and springs begins to disappear. During repeated dry years, some smaller water sources remain dry, even in spring. During drought years in Section A, expect to find water only in Campo, Lake Morena County Park, Boulder Oaks Campground, Laguna Campground, and Warner Springs. Expect Hauser Creek, Cottonwood Creek, Long Canyon Creek, Chariot Canyon, Rodriguez Spur Truck Trail well, San Felipe Creek, and Barrel Spring to be dry.

Conversely, years with normal or heavy precipitation will deposit heavy snows on the San Jacintos, San Bernardinos, and San Gabriels. These often pose a problem through mid-May. The higher Tehachapis, as well, routinely have more than a foot of snow on northern slopes. Hence, the springtime PCT traveler must have a flexible resupply strategy and must be ready to load up tents, gaiters, a warm parka, and an ice ax when needed, and to jettison them in favor of extra water bottles through the dry spells.

Walkers should carry lots of water from Mount Laguna, for it is a long, blistering 23.9 miles to springs in Chariot Canyon. When the water tank at Pioneer Mail Trailhead Picnic Area is in operation, it will deduct 10.1 miles from this leg. An alternative to Chariot Canyon is the well on Rodriguez Spur Truck Trail, 28.1 miles beyond Mount Laguna. In either case, carry a big water container because the next stretch to water at Barrel Spring is a mind-broiling 37.9 miles from Chariot Canyon, and 33 miles from Rodriguez Spur Truck Trail.

PERMITS

A visitor's permit is required for all section hikers to disperse camp within the Hauser Wilderness and on all Cleveland National Forest lands outside the Laguna Mountain Recreation Area. Camping outside a developed campground within 0.5 mile of the PCT could result in up to a $5,000 fine and/or 6-month imprisonment. Permits may be obtained locally from the Descanso Ranger District. There are seasonal limits during thru-hiking season from March until May. (See "Federal Government Agencies," page 25).

SPECIAL CONCERNS

Refer to page 32 for information about rattlesnakes.

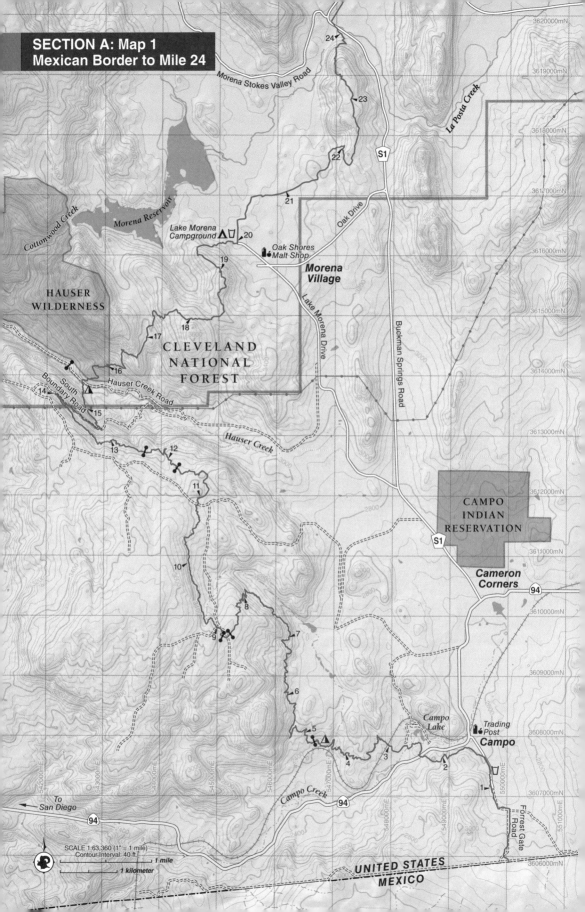

3620000mN

3619000mN

24

Morena Stokes Valley Road

23

3618000mN

La Posta Creek

3617000mN

22

S1

21

Oak Drive

Morena Reservoir

Cottonwood Creek

Lake Morena
Campground ▲ ⌂ 20

Oak Shores
Malt Shop

3616000mN

**Morena
Village**

19

Lake Morena Drive

3615000mN

**HAUSER
WILDERNESS**

18

Buckman Springs Road

17

**CLEVELAND
NATIONAL
FOREST**

3614000mN

16

South Boundary Road

Hauser Creek Road

▲

14

15

3613000mN

Hauser Creek

13

12

3612000mN

**CAMPO
INDIAN
RESERVATION**

11

10

S1

3611000mN

**Cameron
Corners**

94

3610000mN

8

7

9

3609000mN

6

**Campo
Lake**

Trading
Post

3608000mN

Campo

5

▲

3

4

2

1

3607000mN

542000mE

543000mE

544000mE

545000mE

546000mE

547000mE

548000mE

549000mE

550000mE

551000mE

Campo Creek

94

→ To
San Diego

94

3606000mN

Forrest Gate Road

SCALE 1:63,360 (1" = 1 mile)
Contour Interval: 40 ft.

1 mile

1 kilometer

UNITED STATES

MEXICO

MEXICAN BORDER TO WARNER SPRINGS

>>>THE ROUTE

CA 94 leads 50 miles east from San Diego to Campo, where you turn south on Forrest Gate Road, which in one block passes a sprawling U.S. Border Patrol station. The pavement ends beyond Rancho del Campo, and you continue south up the graded road. It jogs east at Castle Rock Ranch, turns south at a T-junction with a poorer road, and then climbs moderately along a telephone line. After passing under a 500-kilovolt power line, you reach a junction with a good dirt road that parallels the Mexican border. This road is patrolled regularly by Border Patrol officers. Now look uphill to the left (southeast) to see the gray PCT monument atop a low knoll at the edge of the wide, defoliated border swath. This swath has a welter of paralleling roads that run alongside the barbed wire border fence.

Walk up a short jeep road to the monument, replaced and reinforced in 2016: an 8-foot-high gray wooden affair constructed of four posts of varying sizes and capped with the soon-to-be-familiar delta-shaped PCT emblem. An inscription reads: SOUTHERN TERMINUS PACIFIC CREST NATIONAL SCENIC TRAIL. ESTABLISHED BY ACT OF CONGRESS ON OCTOBER 2, 1968. MEXICO TO CANADA 2650 MILES. 1988 A.D. ELEVATION 2915 FEET. Fifty feet south of the border monument, another dirt road has been bulldozed, parallel to the border. Its southern verge, the border itself, is protected by a 4- to 6-foot-high fence of metal runway-repair panels. Take the requisite photos, sign the register on the back of the

monument, and then turn north and start your adventure (0.0–2,918').

VIEWS Your first vistas north show the steep southern flanks of the Laguna Mountains on the northern horizon, while the low green dome of Hauser Mountain stands in the northwest. The prominent orange buttresses of Morena Butte overlook its northern shoulder.

To find the start of the PCT, look due north, downhill from the monument, to a lone 12-foot-high scrub oak, just left (west) of the road you just came up and immediately north of the grassy, defoliated border strip. Next to it is a gray sign at the actual start of the trail tread. It announces: PACIFIC CREST TRAIL: LAKE MORENA 19.5 MILES. (There may also be bright-orange cones marking the entrance, as some confused hikers have been known to follow the border road right next to the monument before realizing their mistake and turning around.) The PCT's obvious trail tread starts, heading downhill (north), into high brush. A sandy descent curves to parallel the access road. In a few minutes, you pass under the San Diego Gas and Electric power line and walk northeast across a poor road that subserves the line. Continue gently down, just east of the access road, in a low, arid chaparral of chamise, sagebrush, ribbonwood, and yucca, which is punctuated with protruding boulders of bonsall tonalite—a light-gray granitic rock—and white popcorn flowers.

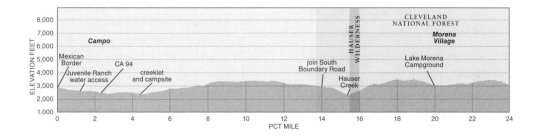

| FIRE | The Border Fire in June 2016 burned more than 7,000 acres near the PCT's beginning in Campo. The stretch of trail that burned has since reopened, but it serves as an early reminder of the flammability of the Southern California landscape.

In minutes, the descent ends as you cross another dirt road (0.3–2,805'); then, at the way marked by 4-by-4-inch posts, swing west on the edge of a large dry meadow dotted with mustard and large canyon live oaks. Just west of the entrance to Castle Rock Ranch, you step across Forrest Gate Road (0.7–2,707') to its west side, where you wind and undulate easily above the now-paved road through stands of feathery, stringy-barked ribbonwood and around granitic blocks.

Soon you note the buildings and exercise yards of Camp Lockett, a World War II Army camp that served as the last home of the Buffalo Soldiers, the elite African American cavalrymen. A state historical landmark, it is now an equestrian center that hosts public and private events. Marked by a post, the path dips to merge with the paved road shoulder across from its entrances. Walk along the road's west shoulder, going north 250 yards, past a cluster of tan-pink bungalows. Just across from Camp Lockett's entrance, and just up Forrest Gate Road from the modern Border Patrol Station, trail tread resumes and veers left (northwest), away from the roadside (1.4–2,586'), via three old concrete steps.

RESUPPLY ACCESS

Before heading off on the PCT, be sure you are adequately provisioned, since the next certain water is at Lake Morena County Park, 18.6 miles away. A post office and ranch-supply store are just two blocks north in sleepy, agricultural Campo. A general store lies 0.3 mile north, at the junction of Forrest Gate Road and CA 94. The next major resupply point is in Mount Laguna, about 41.6 miles away.

Now turning your attention to the trail, you climb gently from the road, pass a lone live oak, momentarily reach a terrace, and then cut obliquely across a road serving the bungalows. Beyond, the sandy path climbs minimally across a brushy slope, then swings southwest at an overlook of CA 94 and Campo Valley. Paralleling the highway, the PCT undulates over a string of low ridges, comes close to a descending jeep road, then descends easily to a PCT-posted crossing (2.3–2,470') of two-lane CA 94. North of it, the PCT leads counterclockwise around a low hill and then descends into a grove of cottonwoods alongside Campo Creek. Just before crossing that attractive but seasonal stream, you ignore a jeep road climbing south. Instead, you follow PCT posts to the northwest bank, then traverse southwest on an alluvial terrace for a few minutes. Presently the route veers uphill, soon to find the San Diego & Arizona Eastern Railroad's tracks (3.0–2,464'). You have a gentle ascent as you continue over the tracks and wind west over the nose of a low ridge. Now in a maze of small gullies and low-rise chamise chaparral, the tread descends gently to a larger ravine, which is just north of the tracks. Here the cool shade of willows and cottonwoods, with an understory of mint and cattails, makes a picturesque lunch spot. Alas, the creeklet here tends to flow only in winter and early spring.

After momentarily coming close to the tracks again, you undertake a longer but still easy climb northwest to a low gap. A minute's walk beyond it, you strike a poor jeep road, which descends in a south-trending valley. Now climbing more in earnest, you swing southwest on Hauser Mountain's broad, sunny slopes, then switchback to find a north-ascending line.

The well-built, alternately sandy and rocky path soon rises high enough to afford fine, clear vistas southeast back to the border and east over a lovely ranch that lies below Hauser Mountain's eastern escarpment. Pleasant, more-or-less level walking leads northwest, and then the trail abruptly switchbacks up to the south to gain a canyon rim. Here the steep slopes yield to the chaparral-covered summit dome of Hauser Mountain. The path continues south, ascending gently and then passing through a pipe gate to a little-used road (8.8–3,361'). Beyond it you climb only minutes more before striking a second jeep road. Next you undertake a contour north, and you can see your trail snaking ahead for over a mile. Umpteen hillside ravines later, you step across an east-descending jeep road (9.0–3,343') before winding up to a scenic point low on the northeast ridge of Hauser Mountain.

VIEWS To the north and west, an impressive vista of Hauser Canyon unfolds. On the northern canyon wall stand the orange granitic pillars of Morena Butte. This area now lies in one of California's smallest wilderness areas, Hauser Wilderness, created in 1984.

The trail now descends northwest along the north face of Hauser Mountain, making a long traverse downcanyon. Presently, you note a road below you and continue out onto the nose of a low ridge to meet it—South Boundary Road 17S08 (14.0–2,939'). The PCT route heads southeast on this little-traveled administrative road, first climbing gently and then descending likewise to a junction (14.7–2,831') with a trail segment. This branches left, dropping rapidly from the road where it begins to bend north on a rocky hillside. To stay on public lands while avoiding unnecessary elevation loss, the PCT makes a rocky descent northwest across the canyon wall via five switchbacks. Finally, the grade moderates to reach a pleasant glade of live oaks and sycamores. In it, the PCT crosses Hauser Creek (15.4–2,317'), which

is usually flowing in winter and early spring but may be dry by April in drought years.

CAMPING A small, flat area just downstream could offer the best first night's camp north of the Mexican border for those who are disinclined to make the 1,000-foot climb to reach Lake Morena County Park. However, beware of pollution of the stream by cattle and of plentiful poison oak. Consider filling up your water here and continuing farther along the trail to dry camp. This will help reduce the physical impacts of camping near the water source, lessen crowding, and benefit wildlife that depend on Hauser Canyon for water.

Just across Hauser Creek, you find Hauser Creek Road, then cross it to begin an earnest, sweaty ascent of the southern slopes of Morena Butte. The first leg of this climb lies in the southeastern corner of Hauser Wilderness, and it consists of a moderate-to-steep grade through straggly chaparral. As the climb progresses, vistas unfold downcanyon to meadows and to Barrett Lake, which is framed by the bluffs of nearby Morena Butte. Switchbacks long and short eventually bring you to a saddle (16.7–3,190') on the granitic southeastern spur of Morena Butte. Now the PCT undertakes a traversing descent north, shortly joining and then leaving a jeep trail, which climbs more directly from Hauser Canyon. Beyond it, you wind for a minute or two along a dry creekbed and then step across its sandy wash to climb moderately north, then east, through lush mixed chaparral. In spring, the heavy perfume of startling lilac-blue ceanothus shrubs hangs heavy in the air, while a number of red-and-yellow-flowered globe mallows line the trailside. After reaching a low ridgecrest, you climb southeast a bit to a fair viewpoint, which gives panoramas north over the southern Laguna Mountains.

Now you drop gently east to find a good jeep road in a saddle (18.2–3,400'). Walk right (east) on the jeep road 50 yards, then leave it to angle first northeast and then north along a view-filled, outcrop-strewn ridge. Eventually the

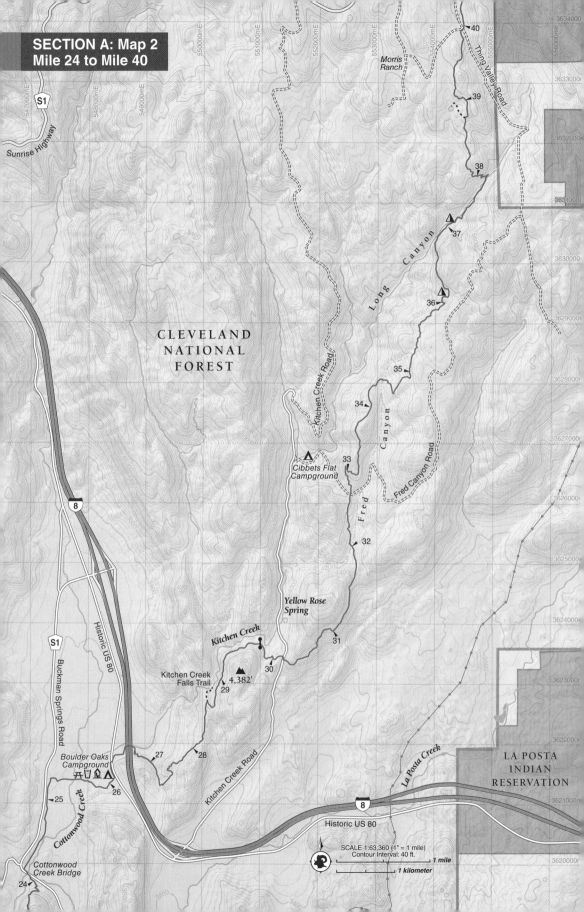

Morris Ranch

Thing Valley Road

40

39

38

37

Long Canyon

36

35

34

CLEVELAND
NATIONAL
FOREST

Kitchen Creek Road

33

Cibbets Flat
Campground

Fred Canyon

Fred Canyon Road

32

Yellow Rose
Spring

31

Kitchen Creek

30

Kitchen Creek
Falls Trail

4,382'

29

8

S1

Sunrise Highway

S1

Historic US 80

Buckman Springs Road

27

28

Boulder Oaks
Campground

26

25

Kitchen Creek Road

La Posta Creek

8

Historic US 80

LA POSTA
INDIAN
RESERVATION

Cottonwood Creek

Cottonwood
Creek Bridge

24

SCALE 1:63,360 (1" = 1 mile)
Contour Interval: 40 ft.

1 mile

1 kilometer

route veers northwest down a chaparral-cloaked nose, then leaves the heights for a descending traverse east to an oak grove and a gate in a barbed wire fence at the corner of Lake Morena Drive and Lake Shore Drive (20.0–3,074'), at a trailhead parking area. Just north is the entrance to Lake Morena County Park.

CAMPING This large facility offers, for a fee, 90 campsites with showers, water, picnic areas, and angling for bass, bluegill, and catfish in Morena Reservoir. There is a designated spot just off the trail for thru-hikers to camp at a discounted rate; check in at the ranger office upon arrival.

RESUPPLY ACCESS

Just 0.3 mile southeast on Lake Morena Drive you'll find a malt shop and market.

The PCT continues from the corner of the two paved roads, following Lake Shore Drive north 80 yards to where one steps through a fence to follow a paved road that traces the campground's perimeter. Beyond the camp area the route becomes trail and continues north to an oak-shaded overlook of Morena Reservoir and its chaparral-cloaked basin. Now walk east and north around the lakeshore on level trail well defined by signs. Ignore the intersecting paths that cross the PCT for lake access. Stay essentially level, and don't head away from the shoreline until PCT emblems mark the way. Only 0.1 mile from the campground, ignore some prominent but rapidly fading paths that fishermen use to continue along the lakeshore.

Rather, just after passing below the last house built in an adjacent cul-de-sac to the east, go right (northeast), uphill through a gated barbed wire fence onto a sandy rolling upland clothed in chamise scrub. The route next crosses many jeep tracks in the open chamise chaparral as it turns east then northeast, climbing gently to a low ridgetop. Now the way drops northeast into a nearby secluded, oak-shaded canyon; hops its seasonal creek; and climbs moderately east, then southeast, to gain a 3,375-foot ridge with expansive vistas west over the reservoir, Morena Butte, and Hauser Mountain. The Laguna Mountains are visible on the northern skyline. You romp easily north on the spine of the ridge in mixed chaparral. After a mile the route makes a descent along the ridge's west flank to a switchback, then to a gate on the ridge's northern nose. You quickly reach Buckman Springs Road S1, which you parallel briefly to its bridge over Cottonwood Creek (24.1–3,065'), which may be dry by spring in drought years. The seasonally swollen creek may require some minor fording in early spring.

Continuing north, the PCT tread soon diverges from the roadbed to wind through a pleasant mile of oak stands and dry meadows, always within earshot of Buckman Springs Road. Abruptly the route then veers east and descends to the sandy-gravelly bed of Cottonwood Creek (25.5–3,107'). Dry most of the year, the creek in winter and spring may be flowing and may be a couple of yards wide. Across it the trail heads east up a ravine and then joins a steadily improving and climbing jeep road that leads through a gate and over a low ridge to reach the equestrian section of Boulder Oaks Campground (26.0–3,183').

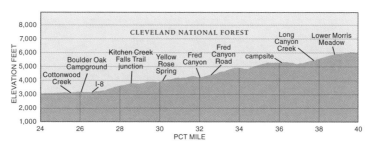

CAMPING This pleasant and little-used facility offers picnic tables, piped water, and toilets among boulders and shady live oaks. Camping here lessens the impact of setting up camp at less-developed sites farther along the trail.

Marked by posts, the PCT winds east across the campground, then momentarily goes north to reach paved, two-lane Old Highway 80 just north of the campground's entrance. Now walk north along the road's west shoulder to the southern verge of Cottonwood Valley's grassy plain, where well-signed PCT tread resumes, leading east.

Soon the route leads north and then east under two concrete spans of I-8 (26.6–3,145'). Just beyond the second bridge, switchbacks climb south to an ascending traverse that heads to a brushy gap. Here the route turns northeast for a long climb on open, sometimes rocky slopes, eventually finding a position some 100 feet above the cool, pooling early-season flow of Kitchen Creek. Arcing north around Peak 4,382, you then switchback up (east) to find paved Kitchen Creek Road (30.2–3,995') on a view-filled pass.

The northbound PCT from atop the pass is found beyond a firebreak east of the pavement. Panoramas expand back to the Mexican border and to Cameron Valley as you ascend gently to moderately along slopes composed of foliated, red-stained gneiss, colored in season with blossoms of white forget-me-nots. After leveling off momentarily on a 4,310-foot saddle, the trail drops, flanked by nodding, brown-flowered peonies and mixed chaparral, to a glade of oaks beside the usually dry creek of Fred Canyon.

CAMPING Now on the west side of the canyon, the trail ascends to

Fred Canyon Road 16S08 (32.6–4,155'), which descends 0.8 mile northwest to Cibbets Flat Campground, with toilets, tables, and water.

Now the path climbs moderately in heavy ceanothus, ocean spray, and chamise cover, switchbacking once around a nose and then climbing to a traverse past Peak 5,036 over to the dry headwaters of Fred Canyon. Next the PCT gains 500 feet, passes a jeep trail east to Fred Canyon Road, and then makes an undulating traverse and a gentle descent into Long Canyon (36.9–5,195').

CAMPING In 0.2 mile a camp could be made a safe distance (at least 200 feet) from a seasonally trickling creek near wild roses.

A gentle ascent in this pretty, meadowed canyon dotted with black oaks finds a ford of Long Canyon Creek, followed by switchbacks and two crossings of a jeep road from Horse Meadow.

At the second crossing (38.8–5,889') you could follow the jeep road northwest 0.3 mile to pretty Lower Morris Meadow, which has a spring and a cozy cluster of Jeffrey pines.

WATER ACCESS

An unsigned trail leads to a water tank with an accessible pipe at Lower Morris Meadow. To get there, leave the PCT at mile 38.8, and walk west to a fence; go through the opening, proceed to a dirt road, head downhill, and look for fence posts. The tank sits to your right.

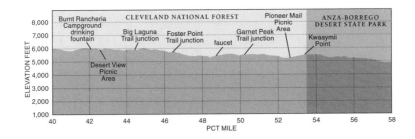

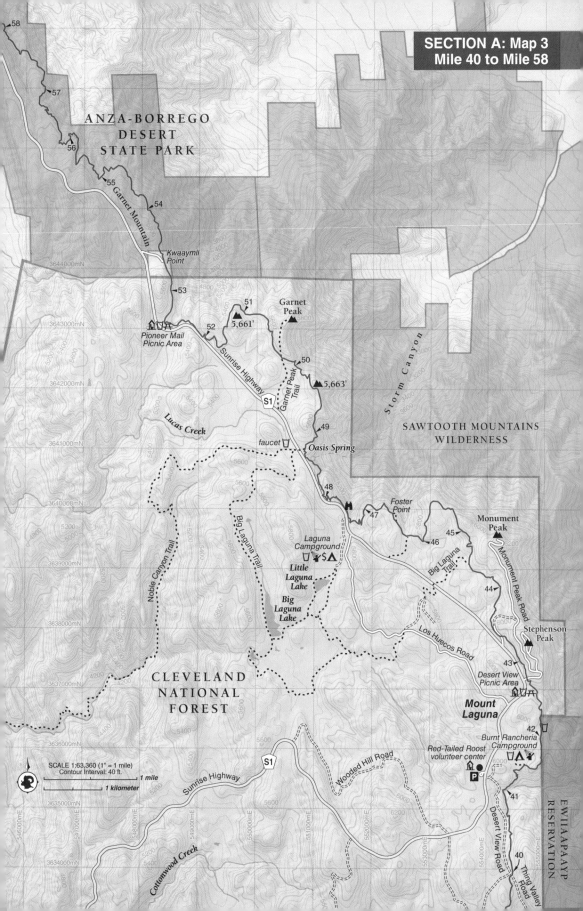

58

57

ANZA-BORREGO
DESERT
STATE PARK

56

55

54

Garnet Mountain

Kwaaymii
Point

53

3644000mN

51
5,661'

Garnet
Peak

52

Pioneer Mail
Picnic Area

50

3643000mN

Sunrise Highway

Garnet Peak Trail

S1

5,663'

3642000mN

Storm Canyon

49

Lucas Creek

faucet

Oasis Spring

SAWTOOTH MOUNTAINS
WILDERNESS

3641000mN

48

Foster
Point

47

Monument
Peak

46

45

3640000mN

Noble Canyon Trail

Big Laguna Trail

Laguna
Campground

Big Laguna Trail

44

Monument Peak Road

3639000mN

Little
Laguna
Lake

Big
Laguna
Lake

Los Huecos Road

Stephenson
Peak

43

Desert View
Picnic Area

3638000mN

CLEVELAND
NATIONAL
FOREST

Mount
Laguna

42

Burnt Rancheria
Campground

3637000mN

Red-Tailed Roost
volunteer center

EWIIAAPAAYP RESERVATION

41

SCALE 1:63,360 (1" = 1 mile)
Contour Interval: 40 ft.

1 mile

1 kilometer

Sunrise Highway

S1

Wooded Hill Road

Desert View Road

40

Thing Valley Road

Cottonwood Creek

3636000mN

3635000mN

3634000mN

546000mE

547000mE

548000mE

549000mE

550000mE

551000mE

552000mE

553000mE

554000mE

Climbing still into the relatively cool Laguna Mountains proper, you alternate between mountain mahogany and Jeffrey pine–black oak forest to cross a saddle, then descend slightly to a crossing of Morris Ranch Road. A few minutes north of the crossing of Morris Ranch Road, the undulating duff-treaded path intersects, then for 80 yards ambles along, a jeep road under open cover of Jeffrey pines and black oaks before clearly branching away to descend. A few minutes' walk leads you to cross a much better road beside shaded La Posta Creek.

WILDLIFE Here you'll see outstanding examples of food caches of acorn woodpeckers—custom-built niches for individual acorns from black oaks and interior live oaks in Jeffrey pine bark. When tasty insect larvae hatch in the stored acorns, the birds return to feast.

Leaving La Posta Creek, the route contours above a pump house. Trekkers should be aware that, in the Laguna Mountain Recreation Area, camping is restricted to campgrounds only; no backcountry camping is allowed. The recreation area stretches from near this site north 10.4 miles to Pioneer Mail Picnic Area.

CAMPING Your trail ascends into the recreation area, passing abandoned wood-rat nests and the first pinyon pines of the trail before reaching the south boundary of Burnt Rancheria Campground (41.5–5,936'), which has toilets, water, and tables. The campground is typically open mid- to late April through late October.

HISTORY Cattlemen began encroaching on the Laguna Mountains in the late 1800s. To halt their advancement, American Indians, called Diegueños by the Spanish padres, burned down a seasonal ranch house—hence the name Burnt Rancheria.

Climbing away from the campground, the PCT does double duty as the Desert View Nature Trail, passing live-forever, pearly everlasting, thistle, yerba santa, and beavertail cacti, all xeric

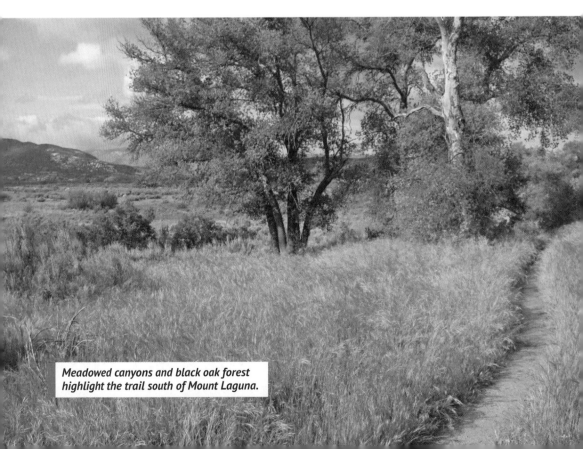

Meadowed canyons and black oak forest highlight the trail south of Mount Laguna.

(drought-tolerant) plants that reflect your proximity to the searing Colorado Desert to the east. Bending north and passing numerous, poorer side trails, your now nearly level path leads back into restful forest, joins dirt Desert View Road, and passes a dirt-road spur leading southwest to Burnt Rancheria Campground (42.1–5,971').

VIEWS From here the PCT climbs north along the Desert View Nature Trail, reaching a spectacular overlook of arid Anza-Borrego Desert State Park, its floor— Vallecito Valley—lying 4,400 feet below you in the rain shadow of the Laguna Mountains. The 35,080-acre Sawtooth Mountains Wilderness, designated in 1994, lies east of and below the PCT as it threads north around Stephenson Peak, Monument Peak, and Garnet Peak. The wilderness was designed to protect the rugged canyons that descend to the Vallecito Valley.

WATER ACCESS

Leaving this overlook, the PCT descends into cooler black oak forest and passes below tables of the Desert View Picnic Area (42.6–5,956'), now with toilets and several water options: the closest is a faucet connected to a metal pipe just south of a small cul-de-sac. There is also a faucet next to the toilets, which is usually shut off in winter.

Northbound hikers should know that once they pass Desert View Picnic Area and the town of Mount Laguna, the next water lies in Chariot Canyon, a 1.8-mile detour from the PCT after a long, usually too-warm, 22.4-mile trek. Less reliable water is found at Pioneer Mail Picnic Area, 10 miles north.

RESUPPLY ACCESS

Hikers in need of supplies can turn left on the road and walk 70 yards west to Sunrise Highway S1, and then south 0.4 mile to Mount Laguna Post Office, a store, phones, restaurants, motels, and a U.S. Forest Service station. The next supply point along the PCT is Warner Springs, 66.9 miles away, though many hikers opt to find rides from CA 78 to the mountain town of Julian or to Stagecoach Trails RV Resort on County Road S2 in Banner.

The trail then switchbacks up to a paved road (42.8–5,981'), which leads to Stephenson Peak and the abandoned Mount Laguna U.S. Air Force Western Air Defense Network Station, now a Federal Aviation Administration navigation-control site.

Continuing on the PCT, you have an easy traverse through high scrub and forest that lie below the golf-ball radar domes on Stephenson Peak. The traverse then ends at a second paved road (43.4–5,915') climbing to the summit. Iris, snowberry, yellow violets, and baby blue eyes lend springtime color to the forest floor as the route skirts north around the Air Force station's boundary. Then it crosses a succession of jeep roads and rises moderately in huckleberry oak, manzanita, and ocean spray chaparral below Monument Peak before dropping easily to a saddle where some jeep roads terminate.

PLANTS A startling contrast of vegetation is presented when the PCT tops the next small ridge. To the east nothing but drought-tolerant, clumped shrubbery survives, while on the Laguna Mountains' summits to the west, a nearly uniform Jeffrey pine and black oak forest stretches from North,

Cuyamaca, and Stonewall Peaks in Cuyamaca Rancho State Park over to hazy mountains above San Diego. A disparity of rainfall maintains these two different life zones, caused by the Laguna Mountains' geography. Warm, moisture-laden air sweeping inland from the Pacific Ocean cools as it rises over the obstructing Lagunas. This cooling causes moisture in the air to condense, bringing rain to nurture pine forests and leaving parched, water-absorbing air to blast down desert slopes in the mountains' lee.

Leaving this instructional vista, the PCT descends through a small burn, crosses bulldozer tracks that encircle it, and then turns west, descending easily into oak-shaded Flathead Flats. Here an obvious patchwork of poor roads leads west 75 yards at the head of Storm Canyon. The trail ascends just under a northwest-trending road, crossing that road in a moment to emerge from shade onto a chaparral-covered nose. Merging with the road, your thoroughfare narrows as it descends, full of views, northwest past rock and chaparral, then turns south to switchback down to a ravine and resume a gently undulating traverse below the Sunrise Highway.

CAMPING In just a moment you reach a dirt spur (47.5–5,422') that descends from the highway and leads to Laguna Campground.

WATER ACCESS

To get water, head west up the road to the highway, and take it south 0.5 mile to Mount Laguna. Laguna Campground, a critical spot for many thru-hikers since backcountry camping isn't allowed, is nearby, across Sunrise Highway at Laguna Meadow Road.

Back on the route, a few minutes' walk leads to a lone switchback that raises you to a

ridgetop pole-line road, which you cross west to descend to a quiet draw and a better dirt road that descends north to Oasis Spring. After you leave this road, live and black oaks, scattered pines, and mountain mahogany line the view-filled way around the spectacular furnace-breathed head of Storm Canyon to reach a closed road (48.7–5,433') on cooler forested land. This intersection is now trail and marks a detour to an occasional water source.

WATER ACCESS

Just beyond a pipe swing gate, there is an unmarked trail junction where the roadbed used to be. As you continue straight (northwest), a spur trail curves gently down and west, then momentarily south, to reach Sunrise Highway S1 in less than 0.1 mile. Here a monument to the Penny Pines reforestation program stands beside a busy trailhead parking area. Directly across two-lane Sunrise Highway S1 is the start of Noble Canyon Trail, which strikes west–southwest only 50 yards to a semireliable water supply. Here lie a freeze-proof cast-iron faucet and a galvanized horse trough in an open stand of black oaks; the water system is powered by portable generator, however, and cannot be relied on year-round. Note that camping is not allowed in this vicinity. A moment farther on is a junction with the southbound Big Laguna Trail, which heads back to Mount Laguna in about 4 miles.

This is the last water source close to your route until Cuyamaca Reservoir, 12.5 miles farther along the PCT and then 1.7 miles along a lateral. Closer but less certain water may be had during late spring and summer at Pioneer Mail Picnic Area, in 3.9 miles. Be sure to filter it. Possibly more convenient to some northbound travelers are the springs in Chariot Canyon, a 1.8-mile detour from the PCT in 14.9 miles, though hikers have reported notable pollution in recent years. The well on Rodriguez Spur Truck Trail, a 1.3-mile detour from your path in 19.8 miles, can also typically be relied on in April and May.

North across the closed fire road, the PCT swings right (north) and then ascends gently east, recrossing the road to climb easily under the Lagunas' steep eastern scarp to a saddle with the end of a jeep road. From there, the route undulates northwest on scrub-bound slopes while keeping just above the rough jeep track. Your path crosses jeep spurs to the summits of Peak 5,663 and Garnet Peak and then strikes another spur at a saddle (50.2–5,491') west of Garnet Peak. The PCT next traverses around Peak 5,661, passing through hoary-leaved ceanothus brush and providing excellent vistas of Oriflamme Mountain to the north. Beyond, the route drops first south and then west to a sandy saddle with a grass-floored pine forest. The route then heads northwest before winding west to shaded Pioneer Mail Picnic Area (52.6–5,274'), which lies at the end of a parking spur coming from Sunrise Highway.

WATER ACCESS

Hikers will find a 1,000-gallon water tank in low brush just 50 feet beyond the trailhead information sign. It is filled intermittently with untreated water. A 4-foot-diameter concrete trough is fed by the tank. Contact Cleveland National Forest's Descanso Ranger District before leaving Mount Laguna, or check pctwater.com, for the tank's status. This tank is often dry by May.

The PCT's continuation north from the picnic area follows the old, unpaved alignment of Sunrise Highway gently up across a cliff at the head of Cottonwood Canyon, where a striking collection of golden-red boulders hold metal and wood plaques honoring deceased loved ones. The path soon reaches a parking area at

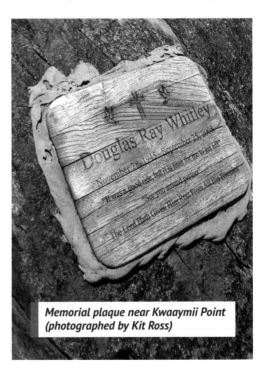

Memorial plaque near Kwaaymii Point (photographed by Kit Ross)

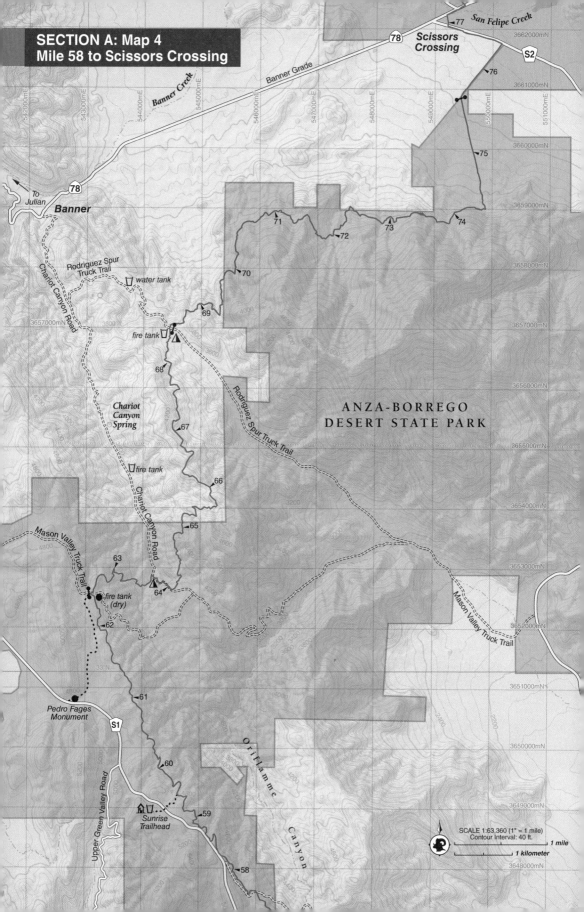

San Felipe Creek

Scissors
Crossing

78

S2

77

76

75

Banner Grade

Banner Creek

543000mE

544000mE

545000mE

546000mE

547000mE

548000mE

549000mE

550000mE

551000mE

3662000mN

3661000mN

3660000mN

78

To
Julian

Banner

74

71

72

73

70

3659000mN

3658000mN

Rodriguez Spur
Truck Trail

water tank

69

4000

Chariot Canyon Road

542000mE

3657000mN

fire tank

68

3800

3600

Rodriguez Spur Truck Trail

3656000mN

**ANZA-BORREGO
DESERT STATE PARK**

*Chariot
Canyon
Spring*

67

3655000mN

fire tank

66

3200

3654000mN

65

3653000mN

Mason Valley Truck Trail

4800

63

Chariot Canyon Road

64

fire tank
(dry)

62

3652000mN

Mason Valley Truck Trail

33 N.

61

3651000mN

Pedro Fages
Monument

S1

60

3650000mN

O r i f l a m m e

59

Sunrise
Trailhead

Upper Green Valley Road

C a n y o n

3649000mN

58

3648000mN

SCALE 1:63,360 (1" = 1 mile)
Contour Interval: 40 ft.

1 mile

1 kilometer

paved Kwaaymii Point Road (53.4–5,472'), just off Sunrise Highway.

Northbound tread recommences a few yards up this road, only 40 yards south of a defunct jeep road climbing Garnet Mountain. Now you contour on the mountain's eastern declivity and enter Anza-Borrego Desert State Park. At the mountain's north end, you drop briskly north on sunny slopes to a jeep road that descends into Oriflamme Canyon.

HISTORY Oriflamme ("golden flame") Mountain, from which the canyon derives its name, received its appellation from numerous sightings, since the 1880s, of burning balls or spirit lights on the mountain's east side. These led to insistent prospecting for gold over the years, but scientists have at least one more-interesting theory—that the lights are static electricity, discharged when dry desert winds blow sand against quartz boulders on the hillside.

The next leg meanders northwest along steep hillsides of light-colored granodiorite—weathered to futuristic knobs—and affords excellent panoramas of seemingly sterile Vallecito Valley.

HISTORY Vallecito Valley was once the site of a Butterfield Overland Mail Stage station. Following an old Spanish trail from Fort Yuma, stages ran from St. Louis to California from 1858 to 1861. The first Europeans to traverse this part of the Colorado Desert, however, were Spanish forces led by Lieutenant Pedro Fages from the San Diego Presidio, who marched through in search of deserters in 1772. Two years later Captain Juan Bautista de Anza, for whom the park is named,

scouted this area for a lifeline trail from Mexico to impoverished Alta California settlements.

Presently the route descends to meet a second road to Oriflamme Canyon. Across it you follow singletrack that soon closely parallels Sunrise Highway. Soon you cross a ridgetop jeep road and then another.

GEOLOGY The rocks lining your route from here to Chariot Canyon are Julian schist—metasediments of the Paleozoic age. This particular schist (a rock, once a shale, that now breaks along paper-thin parallel planes) shows abundant flecks of reflective, glassy mica, and it weathers to a rusty brown containing frequent mineral-stain bandings.

VIEWS A sweeping vista unfolds to the north; green forested Volcan Mountain stands above your unfortunate route down to arid San Felipe Valley and the brown San Felipe Hills. Beyond, Combs Mountain, Thomas Mountain, and the Desert Divide rise to the rugged subalpine splendor of San Jacinto Peak. Over its west shoulder, the bald white alpine cap of San Gorgonio Peak thrusts its height—your next two weeks' work is displayed.

The PCT undulates above Oriflamme Canyon to reach a faint jeep track at a low gap (59.5–4,996').

WATER ACCESS

Thirsty hikers may opt to follow that track west 0.25 mile through a verdant meadow to Sunrise Highway. Cross the street, where there is a parking lot and outhouse. Look

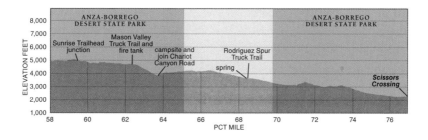

for a tank and horse trough at the barbed wire gate, which may afford a water gift in springtime but must not be relied on.

Returning to your trek, you follow the PCT as it winds north along chaparral-clothed summits to the Mason Valley Truck Trail (62.4–4,694'), just east of a locked gate. Northbound travelers here turn right and curve 100 yards east to a junction with Chariot Canyon Road, now barely distinguishable as a road.

WATER ACCESS

Emergency water is sporadically available 75 yards east of this junction, where a spigot juts out of the hillside below a concrete-box water tank used by fire crews. Don't count on it, though.

Back on the route, the PCT leads north down rocky Chariot Canyon "Road," on a bone-jarring descent that ends at a lupine flat holding the canyon's seasonal creek. **CAMPING** Fair but waterless camping may be found here, by a road junction (63.7–3,864').

WATER ACCESS

If you are low on water, you should detour here and continue north down Chariot Canyon Road in search of that precious desert commodity. But check upstream from the PCT before heading downcanyon to the springs; water is sometimes found there. Otherwise, walk north down the gently sloping sandy, sunny wash. Presently, you pass in and out of stands of cottonwoods and live oaks and leave Anza-Borrego Desert State Park. Beyond, you begin to encounter tailings, mine tunnels, and shacks of some of the many gold mines that dot Chariot Canyon. Hikers commonly find water in the streambed in the next 0.25 mile, relieving them of the full trek down to the main springs.

If not, continue north, cross to the east bank, and presently find a short dirt spur road. It branches right, east, uphill 75 yards to an 18-foot-diameter, buried concrete water tank set in the hillside. This road is marked near its junction by a square concrete valve box. Water can be had from the tank by way of a heavy iron plate set in its top. If you don't find water here, continue downcanyon, recrossing Chariot Canyon Creek twice in quick succession to find permanent springs just short of dirt Ben Hur Mine Road. In severe drought years, however, the springs are dry.

Those who return to the PCT in upper Chariot Canyon should note that their watery treasure must last awhile: the unreliable well on Rodriguez Spur Truck Trail is the next near-route water for the northbound, in 4.9 miles. After that, Barrel Spring, 32.5 blistering-hot miles ahead, has the next on-route water for those bypassing Julian and Banner. Heading south, the next reliable water is on the Noble Canyon Trail, 14.9 long miles up in the Laguna Mountains.

RESUPPLY ACCESS

If the springs are dry, continue out to the road's end on CA 78 at Banner, a small ranch resort with a store, restaurant, phones, and camping. From there it is 7 miles west on CA 78 to beautiful, hiker-friendly Julian, with complete supplies and delicious apple pie. The northbound traveler could get back on route by catching a ride east from Banner to the PCT near Scissors Crossing, in 5 miles.

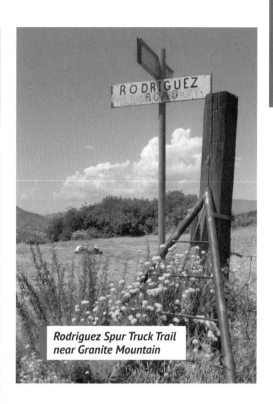

Rodriguez Spur Truck Trail near Granite Mountain

From the road junction in upper Chariot Canyon, you climb steeply east up the Mason Valley cutoff road to a resumption of PCT tread. This branches left (northeast), the junction perhaps marked with a brown-and-white state park sign. Now, a well-built tread snakes gently uphill around the western and northern slopes of rounded Chariot Mountain. Eventually the path skirts briefly northwest along a crest saddle, veers left, and then soon veers northeast across a gap. Just beyond it you get vistas southeast, down desertlike Rodriguez Canyon and into the mirage-wavering, incandescent heart of Anza-Borrego Desert State Park. Thankfully, your way continues north and skirts the hottest regions.

CAMPING A businesslike descent now leads down to the head of Rodriguez Canyon, where you cross Rodriguez Spur Truck Trail (68.4–3,653'). This is a popular, if wind-prone, area to camp.

WATER ACCESS

Continue down Rodriguez Spur Truck Trail a few minutes to find a well, just 40 feet below the road. It is 12 feet high, capped with a plastic barrel. A circular concrete horse trough in a small patch of irrigated grass lies just northwest, only yards below the road. It is often empty or difficult to access in late summer and fall. Check pctwater.com for current information. If the spring north of the trail is not flowing and you don't have enough water to make it to Scissors Crossing, you can opt to continue 2.2 miles down Rodriguez Spur Truck Trail to CA 78. The Banner store is across the highway to the east about 200 feet, and it's often easy to find a ride to Julian from here.

Immediately beyond good dirt Rodriguez Spur Truck Trail, you pass through a pipe gate and angle across an east-curving jeep track; then you, too, swing east. A graded but persistent descent next leads north on the steep, rocky, barren slopes of Granite Mountain, offering impressive panoramas.

North over arid San Felipe Valley, look carefully for the next leg of the PCT, which traverses along the San Felipe Hills, low on the northern horizon. In the far distance, green San Jacinto Peak and glistening, bald San Gorgonio Peak rear above 2-mile heights. Closer by, the rusty headframes of a few old gold mines (part of the once rich Julian mining complex that caused excitement in 1869–70) lie in ravines below you.

After winding down a succession of dry slopes, the PCT turns more east and almost levels just above the gentle, brushy alluvial fans at the foot of Granite Mountain.

First you ascend to a rocky gap on Granite Mountain's north ridge. Next you descend to cross a succession of bouldery washes, then undulate east some more to a second gap (70.3–3,130') behind a prominent light-colored granitic knob. Begin your final descent on four small switchbacks, followed by a descending traverse east. Abruptly, near the base of a cluster of pinnacles below Granite Mountain's northeast ridge, you veer north, emerging onto a sandy alluvial plain. After quickly crossing a jeep track, you proceed almost arrow-straight across northern Earthquake Valley, imperceptibly descending through an open desert association of low buckwheat, rabbitbrush, and teddy bear cholla shrubs, these sprinkled with larger junipers and graceful agave. You eventually pass through a gate in a barbed wire fence, then swing northeast, tracing an old jeep road that is immediately west of the fenceline. This stretch ends at

two-lane County Highway S2 (76.4–2,555') at a spot just west of a white, wooden cattle guard.

A full-service campground and RV park (stagecoachtrails.com) welcomes hikers 4 miles southeast on County Highway S2, with a pool, water, a camp store, and showers. Heavy winds are common in this area.

Now locate a faint trail that turns left (west) near the south shoulder of County Highway S2, just south of a four-strand green barbed wire fence. It winds fairly level past low shrubs, many of them equipped with murderously efficient, thigh-slashing, clothes-grabbing spines. Nearing a junction with CA 78 (77.0–2,278'), find a metal pipe gate and cross County Highway S2, safe from attack by menacing flora but now exposed to the considerable traffic of desert-bound vacationers. This was the route of the Butterfield Stage Line, which carried mail across the western United States, passing this way in the 1850s. Now walk directly north, at first paralleling a wooden-post fence, then drifting vaguely away to the left through catclaw shrubs, beyond which trail tread peters out as you walk down to cross a dry sandy wash. Momentarily, you emerge on a low terrace, just beneath the south shoulder of CA 78. Now head right, northeast, along the shrubby terrace, close beside CA 78, to find another cattle gate adjacent to the concrete bridge where the highway spans San Felipe Creek (77.1–2,257').

WATER ACCESS

San Felipe Creek is nearby but should not be counted on, especially in drought years. Even when present, it is usually heavily contaminated by cattle.

Continuing, step across San Felipe Creek's sandy bed, and resume a parallel course to CA 78—again on a low terrace—where trail tread is flanked by tumbleweeds, mustard, and baccharis. In just a few minutes, you cross CA 78 (77.3–2,261') to find the trail climbing northwest, up from the highway at a junction marked with a CHAINS REQUIRED sign.

WATER ACCESS

Northbound hikers should note that Barrel Spring, the next possible (but not certain) water hole, is still 23.8 potentially scorching miles away. If your water reserves are low, consider walking 1 mile northeast on CA 78 to Sentenac Cienega, a marsh along San Felipe Creek. Water is usually found here all spring. Southbound hikers will find water in Banner too; near the route at Rodriguez Spur Truck Trail, in 8.9 miles; or in Chariot Canyon in 13.6 miles.

Trail angels often place water bottles at the underpass at Scissors Crossing and in the San Felipe Hills during the spring thru-hiking season. However, count on this gracious act at your peril. See page 16 for more on water caches.

RESUPPLY ACCESS

This is also a reasonable spot to detour for supplies, as well as water—delightful and cool Julian is 12.5 miles west up CA 78, while Borrego Springs is about 15 miles east on CA 78.

An alternative way to find water from the Scissors Crossing environs would be to hop on a bus and retreat west up to the cool green haven of Julian. (See "Supplies," page 70.) A San Diego County bus stops at Scissors Crossing each morning and evening via routes 891 and 894. Contact San Diego County MTA at 800-858-0291 for an up-to-date schedule.

Commencing a long, exposed traverse of the San Felipe Hills, the PCT ascends briefly across a cobbly alluvial fan to the southern foot of Grapevine Mountain. Here you cross into Anza-Borrego Desert State Park and, now on rotten granite footing, begin to climb Grapevine Mountain's truly desertlike southwestern flanks. Even in springtime, PCT hikers would do well to attack this ascent in the very early morning, as temperatures over 100°F are commonplace, and most of the next 24 miles are virtually shadeless. Hikers trying to walk the length of the San Felipe Hills in one hot day will be either gratified or frustrated by the extraordinarily gentle grade of the route, which adds many extra switchbacks and a few unnecessary miles to the task.

PLANTS   Early on the walk, however, the easy grade allows one to marvel at the "forest" of bizarre ocotillo shrubs. Standing 10–15 feet tall and resembling nothing more than a bundle of giant, green pipe cleaners, ocotillos are perfectly adapted to their searing desert environment. Much of the year, ocotillos' branches look like spiny, lifeless stalks. But within just two to three days after a rainstorm, the branches sprout vibrant green clusters of delicate leaves along their entire length, allowing renewed growth. Almost as quickly, the leaves wither and die as groundwater becomes scarce. In this manner ocotillos may leaf out six to eight times a year.

The PCT continues to climb imperceptibly in and out of innumerable small canyons and gullies, none of which holds running water

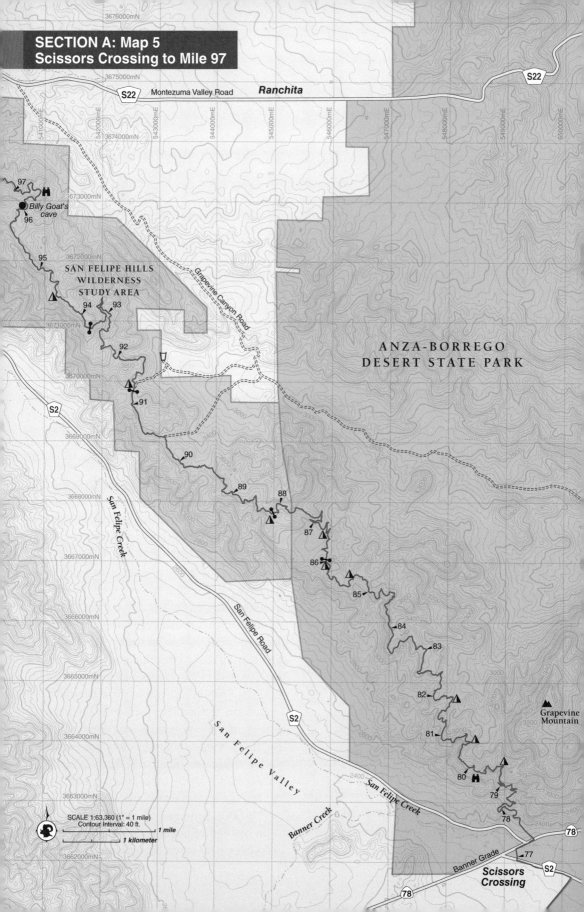

S22

S22   Montezuma Valley Road   *Ranchita*

97

Billy Goat's cave

96

95

SAN FELIPE HILLS
WILDERNESS
STUDY AREA

94   93

92

91

90

89

88

87

86

85

84

83

82

81

80

79

78

77

Grapevine Canyon Road

ANZA-BORREGO
DESERT STATE PARK

San Felipe Creek

San Felipe Road

S2

San Felipe Valley

Banner Creek

San Felipe Creek

Grapevine
Mountain

Banner Grade

*Scissors
Crossing*

S2

78

78

S2

SCALE 1:63,360 (1" = 1 mile)
Contour interval: 40 ft.

1 mile

1 kilometer

except during a rainsquall. Still in a very desert-like association of agave, barrel cactus, and teddy bear cholla, you eventually reach the crest of the San Felipe Hills and cross to their northeastern slopes at a pipe gate (86.0–3,364'). Now the path descends gently into a small, sandy valley that makes for adequate but waterless camping over the next several miles. Now, you cross a dry, sandy wash, which drains the valley. But you can see the trail's switchbacks on the slopes ahead, so navigation is easy.

An ascent of those switchbacks leads gently back to the ridgecrest (88.2–3,596') and several small campsites. The next leg of your journey stays high on the San Felipe Hills' steep southwestern slopes on an undulating course ranging between 3,400 feet and 3,600 feet.

CAMPING Just below a ridge saddle, you pass a junction with an east-branching jeep road, and then your path crosses the next saddle to the north, bisecting another, poorer jeep road (91.2–3,559') just beyond a pipe gate and a small campsite.

WATER ACCESS

Here, trail angels have established an emergency water cache for PCT thru-hikers. It consists of gallon water jugs secured by a nylon cord. This cache is usually replenished throughout the spring peak-hiking season by trail angels, but no one should depend on it. See page 16 for more about water caches.

Pressing on, you begin a long ascent, again on the eastern slopes of the San Felipe Hills, climbing now past dense chamise. An excruciatingly gentle, time-consuming switchback finally brings you back to the ridgetop and a cattle gate (93.8–4,141'). A more interesting part of the trail then traverses the headwalls of two treacherously steep canyons, these plummeting 1,200 feet to linear San Felipe Valley.

TRAIL INFO Across that valley the Volcan Mountains rise in pine-green splendor, an enviably cool contrast to your scorched environs. The San Felipe Hills are dry and brown for the same reason that the Volcan Mountains are lush and green: a rain shadow causes moisture-laden Pacific storms to dump their rain on the higher Volcan Mountains, leaving little for the San Felipe Hills.

Presently you veer northeast through a gap, back into dense chaparral on the east side of the San Felipe Hills. Beginning a long, gentle downgrade, the route winds around minor ridges and into nooks, crannies, and (it seems) every gully in sight. After a few miles, most hikers will yearn for a more direct, if steeper, route. But slowly the PCT loses elevation as it circumnavigates a branch of Hoover Canyon, and you gain vistas northeast over sparsely populated Montezuma Valley to San Ysidro Mountain. After awhile you pass through three gates in quick succession, then just a few minutes later descend under live oak cover to join an unpaved road. Now, perhaps marked by a PCT post, your route goes left, west, just a few yards on the road to find Barrel Spring (101.1–3,482').

CAMPING Here, after the first major spring rains, cool water is

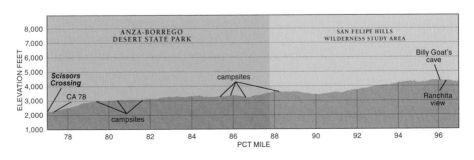

piped from a groundwater spring into a concrete trough. This good water hole and a pleasant, shady stand of canyon live oaks make a hospitable campsite. If you camp here, camp only in existing and impacted sites and try not to expand or further degrade these sites.

WATER ACCESS

If water isn't flowing in the trough, follow the PCT and the feeder pipe back southeast about 100 yards to an old dirt road that angles uphill to the spring's source. Northbound hikers can be assured of reliable water in 8.7 miles at Warner Springs Fire Station.

Southbound hikers have a longer walk to water: 23.8 miles to springtime off-route water at Sentenac Cienega, 32.7 miles to off-route water on Rodriguez Spur Truck Trail, or 37.4 miles to off-route springs in Chariot Canyon.

RESUPPLY ACCESS

If no water is available at Barrel Spring, you can try to catch a ride heading east on Montezuma Valley Road S22 to Ranchita, a small village with a mini store and hiker-friendly yoga retreat that has tent and tepee sites, showers, and hot meals for PCT-ers. You can continue east on S22, 15 miles from the PCT to Borrego Springs, for resupply.

Resuming your northward trek, you follow the dirt road from Barrel Spring down through a gate to a dirt-road pullout just south of paved Montezuma Valley Road S22 (101.2–3,453'). Just across the highway is a poor dirt road, on which you head north just 50 yards to a barbed wire cattle gate. Just beyond it, PCT posts indicate a route leading left (northwest), which quickly crosses the sandy wash of usually dry Buena Vista Creek. The way continues northwest across a sagebrush flat to the southern foot of a ridge. As the trail turns west at the ridge's base, the tread becomes well defined, soon contouring north into a small canyon. Then the trail begins to climb easily, and you are treated to pleasant views west as you ascend to a 3,550-foot ridgetop.

The trail next drops easily west along its northern slope; nearing the southern margin of a narrow, grassy, west-trending valley, the tread abruptly ends. But looking north across the pasture, you'll hopefully spot a PCT post marking the crossing of a jeep road. You'll then note tread immediately north, ascending north along the next low ridge. Climb it, then drop northeast to its base on the edge of another, much larger rolling grassland. Thanks to the efforts of PCTA volunteers, trail tread is well defined and well posted from here to San Ysidro Creek.

Follow the undulating path almost due north across the meadow, passing some well-trod cattle tracks to angle into the shallow mouth of sandy San Ysidro Creek's chaparral-clad valley. Along the way, you'll pass below a trickling hillside spring seep where cattle often congregate. Later, on a level course through a grove of live oaks near the stream's east bank, the path contours north along the canyon's east slopes but soon drops to cross San Ysidro Creek (105.0–3,354'), which usually flows in spring. Like other key points on this trail segment, this crossing is confused by a jeep track just north of the creek. Anticipate the crossing where San Ysidro Creek first bends upcanyon (northeast) under the first white-barked sycamore tree to shade your path.

Across San Ysidro Creek, head straight uphill 20 yards to find the path, which continues upcanyon for only a moment before switchbacking west moderately up out of the shade

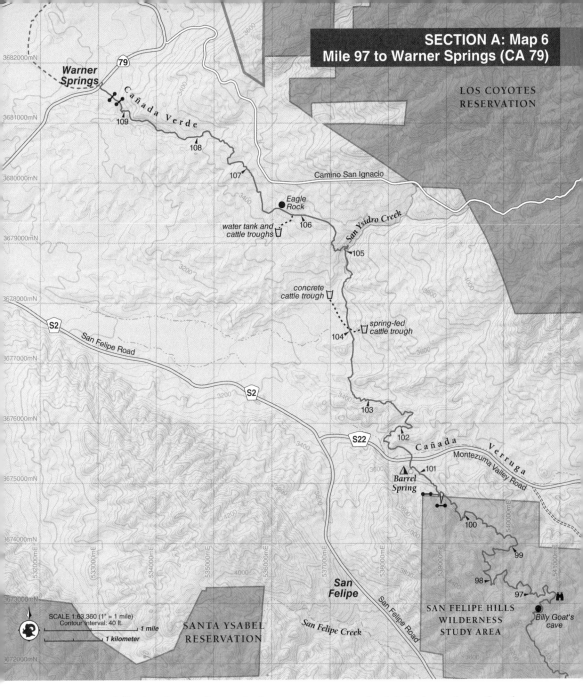

Warner
Springs

79

Cañada Verde

109

108

107

LOS COYOTES
RESERVATION

Camino San Ignacio

Eagle
Rock

water tank and
cattle troughs

106

San Ysidro Creek

105

concrete
cattle trough

spring-fed
cattle trough

104

S2

San Felipe Road

3200

S2

103

S22

102

Cañada   Verruga
Montezuma Valley Road

101

Barrel
Spring

100

99

98

97

SAN FELIPE HILLS
WILDERNESS
STUDY AREA

Billy Goat's
cave

San
Felipe

San Felipe Creek

San Felipe Road

SCALE 1:63,360 (1" = 1 mile)
Contour Interval: 40 ft.
1 mile
1 kilometer

SANTA YSABEL
RESERVATION

onto an open hillside. The tread ascends from San Ysidro Creek, soon turning north to attain the canyon's rim.

VIEWS Here you have views west over Warner Valley to Lake Henshaw, a sag pond along the Elsinore Fault, and to famous Mount Palomar Observatory, on the horizon. After a brief course north the trail turns west and reenters grassland. It leads gently up, then down, to cross a good dirt road (106.2–3,524'). A brief

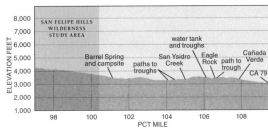

ELEVATION FEET

SAN FELIPE HILLS
WILDERNESS
STUDY AREA

Barrel Spring
and campsite

paths to
troughs

San Ysidro
Creek

Eagle
Rock

water tank
and troughs

path to
trough

Cañada
Verde

CA 79

PCT MILE

detour here leads to Eagle Rock, an outcrop of boulders on a small hilltop that makes a scenic and restful lunch spot. Soon the trail adopts a more northern course as it rolls across a corrugation of ridgelets and dry washes. After crossing a poor jeep trail in one such ravine, the trail climbs through low chaparral and soon crosses a ridgetop jeep road, which served as part of the temporary PCT route for many years.

From the ridge you descend gently past shady canyon live oaks and cottonwoods, which line the pretty valley called Cañada Verde (Spanish for "green ravine"). Soon the PCT closely parallels the southern banks of a small stream that flows until late spring of most years.

BE MINDFUL of bee-infested oaks in this area; hikers have reported attacks by angry hornets as they pass. Several of the guilty trees have small warning signs tacked to their trunks.

You follow the canyon bottom almost a mile and then, near Cañada Verde's mouth, pass through two pipe gates, the second one at a jeep road. Across the jeep road you continue

northwest just south of Cañada Verde's banks, and in 0.25 mile find the concrete bridge of two-lane CA 79 (109.5–3,045'), just west of Warner Springs Fire Station. Although the PCT actually heads under the highway, the bridge clearance is too low for horses, so a pipe gate allows access to the highway. Warner Springs Post Office lies 1.2 miles northeast along the highway, though hikers are encouraged to follow the marked trail from the Warner Springs Community Resource Center. This hiker-friendly property has an indoor lounge, water, and a resupply store—it is just across the road from the fire station. Check the website or call to ensure the center is still open.

WATER ACCESS

Water is available at both the fire station and the community center. The next possible water source for northbound hikers lies in Agua Caliente Creek, in 5.2 miles. Southbound hikers can obtain water at Barrel Spring, 8.4 miles away.

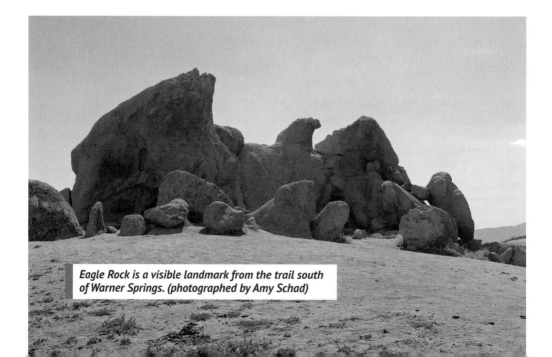

Eagle Rock is a visible landmark from the trail south of Warner Springs. (photographed by Amy Schad)

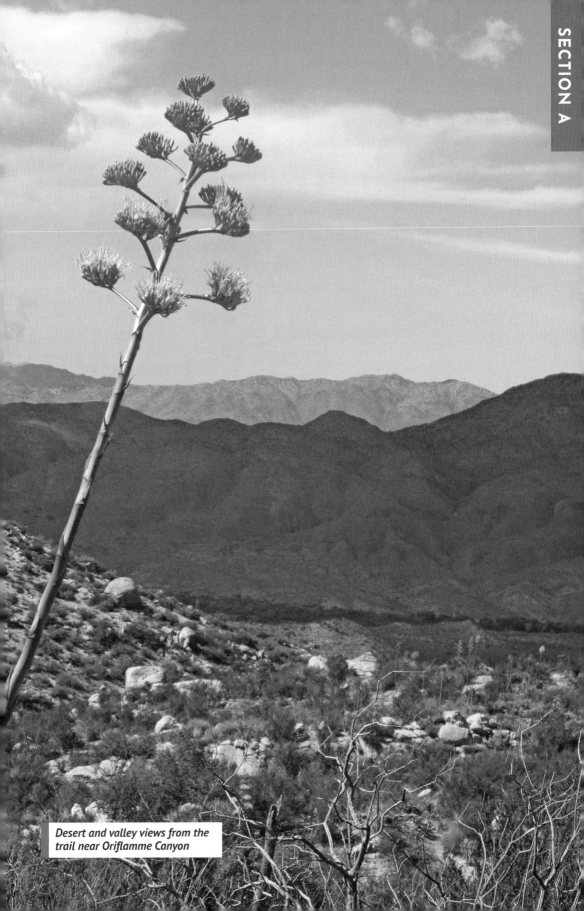

*Desert and valley views from the
trail near Oriflamme Canyon*

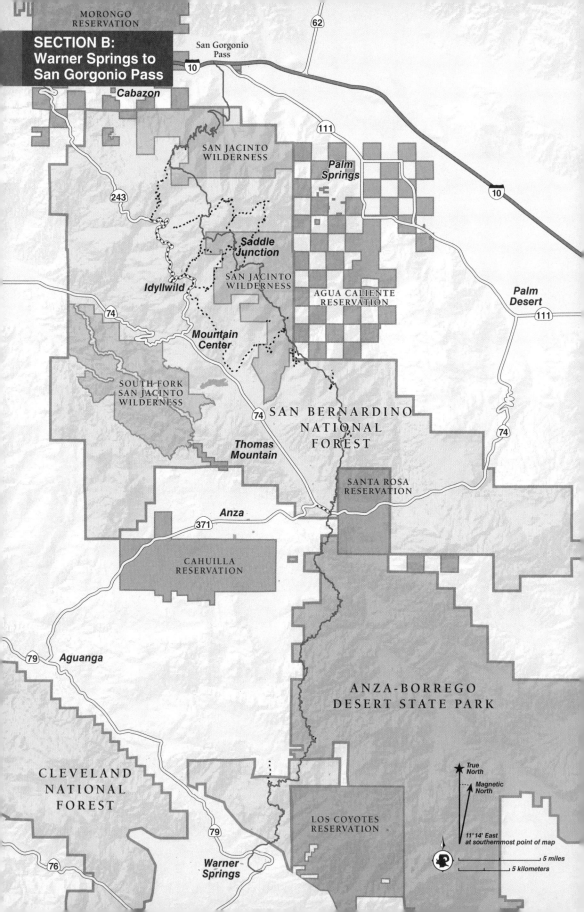

MORONGO
RESERVATION

San Gorgonio
Pass

62

10

Cabazon

111

SAN JACINTO
WILDERNESS

*Palm
Springs*

243

**Saddle
Junction**

SAN JACINTO
WILDERNESS

Idyllwild

AGUA CALIENTE
RESERVATION

*Palm
Desert*

111

10

74

**Mountain
Center**

SOUTH FORK
SAN JACINTO
WILDERNESS

SAN BERNARDINO
NATIONAL
FOREST

74

*Thomas
Mountain*

74

SANTA ROSA
RESERVATION

Anza

371

CAHUILLA
RESERVATION

79

Aguanga

**ANZA-BORREGO
DESERT STATE PARK**

CLEVELAND
NATIONAL
FOREST

LOS COYOTES
RESERVATION

★ True
North

↑ Magnetic
North

11°14' East
at southernmost point of map

5 miles

5 kilometers

79

*Warner
Springs*

76

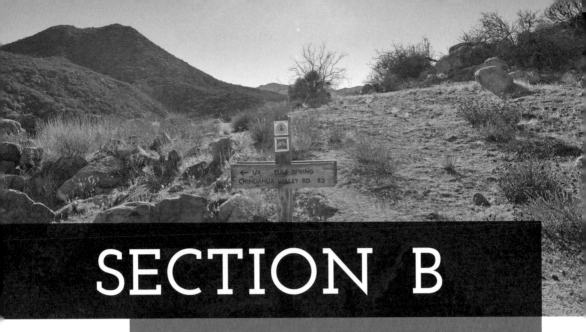

SECTION B

Warner Springs to San Gorgonio Pass

THE SAN JACINTO MOUNTAINS are the high point—and the highlight—of the Pacific Crest Trail's (PCT's) excursion through the northern Peninsular Ranges, and they afford the first true high-mountain air and scenery of your journey. But this section of trail also includes many miles of walking under shady live oaks and through the shadeless chaparral community (see "Special Concerns" on page 102). On the Desert Divide, where you have your first taste of the San Jacinto Mountains, you find an interesting combination of pine forest, chaparral, and desert species. Leaving the San Jacintos, the PCT plunges almost 8,000 feet down to arid San Gorgonio Pass, and in so doing passes through every life zone in California save for the alpine zone.

The Peninsular Ranges stretch from the southern tip of Baja California, paralleling the coastline, some 900 miles north to San Gorgonio Pass, which truncates the range along the Banning Fault and lesser faults. The

Above: Near Tule Spring crossroads

ranges' core, forming the Laguna Mountains, the Anza Upland, and the San Jacinto Mountains, where the PCT winds, is made of crystalline rocks— granite and its relatives—which were first intruded in a liquid state several miles beneath the surface and then later solidified. These rocks are similar in age and type to the granitic rocks of the Sierra Nevada.

Your walk from Warner Springs to San Gorgonio Pass treads mostly upon these rocks, which are usually fine-grained, gray to creamy in color, and strongly resistant to weathering, as demonstrated by obdurate mono-liths around Indian Flats and Bucksnort Mountain; by outcrops jutting from the alluvium of Terwilliger and Anza Valleys; and by the jagged, saurian spine of the San Jacinto Mountains, as on Fuller Ridge. The remainder of the terrain you tread is across either sand and gravel weathered from the granite, found in basins, or metamorphic rocks. These rocks are seen in Agua Caliente Creek's canyon and along much of the Desert Divide.

Section B ends at San Gorgonio Pass, a broad, cactus-dotted trough running east–west, flanked by the San Bernardino and San Jacinto Moun-tains to the north and south, respectively. Once a major corridor of Ameri-can Indian traders, San Gorgonio Pass is bounded by faults on either side. It lies some 9,000 feet below the summits of San Jacinto and San Gorgonio, each standing just a few air miles to one side.

Proof that awesome geologic processes are at work today can be seen right at the start of this section, at Warner Springs. Now a work-in-progress resort but used for centuries by neighboring Cahuilla and Cupeño tribes, the hot springs here bubble up from deep within the earth's crust and escape along the Aguanga Fault, which cuts just yards behind this small resort community. Warner's hot springs also served Kit Carson in 1846 and was an overnight stop on the Butterfield Stage Line from 1858 to 1861.

Section B also traverses the crown jewel of the Peninsular Ranges—
Santa Rosa and San Jacinto Mountains National Monument. Created in
October 2000 to protect 272,000 acres of mountains along the vast eastern
sweep of those ranges, the monument stretches from the Anza-Borrego
Desert State Park boundary on the south to the San Gorgonio Pass on the
north. National designation will hopefully give added protection to the
natural, historical, and cultural resources found along this rugged mountain
crest and help the diverse agencies that share jurisdiction over the varied
landscape coordinate their efforts.

DECLINATION 11°14'E

USGS MAPS

Warner Springs	Anza	Idyllwild
Hot Springs Mountain	Butterfly Peak	San Jacinto Peak
Bucksnort Mountain	Palm View Peak	White Water
Beauty Mountain		

POINTS ON THE TRAIL, SOUTH TO NORTH

	Mile	Elevation in feet	Latitude/Longitude
Warner Springs, first crossing of CA 79	109.5	3,045	N33° 16' 24.660" W116° 38' 41.820"
Lost Valley Spring	119.6	4,349	N33° 20' 34.380" W116° 38' 19.680"
Chihuahua Valley Road	127.3	5,057	N33° 22' 53.760" W116° 35' 42.660"
Tule Canyon Truck Trail to Tule Spring and Anza	137.0	3,620	N33° 27' 36.480" W116° 35' 59.580"
Table Mountain Truck Trail to Anza	147.0	4,909	N33° 31' 41.480" W116° 35' 26.820"
CA 74/Paradise Valley Cafe	151.9	4,924	N33° 33' 47.280" W116° 34' 36.300"
Trail junction to Live Oak and Tunnel Springs	158.4	5,952	N33° 37' 23.160" W116° 33' 50.460"
Cedar Spring trail junction (to camping and CA 74)	162.6	6,775	N33° 39' 58.500" W116° 34' 31.080"
Fobes Ranch Trail junction (to CA 74)	166.5	5,994	N33° 41' 24.240" W116° 36' 34.440"
Spitler Peak Trail	168.6	7,009	N33° 42' 36.030" W116° 37' 21.060"
Tahquitz Valley Trail	177.3	8,134	N33° 45' 38.540" W116° 39' 56.230"
Saddle Junction to Humber Park/Idyllwild	179.4	8,114	N33° 46' 27.420" W116° 40' 22.980"
Fuller Ridge Trail	190.5	7,746	N33° 50' 20.640" W116° 44' 10.680"
Snow Canyon Road (water spigot)	205.7	1,730	N33° 52' 41.240" W116° 40' 44.420"
I-10, Cabazon	209.5	1,337	N33° 55' 27.240" W116° 41' 40.380"

SECTION B

CAMPSITES AND BIVY SITES

Mile	Elevation in feet	Latitude/ Longitude	Number of tents	Feature	Notes
115.0	3,235	N33° 18' 39.600" W116° 37' 39.300"	4	Agua Caliente Creek	Near dry creekbed
123.8	5,020	N33° 21' 10.740" W116° 36' 33.420"	4	Lost Valley	Small campsites amid large boulders
129.2	5,592	N33° 23' 47.100" W116° 36' 04.860"	>8	Combs Peak	Surrounded by small boulders, wind-prone, spectacular views
140.2	3,347	N33° 28' 49.800" W116° 34' 27.660"	>5	Nance Canyon	Several sandy campsites near seasonal water, downstream from trail
155.9	5,182	N33° 35' 44.220" W116° 34' 16.860"	>5	North of CA 74	Shade
161.0	6,820	N33° 38' 54.060" W116° 34' 00.420"	>5	Penrod Canyon	Shade, seasonal creekbed
168.6 (alt.)	4,427	N33° 40' 46.020" W116° 40' 56.100"	130	Hurkey Creek Park	Restrooms, drinking water, fire rings, coin-operated showers
175.4	8,231	N33° 45' 39.000" W116° 38' 39.900"	6–8	Little Tahquitz Valley	Established campsites and water
179.5	8,169	N33° 46' 32.570" W116° 40' 27.000"	>10	Saddle Junction/ Chinquapin Flats area	Several campsites near the intersection with Devils Slide Trail
183.3	8,107	N33° 46' 57.360" W116° 42' 09.600"	>5	Strawberry Junction Camp	Only designated campsite in the SJSP Wilderness Area
193.6	6,463	N33° 51' 20.340" W116° 43' 31.740"	4	West Fork Snow Creek	
193.9	6,393	N33° 51' 18.420" W116° 43' 21.480"	4	West Fork Snow Creek	0.2 mile off PCT on unmarked trail, seasonal water and flat clearing for camping
195.4	5,658	N33° 51' 53.880" W116° 43' 02.220"	2	Snow Canyon	Amid boulders
197.2	4,908	N33° 52' 16.140" W116° 42' 41.220"	2	Snow Canyon	Amid boulders
201.1	3,351	N33° 52' 17.760" W116° 41' 37.260"	2	Snow Canyon	Amid boulders
201.7	3,259	N33° 52' 03.300" W116° 41' 30.660"	2	Snow Canyon	At saddle
204.8	2,109	N33° 52' 50.820" W116° 41' 02.400"	2	Snow Canyon	Near dry creekbed

WEATHER TO GO

Traversing the lower, dry chaparral in the southern half of this section is most enjoyable before mid-May and can be especially enjoyable and temperate in winter. After May, it is uncomfortably hot, with springs and creeks rapidly diminishing. The heights of the San Jacinto Mountains, however, can still contain deep snowdrifts, and further snowstorms (however brief) can threaten until late May of most years. San Gorgonio Pass, at the end of this section, is uncomfortably warm except in winter.

SUPPLIES

Warner Springs Ranch was once a 2,500-acre private family resort centered around natural hot springs. Established by John Warner in 1844 on the site of a Cupeño Indian village, the ranch became an important stop for the historic Butterfield Overland Stage. Subsequent visitors have included a long roster of presidents and Hollywood notables. The resort closed in 2012, but new owners have since reopened the golf course, cabins, and a grill that lures hikers with fresh California cuisine and an outdoor patio. Call or check the website for updates: 760-782-4271, warnerspringsranchresort.com. It is located just south of the post office.

Just off the trail, the volunteer-run Warner Springs Community Resource Center (760-782-0670, wscrcenter.org) welcomes hikers most of the year. There's a small resupply store and a communal room with tables and couches, internet access, maps, and books. Hikers can also borrow computers and charge phones. Check the website or call for hours and to ensure the center is still open.

Resupply boxes may be mailed to Warner Springs Post Office, located 1.2 miles northeast of the start of this section on CA 79. Your best bet for amenities is to continue to the larger town of Anza, a 6-mile detour from the route 42.4 miles beyond the section's start, for a post office, stores, and restaurants.

The Paradise Valley Cafe (61721 CA 74, Mountain Center, CA 92561; 951-659-3663; theparadisevalleycafe.com), 1 mile west of the PCT's intersection with CA 74, welcomes hikers with hearty meals, water refills, and a trail register. It also accepts hiker resupply packages via USPS, UPS, and FedEx.

Farther along at Saddle Junction, high in the San Jacinto Wilderness and 69.9 miles from the start of Section B, most hikers choose to descend the historical Devils Slide Trail to Idyllwild. This restful mountain resort community has a complete range of facilities, including a mountaineering supply shop with a knowledgeable staff and everything for the PCT trekker. PCT travelers are welcome at the San Jacinto Wilderness State Park's Hike and Bike campsite (for a nominal fee) at 25905 CA 243, near the ranger station in Idyllwild; it's just a minute from downtown.

Ending this section in Whitewater, a tiny community without any supplies, you have a choice of supply stations. Here, about 100 miles from the start, you can hitchhike east 12.5 miles via I-10 and CA 111 to revel in the fleshpots of Palm Springs, that famous movie-star and golf-course-studded desert oasis. It offers complete facilities, including a restaurant and an aerial-tram ride from Palm Springs up 6,000 feet to the subalpine shoulder of San Jacinto Peak.

Alternatively, hikers may elect to hitchhike west on I-10 from West Palm Springs Village. From the Haugen-Lehmann Way exit you go 4.5 miles on I-10 to the Main Street exit of Cabazon, a small community with a post office and store. Hadley's, a backpacker's dream market, lies 2 miles farther west next to the high-rise Morongo Casino Resort, and it sells an astounding variety of dried fruits and nuts, along with date shakes and ice cream. Near Hadley's is a truly enormous outlet mall, affording the hiker with money to burn a chance to purchase the latest in hiker couture, sports shoes, and electronic gadgetry, or to refuel at some nice chain restaurants.

WATER

Water remains scarce in the southern reaches of Section B. Except high in the San Jacinto Wilderness, or at springs where wells have been dug for livestock, do not expect to find water away from civilization. Once you reach the cooler, higher Desert Divide, however, water becomes more plentiful. In fact, many would-be PCT thru-hikes have been ended prematurely by thigh-deep spring snows on the southern flanks of the San Jacinto Mountains. Keep an eye on the weather, and be prepared for rough going.

PERMITS

The San Jacinto Wilderness consists of two units: the national-forest wilderness and the state-park wilderness. If you are a section hiker and camping in only one of these, you need a permit only for it; if you are camping in both, you need two permits. Obtain the wilderness permit online at fsva.org or by writing the U.S. Forest Service (USFS), Box 518, Idyllwild, CA 92549. You can also pick one up at the station, at 54270 Pine Crest Highway in Idyllwild; for hours and more information, call 909-382-2921. Obtain the state-park permit by writing Mount San Jacinto Wilderness State Park, Box 308, Idyllwild, CA 92549, or by going to the station (951-659-2607) 200 yards down the road and across the street from the USFS station. Day permits may be acquired at both offices as well. No dogs or fires are ever allowed within the state park. Rangers at both stations know the trails and their conditions well; calling them ahead of your hike or stopping in on a zero day in Idyllwild is recommended.

SPECIAL CONCERNS

Hikers along the California PCT cannot help but become familiar with the chaparral, that community of typically chest-high, tough, wiry, calf-slashing shrubs and small trees that you meet first by the Mexican border. Draped like a green velvet blanket over most of that part of Southern California reached by ocean air, and extending from close beside the sea up to about 5,000 feet, where it mingles with conifers and oaks, chaparral lines most of the PCT south of the Sierra. Chaparral surrounds Warner Springs, at the beginning of this section.

Named by early Spanish Californians, who were reminded of their *chaparro,* or live oak scrub from Mediterranean climes, the California chaparral is a unique assemblage of plants—mostly shrubs—that find this region's long, rainless summers and cooler, wet winters ideal for growth. Chamise, also known as greasewood because of its texture and its almost explosive flammability, is the most widespread species, but several species of ceanothus (mountain lilac, buckbrush, tobacco brush, and coffee brush), plus ribbonwood, ocean spray, sumac, sagebrush, mountain mahogany, hollyleaf cherry, and yerba santa, also rank as major members of chaparral, depending on topographic and soil conditions.

All true chaparral plants have small, thick, stiff evergreen leaves, and many have leaves with waxy outer surfaces. The plants' roots are long, enabling them to reach deep into rocky

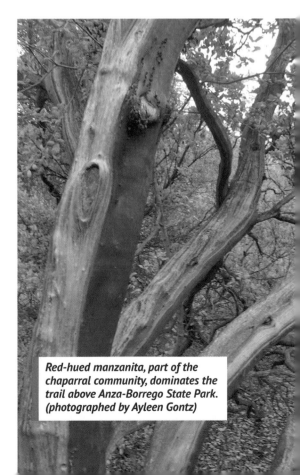

Red-hued manzanita, part of the chaparral community, dominates the trail above Anza-Borrego State Park. (photographed by Ayleen Gontz)

subsoil for scarce water. Chaparral plants are suited to survive not only the protracted rainless, hot months but also a low annual rainfall and a rapid runoff from the thin, poorly developed soils. The plants' main defense against loss of precious water is near dormancy during the hot, dry summer spells. Almost all photosynthetic activity ceases during this time, but the stiff evergreen leaves are ready to resume photosynthesis within minutes of a rainfall, unlike plants that lose their leaves or wilt in the face of heat. The small size of the leaves themselves, along with a waxy coating or a hairy insulating cover and the presence of relatively few evaporative stomata, greatly reduces water loss.

Not only can chaparral plants vie successfully for, and conserve, scant water resources, but they also win out by thriving in the face of fire. All of the most widespread species are adapted to reproduce well in the aftermath of fast-moving range fires that are a hallmark of Southern California wildlands. In fact, fires actually benefit these species, and most of them contain highly flammable, volatile oils that promote fires. Before the arrival of Spanish settlers, American Indians purposely burned the Southern California chaparral every five to eight years to meet their needs for survival and growth.

Not only does fire exterminate encroaching species, but it also returns valuable nitrogen to the soil, thus promoting growth. Some of the species, like scrub oak and ceanothus, need fire to weaken their seeds' coatings to allow germination. Most of the other chaparral plants circumvent the ravages of fire by resprouting—in as little as 10 days—from tough root crowns or by putting out so many seeds that at least some will survive any fire. Chaparral is also unusual in that it succeeds itself right after a fire, unlike other plant communities, such as pine forests, which pass through one or more vegetational stages before returning to the final, climax stage.

WARNER SPRINGS TO SAN GORGONIO PASS

>>>THE ROUTE

WATER ACCESS

Before leaving Warner Springs, northbound hikers must be sure to stock up on water. The next likely source along the route, barring the seasonal flow of Agua Caliente Creek (reached in 5.2 miles), is the permanent water tank just outside a trail angel's property on dirt Chihuahua Valley Road, a 17.8-mile trek away.

Pedestrians can start north on Section B's PCT by simply crossing CA 79 at the fire station to a gate and PCT marker (109.5–3,045'). Your trail departs west away from the Cañada Verde wash, quickly crosses a jeep road, and curves gently down into spring-wildflower meadows. Well marked by posts with well-defined tread, the PCT soon recrosses the jeep road.

Next your trail skirts the flanks of low Knob 3,009, then turns north across sandy flats speckled with mature canyon live oaks to cross the usually dry bed of Agua Caliente Creek. In just a minute or two, your deep-sand trail recrosses the creek to its east bank and then climbs east a few yards into a cozy oak grove and to a long-abandoned campground with a few nonworking faucets and numbered signs posted at weed-choked sites (111.1–2,926'). Here the PCT momentarily joins a dirt road, and then

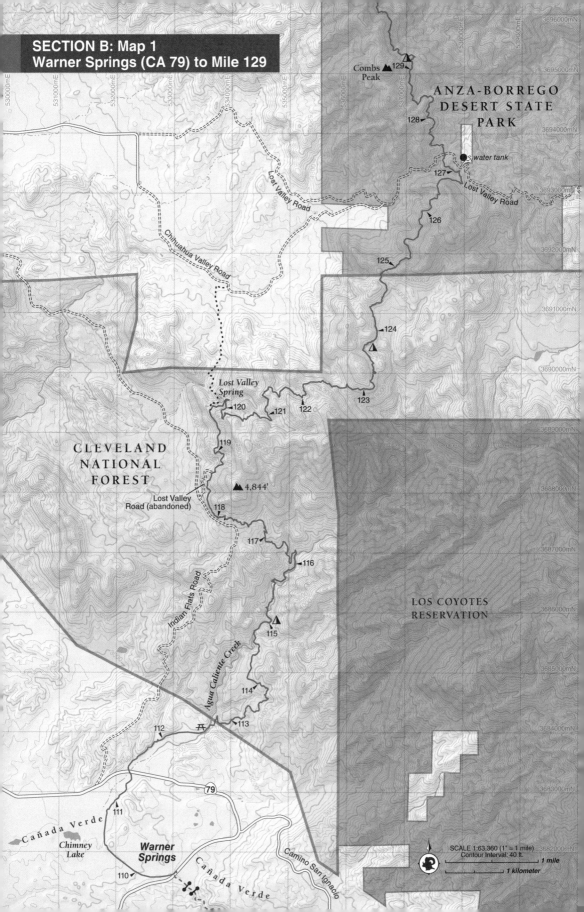

Combs ▲▲ 129 ⚠
Peak

ANZA-BORREGO
DESERT STATE
PARK

128

● water tank

127
Lost Valley Road

Lost Valley Road

126

Chihuahua Valley Road

125

124
⚠

4600

Lost Valley
Spring

120   121   122   123

119

CLEVELAND
NATIONAL
FOREST

▲▲ 4,844'

Lost Valley
Road (abandoned)

118

117

116

Indian Flats Road

LOS COYOTES
RESERVATION

⚠
115

Agua Caliente Creek

114

112   ⛫ 113

79

111

Cañada Verde

Chimney
Lake

*Warner
Springs*

Camino San Ignacio

Cañada Verde

110

SCALE 1:63,360 (1" ≈ 1 mile)
Contour Interval: 40 ft.

1 mile

1 kilometer

it turns northward before branching left to cross another usually dry streambed in Cañada Agua Caliente. Moments later, the PCT passes under CA 79 (111.4–2,929') via a concrete bridge while simultaneously crossing Agua Caliente Creek, which often flows lazily here.

WATER ACCESS

Sure water can be found at the Warner Springs Fire Station and the Community Resource Center. Both of these oases are right on CA 79 near the trail. The community center's hours can vary, but you'll find a 24-7 water fountain and restrooms across the parking lot. Check the website or call to ensure the center is still open.

North of the highway, the PCT leaves the western margin of Agua Caliente Creek's sandy bed. The trail clambers up to pass through a gate and then, ignoring a right-branching path back down to the stream, climbs from a fringe of trees onto a nearly level alluvial terrace covered with sagebrush and dotted with massive live oaks. Follow the terrace upcanyon (northeast), staying some 30 feet above Agua Caliente Creek, which usually flows in this vicinity, if only as a trickle. The PCT dips momentarily in a north-trending wash (ignore a prominent trail down to the creek), then shortly merges with a wider path (an old jeep road) that continues upcanyon (east), well marked by PCT posts. A few minutes' walk leads to a junction with a dirt

road that crosses from the southwest. Beyond this junction the trail, indicated by PCT posts, continues ahead, now paralleling the aforementioned road to its right and coming slowly closer to the cut banks of Agua Caliente Creek.

In a short while, the trail strikes the dirt road at its end, where you find a picnic table (112.6–2,990'). It's a pleasant, sunny spot to stop and rest, all just a few feet from the cool, trickling stream.

The trail resumes at the upstream end of the camp and descends momentarily to cross via rocks 15-foot-wide Agua Caliente Creek, here burbling among baccharis shrubs, sycamores, and cottonwoods. Across the stream, the route climbs north and east away from the creek.

Chia, white forget-me-nots, and beavertail cacti line the moderate ascent across the Cleveland National Forest border to a terrace, along which the sandy path winds north through ribbonwood chaparral. Then you soon descend to cross Agua Caliente Creek (114.7–3,189'), where tall grasses, squawbush, brodiaea, and forget-me-nots grow below oaks, sycamores, and willows in the narrow, usually watered canyon—a refuge for mourning doves and horned lizards. Particularly in winter and spring, ticks also inhabit the grasses and shrubs, so you should check your legs often. You cross Agua Caliente Creek several times in the next mile, alternating shady, cool creekside walking with hot, yucca-dotted Paleozoic Julian schist hillsides. A final, shaded traverse north of the seasonal stream leads to a switchback in a side canyon, after which the moderately ascending route winds northwest in chaparral laced with deer brush and white sage. Soon the grade eases to contour west, then north, below Peak 4,844 and

SECTION B

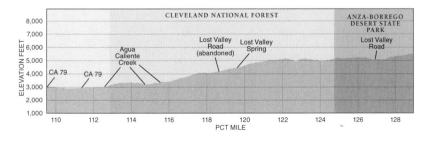

above Indian Flats Road. Here the trail affords good views southwest across Warner Valley to Lake Henshaw, a large sag pond on the Elsinore Fault, and northwest to weathered tonalite outcrops near Indian Flats.

Continuing north, the PCT turns right onto poor Lost Valley Road and ascends it to reach a spur road (119.5–4,349') marked by a cement post and sign.

WATER ACCESS

From here, Lost Valley Road descends north 0.2 mile to reach Lost Valley Spring. The spring often has flow well into all but the driest summers; be sure to treat it before drinking.

From this junction, the PCT climbs northeast above the spring along a 0.3-mile spur—an overgrown jeep track—to reach a continuation of trail tread where the spur ends in a ravine. You ascend briskly south to find excellent views back over boulder-dotted Indian Flats and south over Valle de San Jose. Soon the way swings east on a gentle, sandy ascent through chaparral and past scattered Coulter pines. After climbing over three low ridges, you drop moderately east to a saddle that lies along the northwest-trending Hot Springs Fault. To the southeast, Hot Springs Mountain's lookout tower rises above tree-lined Agua Caliente Creek.

The PCT ascends east a bit, then turns north to undulate through dry brushland—often sparingly shaded by oaks and Coulter pines—to the east of a boulder-castellated ridge. About 2 miles

from the saddle, you pass into Anza-Borrego Desert State Park, then cross a gap to the sunnier west slopes of the ridgeline. With vistas west over Chihuahua Valley, you contour generally north to yet another gap, then descend quickly east, cross a ravine, and traverse northwest to strike nearby Chihuahua Valley Road (127.3–5,057'), which drops west into Chihuahua Valley.

WATER ACCESS

Detour here for water: just before Chihuahua Valley Road, look for a spur trail to the right, which may be marked by a small WATER AND SHADE sign. Follow the trail flanked by waist-high brush uphill briefly to a dirt road. Signs lead the way from here to a 20-foot-high, silver water tank with a valve at its base. The owner is a big supporter of the PCT and welcomes hikers to stay on the property after tanking up. Be sure to close the tank's valve. Check with the Warner Springs Community Center to verify that the tank and property are still open to hikers before setting off.

CAMPING Directly across the dirt road, the PCT starts a sustained ascent along Bucksnort Mountain's east slopes. The climb ends at the east shoulder of Combs Peak (129.2–5,592'), where nicely arranged boulders, outstanding vistas, and the first level

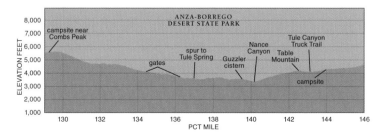

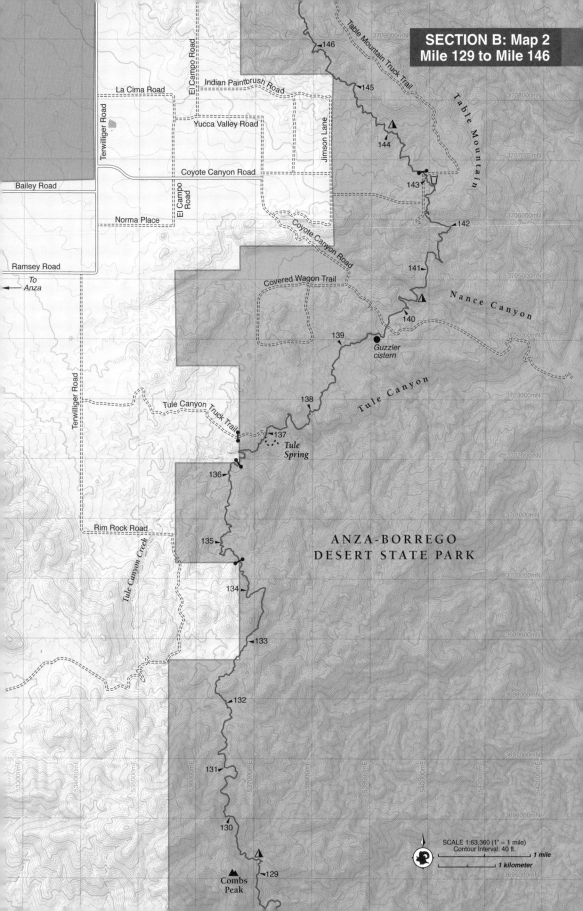

146

145

Table Mountain Truck Trail

Table Mountain

144

143

142

141

Nance Canyon

140

Covered Wagon Trail

Coyote Canyon Road

Jimson Lane

139

Guzzler cistern

138

Tule Canyon

Tule Canyon Truck Trail

137

Tule Spring

136

Rim Rock Road

135

Tule Canyon Creek

134

ANZA-BORREGO
DESERT STATE PARK

133

132

131

130

129

Combs Peak

La Cima Road

El Campo Road

Indian Paintbrush Road

Yucca Valley Road

Terwilliger Road

Coyote Canyon Road

El Campo Road

Bailey Road

Norma Place

Ramsey Road

To Anza

Terwilliger Road

SCALE 1:63,360 (1" = 1 mile)
Contour Interval: 40 ft.

1 mile

1 kilometer

533000mE
534000mE
535000mE
536000mE
537000mE
538000mE
539000mE
540000mE
541000mE
542000mE

3709000mN
3708000mN
3707000mN
3706000mN
3705000mN
3704000mN
3703000mN
3702000mN
3701000mN
3700000mN
3699000mN
3698000mN
3697000mN
3696000mN
3695000mN

spot for miles combine to make a nice, if water-less, campsite. Be sure to practice Leave No Trace principles: set up tents only in impacted sites, dispose of waste properly, and leave all rocks and plants as you find them.

VIEWS The 180-degree panorama here encompasses a sizable chunk of Southern California real estate. To the north, distant, seasonally snowcapped San Gorgonio Peak peers over the west shoulder of nearer, sometimes snowy San Jacinto Peak. Closer in the north, Thomas Mountain stands behind sprawling Anza and Terwilliger Valleys. The rocky spine descending right (southeast) from San Jacinto Peak is the PCT-traversed Desert Divide. To the east–northeast, the dry summits of the Santa Rosa Mountains loom above desert-floored Coyote Canyon, while you spy to the east the vast Salton Sea beyond Anza-Borrego Desert State Park.

HISTORY The park and the town of Anza to the north both com-memorate Captain Juan Bautista de Anza, who in 1774 rejoiced upon entering the valley now bearing his name. He had struggled through the Borrego Desert and Coyote Canyon with a couple of dozen men—mostly soldiers—while scouting a route from Sonora, Mexico, to San Francisco. He returned a year later, leading more than 200 settlers and many cattle.

The northbound PCT contours across the steep east face of Bucksnort Mountain, then begins to descend in earnest, on rocky, sandy tread in low chaparral, crossing a couple of pipe gates and private, gated farms.

You eventually cross a usually dry creekbed at the head of Tule Canyon.

From here your way becomes less steep and rolls north into a tall brushland dominated by ribbonwood and chamise. The PCT rounds the canyon's eastern slopes, drops easily to a broad saddle, then climbs gently north to gain the west end of a low ridge. A few minutes of gentle downhill walking leads to a trail junction (131.9–4,681').

You take the newer tread, which first con-tours east and then drops moderately on a northward tack. After traversing east-facing slopes, the PCT descends across to the west side of a small saddle, descends southwest, and soon levels to momentarily strike a fair dirt road (134.2–4,107') at the Anza-Borrego Desert State Park boundary. Northwest across it the path resumes, making an easy but shade-less descent. After a switchback the way bends north, still descending.

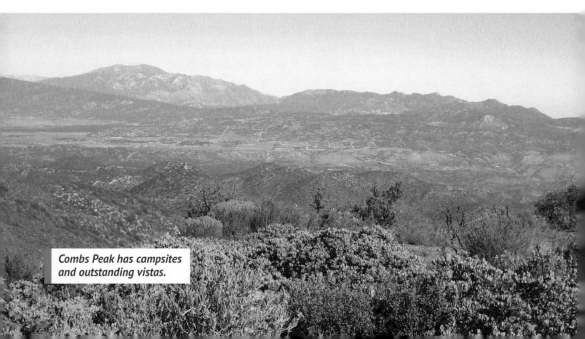

Combs Peak has campsites and outstanding vistas.

Continue north, past a white-pipe post marking a section's corner. You then drop for a moment to a shallow, hop-across ford of Tule Canyon Creek (3,590'). Water usually flows here, sometimes merely at a trickle, for most of the year. It is more reliable downstream at Tule Spring. Due to land-ownership constraints, the PCT is forced to climb very steeply (if briefly) up the sandy hillside north of Tule Canyon Creek. Afterward it side-hills gently northeast, downcanyon, soon to cross good Tule Canyon Truck Trail (137.0–3,620').

WATER ACCESS

Just 0.25 mile southeast down this dirt road is Tule Spring. There is a metal-handled spigot 50 feet below the 10,000-gallon water tank, on the edge of Tule Canyon creek's high cut bank. Should the water tank or spigot not be operational for some reason, check in the high grass to the left of the tank—a seep is almost always present, though it may be dry in drought years.

In the morning quiet, among the lovely cottonwoods, one may see desert bighorn sheep watering here, having escaped the scorching heat of the Borrego Sink.

RESUPPLY ACCESS

One may also choose to resupply at Anza from Tule Spring. Ascend Tule Canyon Truck Trail past the PCT, reaching a locked gate 0.3 mile west of the trail, at the boundary of Anza-Borrego Desert State Park. Continue up the sandy, rutted road, which steadily improves, past

a home or two to a junction with larger dirt Terwilliger Road. Turn right (north) and follow this busier way past numerous smaller junctions and a handful of homes to a T-junction with larger dirt Ramsay Road. Now swing right (east) to the paved continuation of Terwilliger Road. Swing left (again due north) on the shoulder of Terwilliger Road to paved Bailey Road. Find the town of Anza as described in more detail in the next "Resupply Access" section on page 110.

Return to the PCT's northward continuation on a sandy, hillside traverse, undulating through rocky ravines. It overlooks the environs of Tule Spring and then bends northeast. After dipping to a broad valley, the trail climbs to a small pass with a self-replenishing guzzler water tank (often dry late in the season), then drops on sandy, indistinct tread to nearby Coyote Canyon Road (139.7–3,510').

CAMPING Across it you continue down a ravine to a single switchback leading to the pleasant grassy floor of Nance Canyon. Step across its seasonal creeklet (140.2–3,347') to find some small flat spots that offer potential dry camping.

Ignore a spur trail going right (downstream) after crossing the creek; instead, go left (upstream). Beyond, a moderate grind leads up around a low knob, then across a rugged bluff. This route offers panoramas south and east over Anza-Borrego Desert State Park's wild, northern canyons, which are visible through a haze of heat waves and salt particles from the Salton Sea. Continue the ascent, making two small switchbacks and passing a faint use trail through a chain-link fence to reach a chamise-covered gap on the south end of Table

Mountain. Now you wind north and descend gently to a narrow, very sandy jeep road (143.1–4,086'). Table Mountain Truck Trail is now obscured by a wider dirt road. The PCT passes a large water cache (that in recent years has also boasted a little free library) just before striking a swing gate in a barbed wire fence (see page 16 for more about water caches). A few feet later, the trail reaches old Table Mountain Truck Trail, followed left (west) a few feet to the new, wider Table Mountain Truck Trail. On it, turn back right (north) 15 yards to the obscure resumption of PCT tread, branching left (northwest), downhill of a 10-foot plastic post.

RESUPPLY ACCESS

This jeep road is so important because it leads to Anza, a logical resupply site. To reach Anza, turn left onto Table Mountain Truck Trail, following it due north up to a junction with a dirt road. Head right (west), undulating down across a hillside on Table Mountain Truck Trail, passing south-branching, dirt Old Cattle Trail in 0.4 mile and then a more obscure merger with the old Table Mountain Truck Trail in another 0.5 mile. A 0.1-mile westward ascent leads to a good dirt road, signed HIGH COUNTRY TRAILS. Turn right on it, and walk north 0.25 mile easily up to a broad road, Sunset Sage

Trail, branching left (west). Take this dirt road 0.75 mile down past numerous north-branching dirt roads and several homes to its end at Yucca Valley Road. Turn left and follow this dirt road briefly south to a four-way junction. Here Coyote Canyon Road heads south and west. Follow this road right (west) across the arid, level grassland, finally making a small dogleg before ending at paved Terwilliger Road.

On Terwilliger Road, you can walk north to Wellman Road. Take it west to Kirby Road, then take Kirby north to Cahuilla Road (CA 371). Turn left (west) and head to the small town of Anza, which has a post office, market, and restaurants.

If you don't want to backtrack from Anza to the PCT at the far eastern part of Terwilliger Valley, walk east back along Cahuilla Road, passing Kirby Road and later crossing a 4,855-foot summit just before reaching a junction with Pines-to-Palms Highway (CA 74). Then go southeast on this highway, which starts southeast and then climbs gently through a grassy valley to reach the PCT just short of a dirt parking turnout.

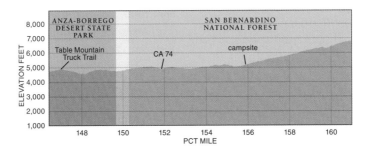

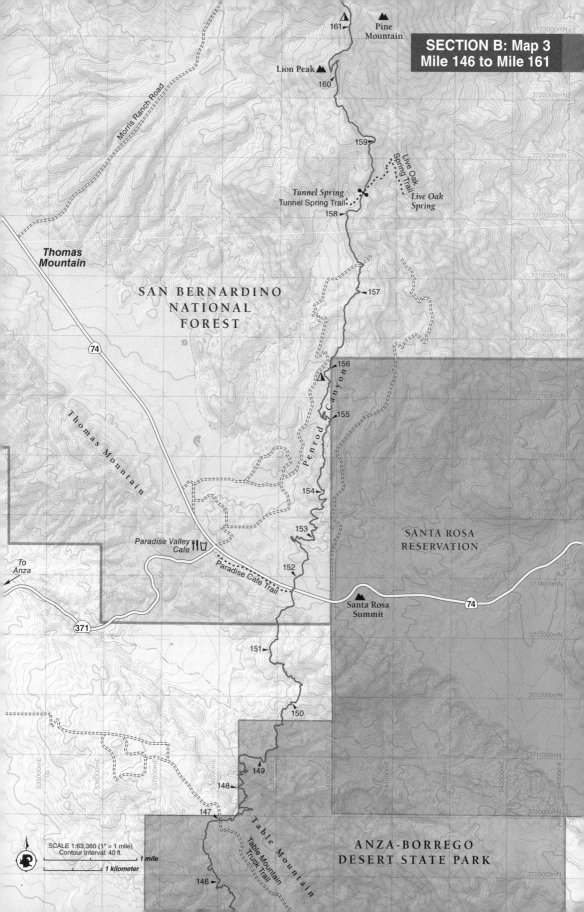

Pine
Mountain

161

Lion Peak

160

159

Live Oak
Spring Trail

Tunnel Spring
Tunnel Spring Trail

*Live Oak
Spring*

158

Morris Ranch Road

**Thomas
Mountain**

157

**SAN BERNARDINO
NATIONAL
FOREST**

74

156

Penrod Canyon

155

Thomas Mountain

154

153

**SANTA ROSA
RESERVATION**

*Paradise Valley
Cafe*

152

Paradise Cafe Trail

To
Anza

Santa Rosa
Summit

74

371

151

150

149

148

147

535000mE
536000mE
537000mE
538000mE
539000mE
540000mE
541000mE
542000mE
543000mE
544000mE

3723000mN
3722000mN
3721000mN
3720000mN
3719000mN
3718000mN
3717000mN
3716000mN
3715000mN
3714000mN
3713000mN
3712000mN
3711000mN
3710000mN
3709000mN

Table Mountain

Table Mountain Truck Trail

**ANZA-BORREGO
DESERT STATE PARK**

146

SCALE 1:63,360 (1" = 1 mile)
Contour Interval: 40 ft.

1 mile

1 kilometer

From the obscure jeep-road junction at the far eastern part of Terwilliger Valley, the PCT ascends indistinctly northwest for a moment before good tread resumes. It leads moderately and persistently uphill, in an ascending traverse along the granitic, boulder-strewn southwestern flanks of Table Mountain. You gain excellent views over Terwilliger Valley and south to your PCT route along Bucksnort Mountain. On a breezy day this stretch is quite enjoyable, particularly in spring when it's likely to be flanked by clusters of California poppy, purple chia, baby blue eyes, and feathery green ribbonwood shrubs among white boulders. At one point, you pass a side trail that leads south to a dirt road serving some hillside homes. Beyond, your climb continues, eventually rising to top Table Mountain's shoulder. You cross Table Mountain Truck Trail (147.0–4,909'), a dirt road at a point just northwest of the long mountain's highest point.

The route drops and leads into a narrow ravine, switchbacks once to cross it, then descends to the bottom of the dry head of Alkali Wash. A steep, rocky, and sometimes hot quintet of switchbacks accomplish the ensuing ascent of the far slope. They lead to a chaparral ridge, where your trail swings east over a low saddle into a grassy flat. Now the path winds north, along the raw, precipitous lip of Horse Canyon.

Walk along a narrow divide, enjoy views, then push on across the flanks of Lookout Mountain. Eventually the trail finds a low pass on the peak's northwestern shoulder, and you have a delightful panorama north over the San Jacinto Mountains. In the leftmost distance the rounded form of lofty San Jacinto Peak reigns, usually with a regal coat of snow in spring. Leaving the gap, you descend into San Bernardino National Forest. The trail levels and then turns north across a sandy, sagebrush-matted valley to quickly strike two-lane Pines-to-Palms Highway (CA 74) (151.9–4,924') at a point just west of Santa Rosa Summit.

WATER ACCESS

Water may be obtained by taking a detour left (northwest) 1 mile to the hiker-friendly Paradise Valley Cafe at the junction of CA 74 and Cahuilla Road (CA 371). There's also a trail register here.

Across Pines-to-Palms Highway (CA 74), you skirt a dirt trailhead parking area and ascend through brushland to a mileage sign and a 6-foot stone monument with a faded diagram of the PCT's route through the San Jacintos. Beyond,

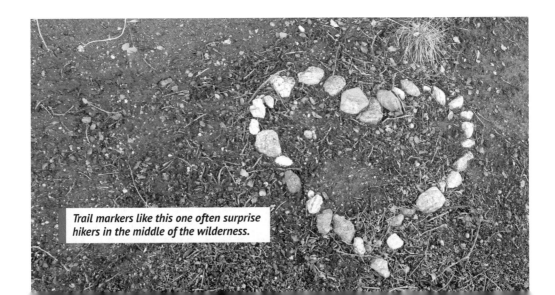

Trail markers like this one often surprise hikers in the middle of the wilderness.

you walk north to a ridgetop, then switchback once down its north side, soon engaged in a sandy, fitful ascent into and out of numerous small ravines and around picturesque blocky cliffs of crumbling granite. You pass close along the western face of a low ridge, then descend short switchbacks to hop across the usually dry creek that drains Penrod Canyon (155.6–5,098').

CAMPING In 0.3 mile, a comfortable waterless camp (out of sight of the PCT) could be made under Coulter pines and live oaks.

The track winds upcanyon, crossing the streambed twice more, then climbs to sunnier chaparral for a contour of the canyon's eastern slopes. Resume the ascent, now steeper, along Penrod Canyon's east wall. Thomas Mountain and Bucksnort Mountain are visible on this stretch, just before you swing east around a nose to abruptly encounter marble bedrock. The first leg of the PCT's climb into the San Jacinto Mountains ends soon, as you first go through a stock gate, and then in 50 yards top out at a saddle on the Desert Divide (158.4–5,952'). Here are junctions with Live Oak Spring Trail 4E03, right, and the unmarked Tunnel Spring Trail, left. Here, too, you reach the boundary with the Santa Rosa and San Jacinto Mountains National Monument, whose western edge is defined by the crest of the Desert Divide. You will pop into and out of this reserve, until you finally descend into San Gorgonio Pass, at the end of this section.

WATER ACCESS

If you're low on water, go to Live Oak Spring if you also plan to break for lunch. Live Oak Spring is reached by a sunny 1-mile, well-graded path that descends east from the saddle, eventually reaching an enormous gold-cup oak, box elders, and reliable water in a circular concrete trough.

Tunnel Spring Trail descends southwest from the PCT atop the gap and should be used for emergency water only. Steep, rocky tread leads down 0.3 mile to where the trail moderates in a grove of oaks and four tall Coulter pines, which have scattered their huge, clawed cones on the ground. Now look right (north) to a shallow streambed and a faint trail along a black PVC pipe. This goes up a few yards to the metal cattle trough at Tunnel Spring, shaded by box elders.

Resuming your northbound trek, you turn north along the east face of the Desert Divide. Shady interior live oaks and Coulter pines alternate with xeric chaparral areas (look for shaggy Mojave yuccas) as the trail ascends gently across Julian schist to the east slopes of Lion Peak. Expect to cross a few bulldozed jeep roads on this traverse—the area south of Lion Peak is private property, used as a cattle range. You get sporadic vistas down Oak Canyon to subdivided upper Palm Canyon; then a rough switchback leads to the ridgetop north of Lion Peak. For the next 2 miles the route remains on or near the divide, traversing gneiss, schist, quartzite, and marble bedrock and skirting past low chaparral laced with rabbitbrush and cacti. Little Desert Peak (6,883') offers panoramas east and north to the Coachella Valley and Palm Springs, and west to coniferous Thomas Mountain and pastoral Garner Valley. Moments later, a short descent ends at a saddle where you cross the Cedar Spring Trail 4E17 (162.6–6,775').

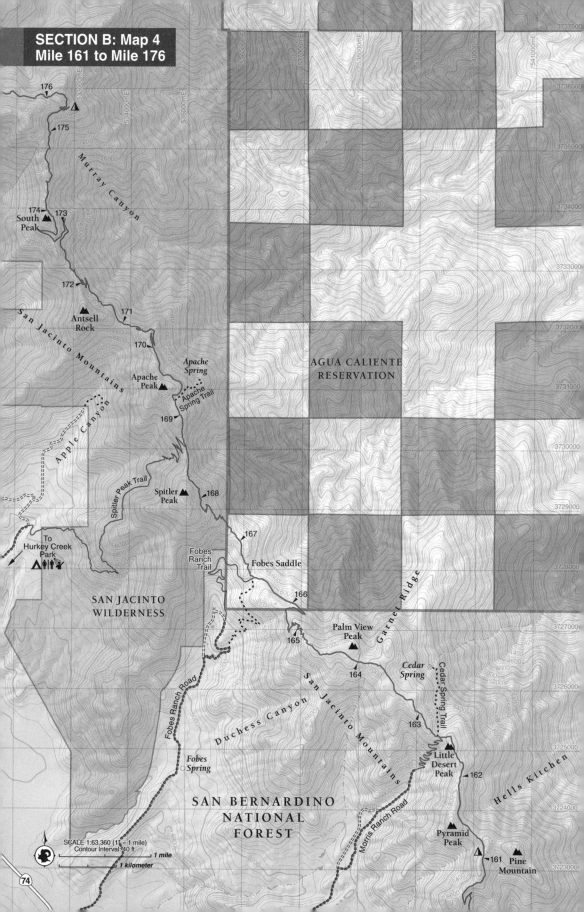

176

175

Murray Canyon

174 — South Peak ▲▲ 173

172

San Jacinto Mountains

Antsell ▲ Rock

171

170

Apache Spring

Apache ▲ Peak

Apache Spring Trail

169

Apple Canyon

Spitler Peak Trail

Spitler ▲ Peak

168

To Hurkey Creek Park ⛺🚻

167

Fobes Ranch Trail

Fobes Saddle

166

SAN JACINTO WILDERNESS

SAN JACINTO WILDERNESS

165

Palm View Peak ▲

Garnet Ridge

Fobes Ranch Road

164

Cedar Spring

Cedar Spring Trail

163

San Jacinto Mountains

Duchess Canyon

Fobes Spring

Little Desert Peak ▲

162

Hells Kitchen

SAN BERNARDINO NATIONAL FOREST

Morris Ranch Road

Pyramid ▲ Peak

△ 161 Pine Mountain

AGUA CALIENTE RESERVATION

SCALE 1:63,360 (1" = 1 mile)
Contour Interval: 40 ft.

1 mile

1 kilometer

WATER ACCESS

Most hikers ignore the southern branch of this good trail, which switchbacks southwest to Morris Ranch Road. Instead, head north a mile down to delightfully shaded flats and clear water at Cedar Spring (6,330')—the only permanent water along the southern Desert Divide. Be sure to carry a full load of water away from Cedar Spring; the day's ridgetop walk is hot, sunny, and entirely waterless.

ALTERNATE ROUTES In the face of high snowpack or early-spring snowstorms on the Desert Divide, northbound hikers should consider leaving the PCT via Cedar Spring (6 miles) or Spitler Peak Trails (7.3 miles), exiting south to the Pines-to-Palms Highway (CA 74), then going north to Idyllwild and Cabazon. Another route to Idyllwild is the 1.6-mile singletrack Fobes Ranch Trail to unpaved Fobes Ranch Road until its intersection with CA 74 in 4 miles. From here it's 1.8 miles south to Garner Valley Fire Station, which has round-the-clock water and a picnic table. In the face of severe storms, another option would be to catch a ride east on the Pines-to-Palms Highway to Palm Springs and then northwest to Whitewater.

The PCT route steeply ascends the ridgecrest, then briefly descends to another saddle. Continuing northwest, you soon pass Trail 4E04, which starts east from near Palm View Peak then drops north toward Garnet Ridge. Past a 7,123-foot summit, you descend, often steeply, on a rocky tread back into a cooler environment of white firs growing at the head of the spectacular West Fork Palm Canyon.

WATER ACCESS

Presently the route emerges on brushy Fobes Saddle and meets Fobes Ranch Trail 4E02 (166.5–5,994'), which descends 0.5 mile west to a 70-gallon plastic tub filled by a spring-fed spigot and hose near seasonal Scovel Creek. From here it's about a 4-mile descent along dirt Fobes Ranch Road to Pines-to-Palms Highway.

TRAIL INFO Thru-hikers often reach the San Jacinto Mountains in early spring, when snow and ice may still cover parts of the trail. Rockslides may occur at any time and make the trail impassable. Check trail reports and pcta.org frequently for status reports between Apache Peak and Fuller Ridge,

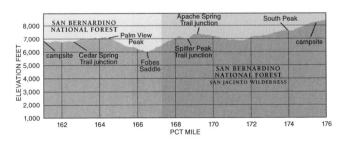

or contact the Idyllwild ranger station for up-to-date information regarding weather conditions and closures.

The PCT north from this saddle ascends steeply to the upper slopes of Spitler Peak, where a series of fires between 1980 and 2018 has turned this area into a charred forest of black oak, white fir, incense cedar, and Jeffrey pine. You will find evidence of it all the way to Red Tahquitz.

Along your climb you enter San Jacinto Wilderness, and then beyond some very steep pitches, the PCT levels to wind around to the north of Spitler Peak and meet the Spitler Peak Trail (168.6–7,009'). It then descends just east of the rocky spine that forms the ridge between Spitler and Apache Peaks. Gaining this knife-edge saddle, where the PCT was widened by firefighters to form a fuel break, the trail wastes no time in attacking the next objective: Apache Peak. Steep rocky, sandy tread leads up its southern slopes to emerge on a blackened summit plateau.

WATER ACCESS

Here a sign marks the Apache Spring Trail (169.2–7,352'), which descends steeply east 0.5 mile to Apache Spring, which has been unreliable as a water source in recent years. From the junction a short use trail ascends northwest to the view-filled summit of Apache Peak.

ALTERNATE ROUTE Keep in mind that snow often begins on the north side of Apache Peak and continues through Fuller Ridge. If you reach Apache Peak and it's impassable, you can backtrack 1 mile to Spitler Peak Trail and follow the Idyllwild alternate down to CA 74. It's a steep 3-mile descent down Apple Canyon Road to Hurkey Creek Park, which has campsites, toilets, and showers. From there, hikers may opt to road walk or find a vehicle to take them the remaining 11 miles to Idyllwild.

The PCT now begins to descend gently along the eastern flanks of Apache Peak, passing through a forest of manzanitas. After a 0.2-mile switchback, you reach a fine overlook of the northern Coachella Valley and of Joshua Tree National Park, which lies well beyond the valley in the Little San Bernardino Mountains. A well-constructed stretch next leads west along a cliff face to a gap, where you can dry-camp, at the head of Apple Canyon. To circumvent the granitic ramparts of Antsell Rock, the PCT's next leg follows a dynamited path under its sweeping northeast slopes. This area sometimes has dangerously icy conditions for springtime PCT thru-hikers—use caution and an ice ax. Once north of Antsell Rock's major buttresses, you take switchbacks for a 400-foot elevation gain to reach the San Jacinto's crest at a pleasantly montane gap. Rockslides are common in this area; use good judgment and exercise extreme caution. Check conditions in advance if possible.

Big-cone spruce, a relative of Douglas-fir, plus white fir and mountain mahogany, provide pleasant cover as the often-dynamited path ascends another 400 feet, first on the east and then on the southwest slopes of South Peak. Notice Lake Hemet, lying just east of the active Thomas Mountain Fault, at the head of Garner Valley, to the southwest.

North of South Peak the rocky PCT is dynamited to traverse under precipitous, granitic gendarmes, and the ascending hiker can gaze northwest to Tahquitz Peak and north to Red Tahquitz, or east down rugged Murray Canyon.

The ascent ends above Andreas Canyon's deep gorge, where your route turns west to descend gently on duff and sand.

Eventually it crosses South Fork Tahquitz Creek in a forest and then joins, moments later, the south end of Tahquitz Valley Trail (177.3–8,134').

WATER ACCESS

This trail descends north 0.3 mile to water in Little Tahquitz.

From that junction the PCT climbs southwest through groves of lodgepole pines to manzanitas and western white pines, which grow on gravelly slopes of decomposed granite. Soon you come to a junction with the Tahquitz Peak Trail 3E08 (178.0–8,619'), which offers a 0.5-mile side trip up to the peak's airy summit lookout.

SIDE TRIP This trip is well worthwhile because from the 8,846-foot summit you can get an idea of how steep canyons, such as Strawberry Valley below, are eroding back into the high, rolling landscape that lies between Red Tahquitz and San Jacinto Peak. Tahquitz Peak commemorates a legendary Cahuilla Indian demon who lived hereabouts, dining on unsuspecting Indian maidens and, when displeased, giving the weather a turn for the worse.

Those who need to press on will turn north and ease down the PCT to Saddle Junction (179.4–8,114'), the crossroads for three other trails into the San Jacinto Wilderness.

SECTION B

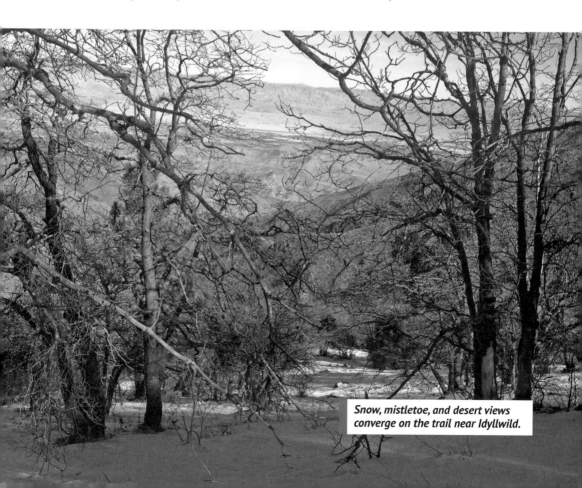

Snow, mistletoe, and desert views converge on the trail near Idyllwild.

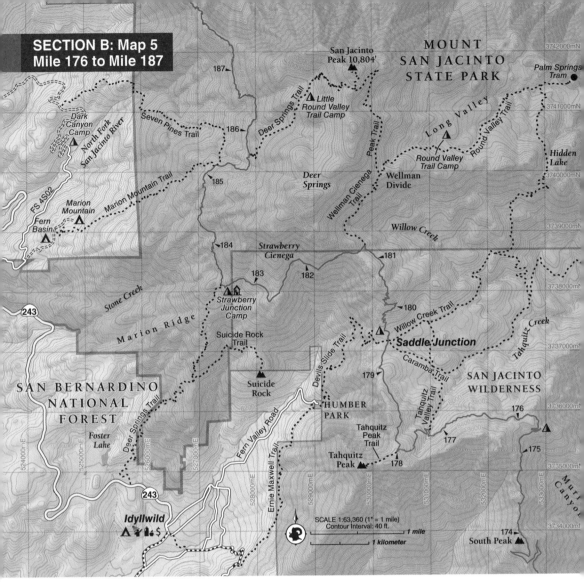

MOUNT
SAN JACINTO
STATE PARK

San Jacinto
Peak 10,804'

Palm Springs
Tram

187

Little
Round Valley
Trail Camp

Long Valley

Hidden
Lake

Dark
Canyon
Camp

North Fork
San Jacinto River

Seven Pines Trail

186

Deer Springs Trail

Peak Trail

Round Valley Trail

Round Valley
Trail Camp

185

Marion Mountain Trail

Deer
Springs

Wellman
Divide

FS 4S02

Marion
Mountain

Wellman Cienega Trail

Willow Creek

Fern
Basin

184

Strawberry
Cienega

181

243

Stone Creek

183

182

180

Marion Ridge

Strawberry
Junction
Camp

Willow Creek Trail

Saddle Junction

Tahquitz Creek

Suicide Rock
Trail

Caramba Trail

Devils Slide Trail

SAN JACINTO
WILDERNESS

SAN BERNARDINO
NATIONAL
FOREST

Deer Springs Trail

Suicide
Rock

179

176

Foster
Lake

Fern Valley Road

HUMBER
PARK

Tahquitz
Peak
Trail

Tahquitz Valley Trail

177

175

Ernie Maxwell Trail

Tahquitz
Peak

178

Muir Canyon

243

Idyllwild

SCALE 1:63,360 (1" = 1 mile)
Contour Interval: 40 ft.

1 mile

1 kilometer

174
South Peak

RESUPPLY ACCESS

From the saddle, Devils Slide Trail descends 2.5 miles west to Humber Park and Fern Valley Road. The mountain-resort community of Idyllwild—a good place to resupply and take a layover day—lies 2 miles down this road. Also leaving the saddle are two more trails, the Willow Creek Trail branching northeast to Long Valley, and the Caramba Trail heading southeast back to Tahquitz Valley.

The PCT continues north, soon switchbacking out of the forest to slopes that offer excellent over-the-shoulder vistas toward Tahquitz (Lily) Rock, a magnet for Southern California rock climbers. Almost 1,000 feet higher than Saddle Junction, the PCT levels to turn left from a junction with the Wellman Cienega Trail (181.2–8,992'), just within the confines of Mount San Jacinto State Park.

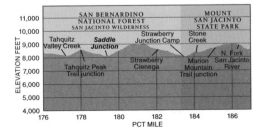

CAMPING Please note that all camping within the state park is restricted to designated sites. Along the PCT there is only one approved campsite: Strawberry Junction Camp. USFS wilderness permits are *not* valid for camping in the state park; get a separate camping permit for a specific date to use these campsites, even if you possess a PCT thru-hiking permit. No dogs or fires are ever allowed within the state park.

SIDE TRIP The Wellman Cienega Trail arcs northwest, then northeast for 1 mile to meet the Round Valley Trail, which leads to Round Valley Trail Camp in 1 mile. Beyond that junction, the Peak Trail continues north another 2.4 miles to 10,834-foot San Jacinto Peak, a recommended side trip.

From the junction the PCT immediately leaves the state park and descends on a generally westward bearing above Strawberry Valley's steep headwall to Strawberry Cienega (182.1–8,597'), a trickling, sphagnum-softened freshet and a lunch stop with a great view. *Cienega* is a Spanish word, often seen in Southern California, meaning "swamp" or "marsh." Further descent leads to a forested junction with Deer Springs Trail 3E17 (183.5–8,047').

CAMPING Just before this junction, look for Strawberry Junction Camp on a small ridge south of the trail, a pleasant but waterless camp with views. There may be some trickles of water until midsummer in heads of canyons nearby.

SIDE TRIP As an alternative to the Devils Slide Trail, you can use the Deer Springs Trail to descend 4.3 miles to CA 243, just 0.5 mile west of downtown Idyllwild. Multiple dry flats in open pines and firs 2–3 minutes below the

PCT's junction with the Deer Springs Trail could also offer dry camping.

Now out of the federal wilderness and back in Mount San Jacinto State Park, the PCT turns north to ascend Marion Mountain's pleasant mixed-conifer slopes and eventually passes two closely spaced trail junctions (185.1–8,706').

SIDE TRIP At the first junction, Marion Mountain Trail descends west–southwest to the environs of Marion Mountain and Fern Basin—first-come, first-serve campgrounds open late May–mid-November. The second, the Seven Pines Trail, descends generally northwest, then west to a saddle, from which FS 4S02 switchbacks almost 2 miles down to seasonal Dark Canyon Campground.

WATER ACCESS

Soon after the second lateral your trail heads up along a marshy, dank creek: the reliable North Fork San Jacinto River, which you cross (8,830') below Deer Springs. Before leaving, restock your water bottles; the next water along the route is from Snow Creek, at the northern base of the San Jacinto Mountains, a punishing 19.5-mile descent away.

A minute beyond the infant San Jacinto River, you climb to a nearby junction with the San Jacinto Peak Trail (also known as the Deer Springs Trail), which is the return route of the recommended side trip to the peak's summit. From the junction you switchback down to

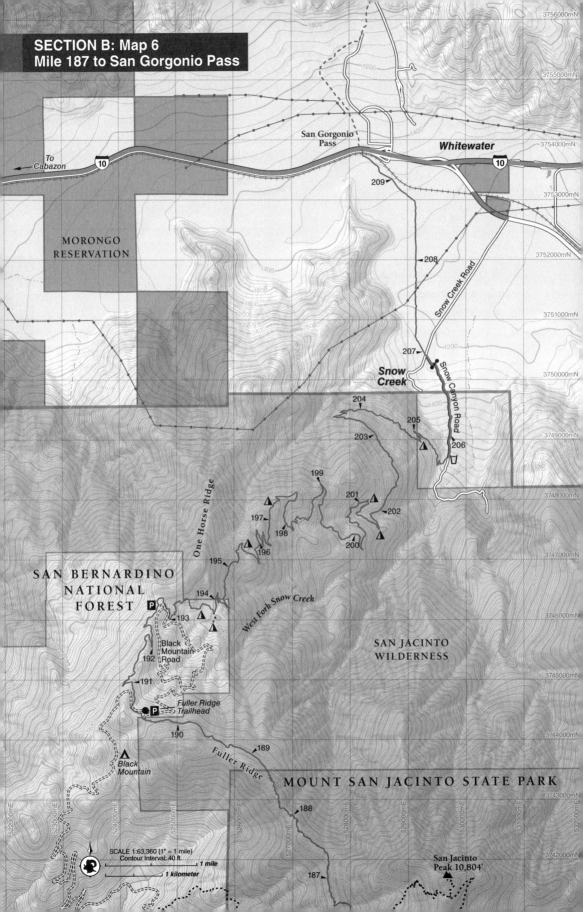

3756000mN

1800

1600

San Gorgonio Pass

Whitewater

1400

10

To
Cabazon

10

209

3754000mN

3753000mN

208

3752000mN

MORONGO
RESERVATION

Snow Creek Road

1400

1600

1800

2000

2200

2400

2600

2800

207

1200

3751000mN

*Snow
Creek*

204

Snow Canyon Road

1400

205

206

3750000mN

3749000mN

203

199

201

202

3748000mN

One Horse Ridge

197

198

195

196

200

3747000mN

SAN BERNARDINO
NATIONAL
FOREST

P

194

193

West Fork Snow Creek

3746000mN

192

Black
Mountain
Road

SAN JACINTO
WILDERNESS

191

3745000mN

*Fuller Ridge
Trailhead*

P

190

189

3744000mN

*Black
Mountain*

Fuller Ridge

MOUNT SAN JACINTO STATE PARK

188

3743000mN

SCALE 1:63,360 (1" = 1 mile)
Contour Interval: 40 ft.

1 mile

1 kilometer

187

San Jacinto
Peak 10,804'

3742000mN

522000mE

523000mE

524000mE

525000mE

526000mE

527000mE

528000mE

529000mE

530000mE

531000mE

532000mE

Fuller Ridge, a rocky, white fir–covered spine separating the San Jacinto and San Gorgonio river drainages.

VIEWS Here northbound trekkers get their first good view of the San Bernardino Mountains' 11,489-foot San Gorgonio Mountain, to the north, which is Southern California's highest point. Separating that range from ours is San Gorgonio Pass, 7,000 feet below you, lying between the Banning Fault and other branches of the great San Andreas Fault (also known as the San Andreas Rift Zone).

The PCT's route along Fuller Ridge is a tortuous one, composed for the most part of miniature switchbacks, alternately descending and climbing, that wind under small gendarmes and around wind-beaten conifers. It can also be as treacherous as it is tortuous when shaded, early-spring snow patches are icy hard. Crampons are often required for safe footing. In a little over 2 miles, though, the route takes to north-facing slopes, and, exchanging state wilderness for a brief stint in the federal wilderness, gently descends to a small dirt-road parking circle at Fuller Ridge Trailhead (190.5–7,746'). The PCT, marked by a post, resumes on the west side of the road loop, heading due north. It rounds northwest above, then drops to cross, well-used Black Mountain Road 4S01 (190.7–7,663'), closed in winter.

The creeks and springs along this stretch, which are often overflowing in spring, cannot be relied upon in summer and fall. The tributary of the North Fork of the San Jacinto River at mile 186.2 is one of the most reliable water sources in the area, but it also can't be counted on year-round.

The trail leaves the road on a gentle to moderate descent north along a ridge clothed in an open stand of mixed conifers. You switchback down three times across the nose of the ridge separating Snow Creek from chaparral-decked Brown Creek.

VIEWS More-open conditions on the west side of the ridge allow for sweeping vistas: hulking San Gorgonio Peak looms to the north, above the desert pass that bears its name, while, stretching to the northwest, the San Bernardino and San Gabriel Valleys, flanked by the lofty summits of the San Gabriel Mountains, extend toward the Los Angeles basin. On a clear day in winter or spring, snow-flecked Mount San Antonio (Mount Baldy) and Mount Wilson are both visible in that range.

Presently your sandy path, lined with lupine and penstemon, meets a switchback in a dirt road, which winds east into a shallow basin. Marked by large ducks, the trail leaves the northwest side of the open gap containing the road, but soon your route turns south to descend alongside and just below that road.

CAMPING You reenter San Jacinto Wilderness, and after a bit your course veers from the road and winds east down dry washes and under the shade of low scrub oaks to a narrow gap (193.9–6,393') in a sawblade ridge of granodiorite needles.

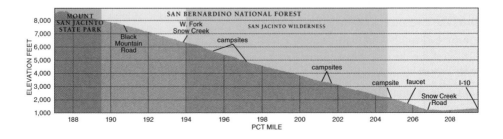

WATER ACCESS

Seasonal West Fork Snow Creek is 0.2 mile south of the trail on an unmarked path just before a small gap. After crossing a dry ravine, look for an old roadbed and follow it down to the bottom of the drainage. There will be a clearing on the right and a stream in the woods straight ahead. There are good camping options nearby.

Four long switchbacks descend the east face of this prominent ridge, depositing you in noticeably more xeric environs.

PLANTS Initially, Coulter pines replace other montane conifers, and then, as the way arcs north in continual descent, you enter a true chaparral: yerba santa, buckwheat, hollyleaf cherry, scrub oak, manzanita, and yucca supply the sparse ground cover, while scarlet gilia and yellow blazing star add spring color. Unlike chaparral communities moistened by maritime air, the desert-facing slopes here force these species to contend with much more extreme drought conditions. As a result, many more of the plants growing here are annuals, which avoid drought by lying dormant as seed, while others, such as yerba santa, wilt and drop their soft leaves to prevent water loss during sustained dry periods.

A continued moderate downgrade and another set of long switchbacks soon allow you to inspect the awesome, avalanche-raw, 9,600-foot north escarpment of San Jacinto Peak, which rises above the cascades of Snow Creek.

GEOLOGY To the northeast the confused alluvial terrain beyond San Gorgonio Pass attests to activity along the San Andreas Fault. Beyond, suburban Desert Hot Springs shimmers in the Coachella Valley heat, with the Little San Bernardino Mountains as the backdrop.

Inexorably, your descent continues at a moderate grade, presently switchbacking in broad sweeps across a dry ravine on slopes north of West Fork Snow Creek.

After striking a small saddle just west of Knob 3,252, the trail, now taking a gentle grade, swings north then northwest down a boulder-studded hillside. A series of small campsites can be found just off the trail as you descend. Note the small village of Snow Creek lying below you at the mountain's base before making three small switchbacks and then heading back southeast toward Snow Canyon. After winding your way through a veritable forest of 20- to 30-foot-high orange granitic boulders, you negotiate a final set of switchbacks before dropping to cross a dry creekbed on the western edge of Snow Canyon. Soon after, you strike narrow, paved Snow Canyon Road (205.7–1,730').

WATER ACCESS

A 3-foot-tall concrete water fountain stands at the trail junction. This permanent water source is a welcome respite after the usually baking-hot descent.

Southbound hikers should note that this water fountain is their last certain water source until North Fork San Jacinto River, a grueling 19.5 miles and a 7,600-foot climb away, high in the San Jacintos. For the northbound, the next water is at Mesa Wind Farm (an emergency source only), 7.7 miles away, or, better, at Whitewater Preserve, a long, hot 13.3 miles away.

Snow Canyon is both a wildlife refuge and a water supply for Palm Springs, so camping here is not allowed.

Make a moderate descent along narrow Snow Canyon Road, which winds north down Snow Canyon's rubbly alluvial fan, often near a small, usually flowing western branch of Snow Creek. This stream may be dry by April in drought years. Eventually the road simultaneously leaves San Bernardino National Forest and its San Jacinto Wilderness at a Desert Water Agency gate, and then it veers northwest to hop across the western branch. Just beyond, your route joins paved Falls Creek Road (207.0–1,235') at the outskirts of the small village of Snow Creek.

Now you briefly follow Falls Creek Road northwest to a junction with Snow Creek Road. From here the PCT route starts a contour northwest. The next 2 miles of PCT winds through well-spaced, head-high, yellow-flowered creosote bushes on a gentle descent. A few minutes' walk leads across a sandy wash, which, at about 1,188 feet elevation, is the PCT's lowest point south of the Columbia Gorge on the Oregon–Washington border. Another few minutes finds your trail intersecting a pair of crossing jeep roads under a high-tension power line. Beyond, the wooden posts continue north, now across a more cobbly desert floor with mixed shrubbery. You cross a good gravel road, then proceed across numerous sandy washes that

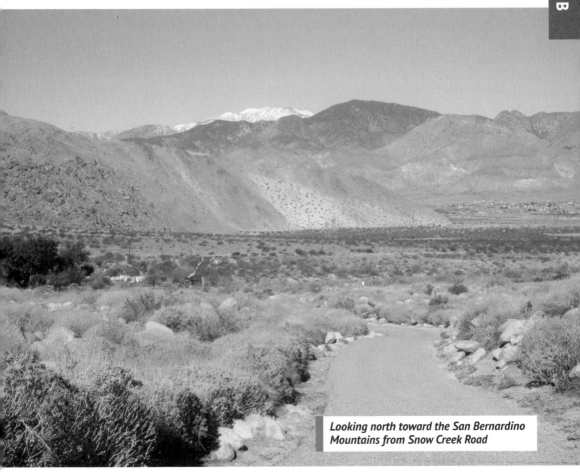

Looking north toward the San Bernardino Mountains from Snow Creek Road

constitute the ephemeral San Gorgonio River. Usually no water is to be found, but often there is a strong westerly wind that throws stinging sand in your face. It also sets hundreds of power-generating wind turbines, standing north across I-10, flapping like alarmed seagulls. In the rainy season, look for purple clusters of sand verbena.

Eventually metal posts indicate a bend northwest in the route, which soon crosses a sandy dirt road. Now you hike left (northwest), slowly diverging from the road, and climb to hike atop a narrow, sinuous, 20-foot-high alluvial bank. It was built to protect the busy railroad that parallels the route just to the north. Shortly, you drop off the north side of the alluvial bank, heading sandily over a level treadless route, marked by 4-by-4-inch posts, west toward a tangle of roads at the mouth of Stubbe Canyon Creek, which could be seen from atop the rise. Here the route emerges from three concrete bridges, one of the railroad and two of I-10 (209.5–1,337').

RESUPPLY ACCESS

To resupply, hitchhike, as recommended under "Supplies," 12.5 miles east to Palm Springs or 4.5 miles west to Cabazon.

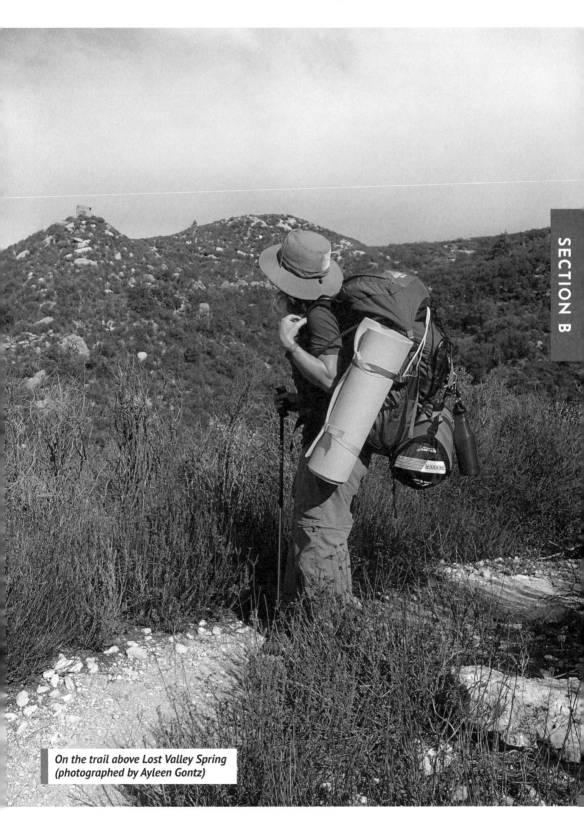

On the trail above Lost Valley Spring
(photographed by Ayleen Gontz)

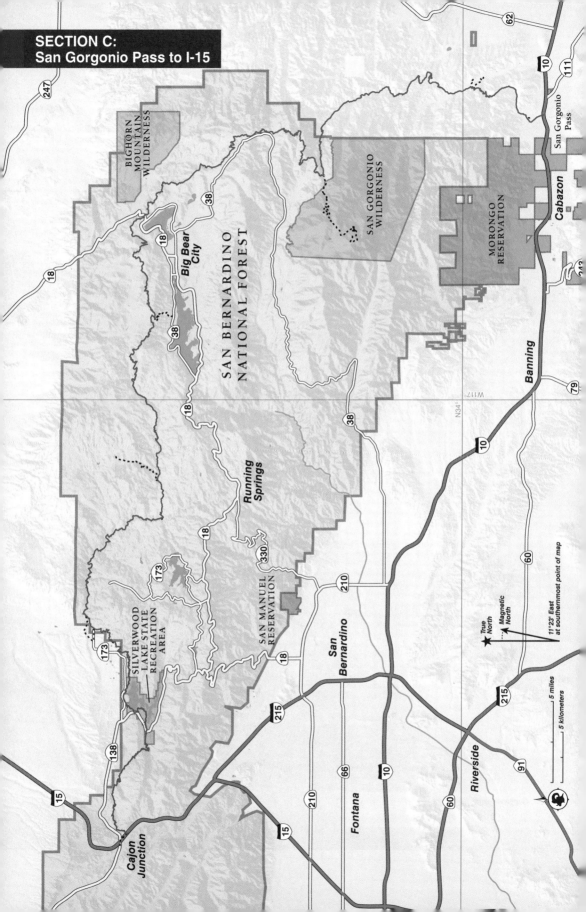

247

62

10

111

BIGHORN MOUNTAIN WILDERNESS

San Gorgonio Pass

Cabazon

38

18

SAN GORGONIO WILDERNESS

Big Bear City

38

MORONGO RESERVATION

18

SAN BERNARDINO NATIONAL FOREST

38

N34°

W117°

18

10

Banning

79

38

Running Springs

60

18

330

True North

Magnetic North

173

210

11°23' East at southernmost point of map

18

SAN MANUEL RESERVATION

San Bernardino

173

SILVERWOOD LAKE STATE RECREATION AREA

18

215

138

215

91

Riverside

5 miles

5 kilometers

15

66

10

60

210

Fontana

15

Cajon Junction

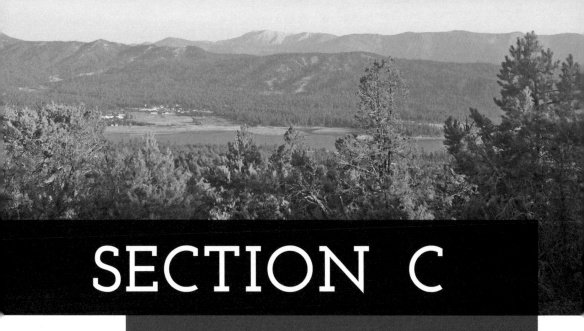

SECTION C

San Gorgonio Pass to I-15 near Cajon Pass

RUNNING THE ENTIRE LENGTH of the San Bernardino Mountains, this long trail section samples most of the diverse ecosystems found there. Beginning in San Gorgonio Pass in the sweltering heat of a typical Colorado Desert (Lower Sonoran Zone) ecosystem, the Pacific Crest Trail (PCT) crosses the San Andreas Fault and then climbs through a sparse chaparral of bayonet-sharp cacti and thorny scrub along the Whitewater River and Mission Creek. Though sprung from subalpine snowbanks high in the San Gorgonio Wilderness, these streams almost all evaporate or sink beneath desert gravel before reaching the foothills.

As you climb higher, small drought-tolerant pinyon pines, which were once a staple of the American Indian diet and are still a food source for various animals, soon border the trail, heralding your passage through the Upper Sonoran Zone. These trees gradually mingle with Jeffrey pines and

Above: A view of Big Bear Lake from the trail

incense cedars until, at about 7,000 feet, you find yourself in the crisp air and enveloping forests of the Transition Zone. Just north of Coon Creek, at the 8,750-foot apex of the PCT in the San Bernardino Mountains, the route touches the Canadian Zone, where isolated snow patches might linger into early summer. Hikers traversing the high San Bernardinos in April or May should expect possible hail or snow and nightly subfreezing temperatures. Bring warm clothing and carry a tent. From the high point, you can turn southwest to scan the San Gorgonio Wilderness' high summits, where hardy subalpine conifers huddle below gale-screening ridges. The PCT was routed around the highest elevations of the wilderness because its backpacker population was already excessive.

The Sand to Snow National Monument, designated by President Barack Obama in 2016, covers 30 miles of the PCT between the San Gorgonio Wilderness to Coon's Creek Jumpoff in the San Bernardino National Forest. The designation offers an extra layer of protection to the trail and its expansive surroundings, which encompass 154,000 acres stretching from the Sonoran Desert floor and the summit of San Gorgonio Mountain, Southern California's highest peak. The monument also includes sand dunes, thousands of American Indian petroglyphs, and two volcanic mesas.

Nearing dammed Big Bear Lake, a popular resort area, the PCT alternates between Jeffrey pine and pinyon forest. In this northern rainshadow of the San Bernardinos, plant and animal life is much more influenced by proximity to the high Mojave Desert, stretching northward, than by the terrain's elevation, which would normally foster a uniform montane Jeffrey pine and fir forest. Instead, Joshua trees, cacti, mountain mahogany, and sagebrush share the rolling hillsides with dry pinyon pine groves, while Jeffrey pines, incense cedars, and white firs grow on the higher summits or in the cold-air microclimates of streambeds.

North of Big Bear Lake the PCT begins to trend west, following the main axis of the San Bernardino Mountains. A part of the Transverse Range

Province, which includes the San Gabriel Mountains and other mountain chains stretching west to the Channel Islands, the San Bernardinos cut conspicuously across the lay of other California physiographic features, which trend northwest–southeast. Long before being intruded by molten rock that solidified to form granitic plutons, the region now straddled by the San Bernardinos had been alternately low land and shallow sea floor. Evidence of this lies in two rock types you will encounter often: Furnace marble, derived from marine carbonates that became limestone; and Saragossa quartzite, derived from sand that became sandstone. The limestone and sandstone were then altered under heat and pressure, perhaps several times, to reach their present metamorphic states.

Near Lake Arrowhead, another reservoir originally constructed to store water to irrigate foothill orange groves, the PCT again veers north, now down Deep Creek, a permanent stream feeding the ephemeral Mojave River.

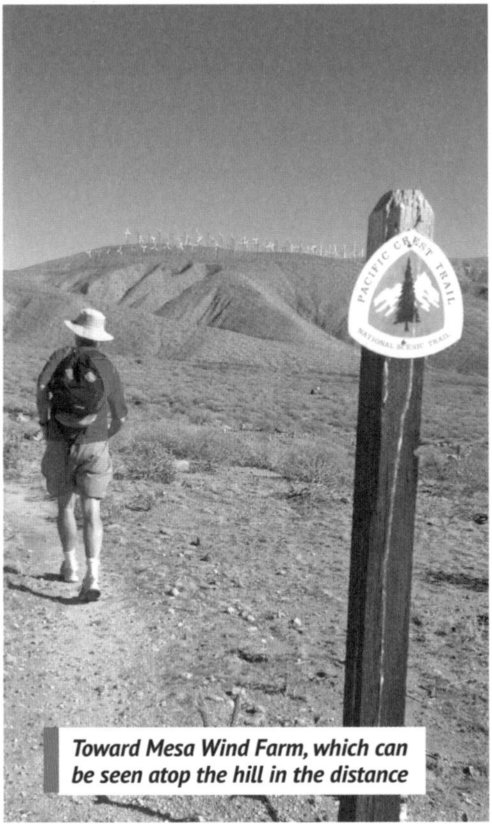

The floral composition of the Mojave Desert, seen here and also later as the PCT skirts Summit Valley, differs strikingly from the lower Colorado Desert flora seen farther south. Bitter-cold, windy winters here account for many of the differences.

Section C ends unremarkably under six-lane I-15 in Cajon Canyon, overshadowed by massive workings of humanity—the freeway, the power lines from the Colorado River, and the multiple railroad

Toward Mesa Wind Farm, which can be seen atop the hill in the distance

tracks. These in turn are dwarfed by an awesome artifact of nature—the cleft of the San Andreas Fault, which slashes through Cajon Canyon and bends west to demarcate the southern base of the San Bernardino Mountains.

DECLINATION 11°23'E

USGS MAPS

White Water	San Gorgonio Peak	Lake Arrowhead
Catclaw Flat	Big Bear City	Silverwood Lake
Onyx Peak	Fawnskin	Cajon
Moonridge	Butler Peak	

POINTS ON THE TRAIL, SOUTH TO NORTH

	Mile	Elevation in feet	Latitude/Longitude
I-10 at San Gorgonio Pass	209.5	1,337	N33° 55' 31.980" W116° 41' 42.240"
Mesa Wind Farm	213.4	2,338	N33° 57' 07.620" W116° 39' 56.760"
Trail junction for Whitewater Preserve (water, camping)	218.5	2,312	N33° 59' 31.140" W116° 39' 51.840"
First Mission Creek crossing	226.2	3,128	N34° 02' 38.350" W116° 39' 27.350"
Onyx Summit/CA 138	252.1	8,531	N34° 11' 30.660" W116° 43' 01.080"
CA 18 near Baldwin Lake	266.1	6,830	N34° 17' 26.700" W116° 48' 09.900"
Van Dusen Canyon Road near seasonal Caribou Creek (to Big Bear City)	275.1	7,264	N34° 17' 19.740" W116° 53' 00.120"
Cougar Crest Trail Junction to Big Bear Discovery Center	277.7	7,674	N34° 16' 51.300" W116° 54' 47.460"
Polique Canyon Road 2N09 to Fawnskin	278.6	7,550	N34° 17' 01.060" W116° 55' 02.090"
Paved Crab Flats Road	292.2	5,469	N34° 16' 31.200" W117° 03' 02.700"
Splinters Cabin Day-Use Area/to Cedar Glen	298.5	4,581	N34° 16' 22.500" W117° 07' 43.680"
Deep Creek Hot Spring	307.9	3,522	N34° 20' 21.360" W117° 10' 37.260"
Mojave Forks Reservoir/detour/road to Hesperia	313.0	3,135	N34° 20' 42.780" W117° 13' 50.040"
Silverwood Lake Recreation Area entrance	329.0	3,397	N34° 17' 16.560" W117° 21' 19.980"
I-15 near Cajon Pass	342.0	2,995	N34° 18' 16.680" W117° 27' 54.720"

CAMPSITES AND BIVY SITES

Mile	Elevation in feet	Latitude/ Longitude	Number of tents	Feature	Notes
218.5	2,208	N33° 59' 31.140" W116° 39' 51.840"	Dozens	Whitewater Preserve	Picnic tables, water, restrooms, a large meadow for PCT camping
226.2	3,128	N34° 02' 38.340" W116° 39' 27.360"	2	Mission Creek	Primitive
229.5	3,955	N34° 04' 14.580" W116° 39' 58.020"	2	Mission Creek	Primitive

CAMPSITES AND BIVY SITES (continued)

Mile	Elevation in feet	Latitude/ Longitude	Number of tents	Feature	Notes
231.4	4,564	N34° 05' 27.300" W116° 40' 22.800"	2	Mission Creek	Primitive, creek nearby
235.5	6,128	N34° 07' 41.520" W116° 42' 31.860"	4	Mission Creek	Dry creekbed, shade
238.7	7,371	N34° 07' 44.640" W116° 44' 27.060"	3	Forested Flats Junction	Seasonal water
239.9	7,968	N34° 07' 32.700" W116° 45' 31.860"	>10	Mission Springs Trail Camp	Outhouse, seasonal spring, and trough nearby
246.4	8,131	N34° 08' 57.660" W116° 42' 38.040"	>10	Coon Creek Cabin Group Camp	Fire ring, no water
256.2	7,605	N34° 12' 53.040" W116° 44' 24.360"	5	Arrastre Trail Camp, Deer Spring	Seasonal stream, picnic table
268.6	6,841	N34° 17' 48.540" W116° 49' 29.460"	5	Doble Trail Camp	0.5 mile off trail, pit toilet, picnic table, 2 faucets with seasonal water
276.6	7,716	N34° 17' 10.560" W116° 53' 59.520"	2	Bertha Ridge	Small campsite near Bertha Peak Trail
285.6	6,577	N34° 18' 04.920" W116° 58' 40.320"	>10	Little Bear Spring Trail Camp	Picnic table, outhouse, corral, faucet with seasonal water, creek nearby (prone to motocross noise)
289.9	6,089	N34° 16' 52.800" W117° 01' 46.860"	>5	Holcomb Creek	
293.2	5,331	N34° 16' 42.540" W117° 03' 48.540"	10	Holcomb Creek	Oak trees, small seasonal stream nearby
294.1	5,215	N34° 16' 37.140" W117° 04' 31.920"	10	Holcomb Crossing Trail Camp	Fire rings, pine trees
294.7	5,185	N34° 16' 41.280" W117° 04' 58.800"	>10	Bench Trail Camp	
317.6	3,371	N34° 18' 57.060" W117° 15' 49.800"	25	Mojave River Forks Campground (run by county)	0.75 mile off trail, showers
318.0	3,331	N34° 18' 44.580" W117° 15' 54.660"	>5	Grass Valley Creek	
319.9	3,595	N34° 18' 21.180" W117° 16' 34.320"	2		
329.0	3,397	N34° 17' 16.560" W117° 21' 19.980"	Dozens	Silverwood Lake Recreation Area	PCT camping in Hike and Bike section, showers, toilets, small store
335.6	3,587	N34° 18' 43.140" W117° 24' 35.040"	>5	Little Horsethief Canyon	Unsheltered, wind-prone, flat

WEATHER TO GO

The San Bernardino Mountains customarily offer clear, warm weather and snow-free trails throughout May and June. By then, however, the lowlands at either end of this section—especially in Mission Creek at the start—typically have daytime temperatures in excess of 100° F. Early spring and fall tend to be some of the best times to explore those areas, if you aren't thru-hiking.

SUPPLIES

The neighborhood of Whitewater, at the beginning of Section C, has nothing for hikers. Supplies may be purchased 4.5 miles west on I-10, in Cabazon, which has a post office, a market, and an enormous designer outlet mall, where almost any conceivable need for clothing, shoes, electronics, or sporting goods can be fulfilled. It also has the Morongo Casino Resort, a gleaming mirage-like complex of gaming, dining, and lodging options, as well as Hadley's, famous for their date milk shakes and mind-boggling array of dried fruits. Fully 10 miles west of the PCT at Whitewater on I-10 is Banning, which has even more complete services than Cabazon. Palm Springs lies 12.5 miles east via I-10 and CA 111. It has several markets, hotels, and fine eateries.

Big Bear City, 3 miles south down Van Dusen Canyon Road from mile 275.1 on the PCT, is the next convenient provisioning stop. It boasts a post office, stores, restaurants, motels, and laundromats beside shallow, picturesque Big Bear Lake. Big Bear Hostel, conveniently located near the village center in the incorporated town of Big Bear Lake, welcomes PCT hikers with free laundry, loaner clothes, and breakfast; it also accepts resupply packages for its guests and often gives hikers morning rides back to the trailhead at CA 18 (see resupply info on page 145).

Fawnskin, another resort community, is located on the northwest shore of Big Bear Lake, and it is 3.7 miles off-route along Polique Canyon Road, about 69 miles from the start. It has a post office, stores, restaurants, and motels. It is also accessible via the Cougar Crest Trail, at the 68-mile point of this PCT section, by way of a 2.7-mile detour.

The next chance for supplies lies in Lake Arrowhead, 3.5 miles from the PCT's crossing of Deep Creek, 89 miles from the start. You'll find them in the Cedar Glen community on the east shore of the lake, which you reach via a popular hikers' access at Splinters Cabin and Hook Creek Road (getting a ride is usually easy, especially on weekends). That road leads up to the convenient Cedar Glen Post Office and nearby supermarket, restaurants, shops, and motels.

Upon descending Deep Creek to Mojave River Forks Reservoir, about 103 miles into this section, walkers may opt to head for the desert community of Hesperia. Arrowhead Lake Road leads north 2.8 miles to Hesperia Lake Park, a delightful enclave with lawn-cushioned camping under deep shade, fishing in a small lake, and a small minimart. Downtown Hesperia lies about 3 miles farther, with a post office and all modern amenities.

Crestline, a mountain village similar to Cedar Glen, also offers similar accommodations for hikers who hitchhike south 10 miles on CA 138 from the 329-mile point of the PCT, at Silverwood Lake State Recreation Area. Travelers with less extensive needs may avail themselves of a small general store a short distance off the trail in the recreation area.

Section C terminates at a road-end just shy of I-15 in Cajon Canyon. This paved spur road leads 0.6 mile northwest to meet CA 138 about 200 yards east of its overpass of I-15 at Cajon Junction. Hikers will find gas stations, two well-stocked minimarts, and a pleasant motel. Also sited there are two of the objects of many hikers' fantasies: a Del Taco restaurant and a McDonald's.

The owners of Cajon Pass Inn (8317 CA 138, Phelan, CA 92371; 760-249-6777), located west of the overpass, offer discounted rates for hikers and will hold supply boxes; they ask that you include your trail name and ETA if possible. This is an excellent option because camping nearby is generally terrible, and, besides, they have a swimming pool and a hot tub! Resupplying here lets you avoid the lengthy descent to Wrightwood. Many prefer, however, to spend time in the charming community of Wrightwood.

From the Cajon Junction overpass, CA 138 continues northwest 8.5 miles to CA 2, which goes 5.5 miles to Wrightwood. This pleasant mountain community has a post office, stores, restaurants, motels, and a laundromat. Those who don't mind a return to true civilization—smog, congestion, street lights, and concrete—may go south 17 miles on I-15 to San Bernardino, which has all the dubious advantages of a hectic metropolis.

WATER

Carry ample water north from I-10 because the Whitewater River and the lower reaches of Mission Creek that the PCT traverses are often dry by June in drought years, though many hikers detour to Whitewater Preserve for 24-7 water. For most of the remainder of this San Bernardino Mountains section, however, water sources are encountered regularly, even if they are not numerous. This situation changes for the last leg, along the rim of the Mojave Desert. Be sure to leave Deep Creek and Silverwood Lake with a few liters of water per person—the stretches of dusty chaparral along Summit Valley, and over to Cajon Pass, are usually bone-dry.

PERMITS

No wilderness permits are required for day or overnight PCT campers in San Bernardino National Forest and the BLM portion of the San Gorgonio Wilderness.

SPECIAL CONCERNS

Refer to page 36 for information about poodle-dog bush and page 34 for ticks.

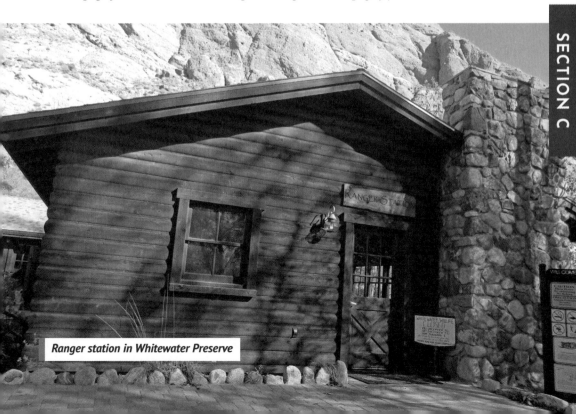

Ranger station in Whitewater Preserve

SECTION C

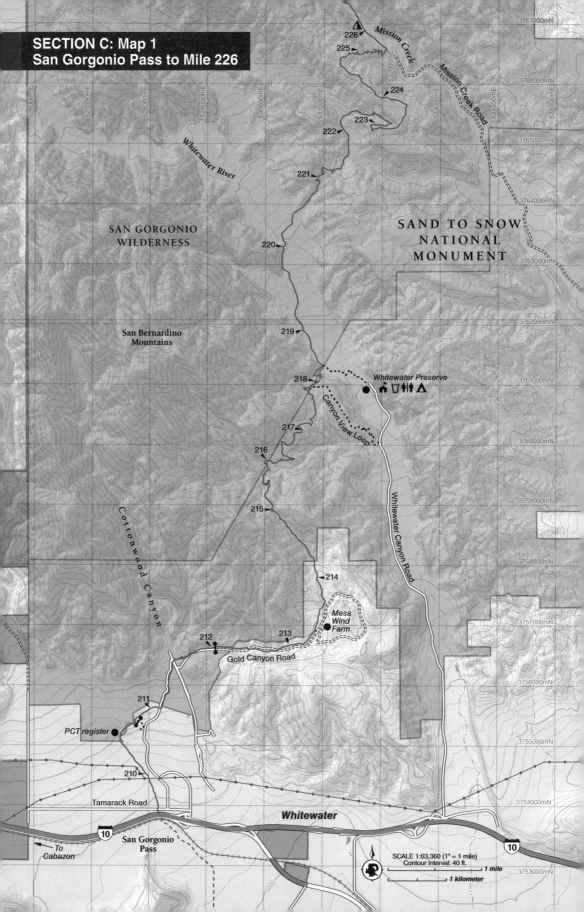

△ 226
225
224 Mission Creek
Mission Creek Road
223
222
221

Whitewater River

SAN GORGONIO WILDERNESS

SAND TO SNOW NATIONAL MONUMENT

220

N34
219

San Bernardino Mountains

218   Whitewater Preserve

Canyon View Loop

217

216

215

Whitewater Canyon Road

Cottonwood Canyon

214

Mesa Wind Farm

212
213

Gold Canyon Road

211

PCT register

210

Tamarack Road

Whitewater

To Cabazon

San Gorgonio Pass

SCALE 1:63,360 (1" = 1 mile)
Contour Interval: 40 ft.

1 mile
1 kilometer

SAN GORGONIO PASS TO I-15 NEAR CAJON PASS

>>>THE ROUTE

Reach the southern terminus of Section C via I-10's Haugen-Lehmann Way exit (209.5–1,337'). Head briefly north to Tamarack Road, which parallels the freeway, and follow it 0.3 mile west to the posted PCT, just west of Fremontia Road.

Passing under these bridges you finally leave Santa Rosa and San Jacinto Mountains National Monument behind.

A quiet neighborhood in Whitewater, West Palm Springs Village is centered 0.3 mile east along Tamarack Road. The village was once the home of legendary trail angels Ziggy and the Bear, who retired in 2016 after a decade of hiker hospitality. Although water is often available at nearby Mesa Wind Farm, the village has no resources for PCT travelers.

Easy-to-follow PCT tread climbs gently north from Tamarack Road, first just west of dry Stubbe Canyon Creek and then on a low levee to its east. You wind past many roads of a small subdivision, then pass under a power line and its attendant road. Across a second such road the tread may be vague, but it is marked by 4-by-4-inch PCT posts, and it runs just west of a wire fence. Beyond it, you wind up to a dirt road over the buried Colorado River Aqueduct. A minute later, you cross a better road and reach a crude sign and trail register.

Keeping to a low bench with knee-high scrub, you traverse a succession of jeep roads, then cross better Cottonwood Road, where you enter the Sand to Snow National Monument. The PCT turns left (north), uphill alongside

Cottonwood Road, keeping within 10 yards of it amid a smattering of silver-flannel-leaved, yellow-flowered brittlebush, a drought-tolerant shrub of the sunflower family. Nearing the mouth of Cottonwood Canyon, the trail passes a dirt parking area and then crosses two side-by-side roads and makes a slightly indistinct ford of the almost always dry stream that drains Cottonwood Canyon. Across it, the way merges with a jeep track to strike east to the mouth of Gold Canyon. Its unusual east–west orientation is due to erosion along the Bonnie Bell fault, a splinter of the great San Andreas rift.

Entering Gold Canyon, your jeep track strikes Gold Canyon Road. In the next long mile, you recross the road, pass through a stock fence at a corral, and then cross the road—now blocked—twice more, all in desert vegetation of Mojave yucca, rabbitbrush, creosote bush, and multiple species of cacti. Presently you see windmills of the hiker-friendly Mesa Wind Farm, and the canyon bends north (213.4–2,338'). Here a sign welcomes you to Section C, and thoughtfully lists the mileages through the San Bernardinos. Next to it, a dirt road junction leads to the wind farm's metal headquarters shed and a few shaded rest options.

WATER ACCESS

Wind-farm workers often leave a cache of water for hikers just off

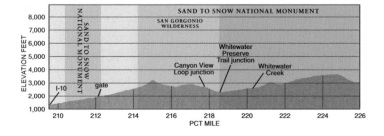

SECTION C

the trail. You can also walk to the large metal building and ask for water. It comes from a well that you walk past: just south of the road, at an electric control panel for the transformer station, a blue-domed cylinder sits atop the well-head, with numerous valves and taps. Camping—in the company of feral cattle—could be done anywhere nearby.

Sometimes vague and trampled by cattle, your path now leads more moderately up a small parallel ravine west of the road. Later you come back alongside the main ravine and momentarily join a rough jeep road. The way leads easily upcanyon, keeping just west of its dry wash and braiding with a network of cattle paths. After passing through a drift fence, the path steepens to climb the head of Gold Canyon. Mostly, the way is unrelentingly shadeless, but occasional small laurel sumac trees offer respite. During the wet season, a profusion of wildflowers may sprinkle the route, including many members of the sunflower family; white, blue, and lavender phacelias; chia; and popcorn flower. Lizards too numerous to count also scurry underfoot. Finally, four small switchbacks help you gain a narrow pass between Gold and Teutang Canyons. This pass is now the approximate southern boundary of the expanded San Gorgonio Wilderness, which the PCT will climb through, until the head of North Fork Mission Creek. The most impressive vistas are southeast, contrasting the granite and seasonal snow of the San Jacinto massif with the Colorado Desert sands of Coachella Valley.

Starting north, you descend moderately to a ridge nose, down which small, tight switchbacks descend. These bring the PCT to a dry crossing of the streambed in Teutang Canyon,

just upstream of a chasm of gray granite. Next you round an intervening promontory to step across another canyon tributary, which has a seasonal spring 0.25 mile upcanyon, then proceed fairly levelly downcanyon. When you gain a narrow ridgetop, your path doubles back on itself to climb northwest, perhaps indistinctly, up an open, grassy slope before resuming a traversing line high above the canyon's floor. This stretch does afford interesting panoramas east over the cleft of Whitewater Canyon to the sun-browned Little San Bernardino Mountains.

Here, a signpost marks the PCT's brief merging with the Canyon View Loop (217.7–2,746'), a popular day hike that begins at Whitewater Preserve. Don't be surprised, after miles of solitude, to encounter groups of day hikers who favor this easy 3.5-mile loop, especially on weekends and holidays. Continue along a ridgelet, rather than following the trail spur that leads east toward Whitewater Canyon Road. Both paths lead to Whitewater Preserve, but the second one avoids a 0.5-mile road walk.

TRAIL INFO The area surrounding the Whitewater River and Mission Creek is prone to flash flooding and trail erosion. Winter rains sometimes create dangerous conditions, and the trail and roads leading to Whitewater Preserve will be closed. Check the preserve's website for the most up-to-date information on flooding and wildfire news: wildlandsconservancy.org.

Eventually you descend, first directly along a ridgelet, then in a sweeping arc that leads to the lip of a canyon. Now on switchbacks that are susceptible to erosion, you drop quickly to the floor of the canyon, where you step across its dry streambed.

The trail now heads sandily downstream and then strikes an old jeep road (218.5–2,312') at the canyon's mouth in Whitewater Canyon, just beneath an impressive conglomerate scarp. Here you turn left (north) on sandy alluvium of the west bank of the Whitewater River, which is a raging torrent true to its name in early season but more often is a burbling brook. A sign here beckons hikers to the Whitewater Preserve, 0.5 mile off the trail, where potable water and camping await. Follow the path south and east as it crosses the river and becomes attractively flanked by small boulders and ribbon-tied posts to reach the preserve.

Southbound trekkers must fill their canteens at the river or at Whitewater Preserve; the next safe, certain on-route water lies across desertlike San Gorgonio Pass at the water fountain by Snow Canyon Road, a little over 13 miles away. The Whitewater River usually has water throughout summer but may be dry by early May in severe drought years. The route winds across sandy washes where the flanking scrub is alive with phainopeplas, which are crested silky flycatchers closely related to waxwings.

To the east, just across the Whitewater River, is a welcoming oasis of trees, water, and meadows. This is the Whitewater Preserve (760-325-7222, wildlandsconservancy.org), formerly a private trout farm that was taken over by the nonprofit Wildlands Conservancy in 2006. It can be a bit jarring to come off the trail and encounter crowds of day-trippers from Palm Springs walking their dogs and eating fast food on picnic tables that dot the property, but it's a welcoming sort of place nonetheless.

CAMPING PCT hikers may camp for free in the large back meadow and sink their aching feet into the cool wading pools. A ranger office has water and emergency phone service when it's open (typically 8 a.m.–5 p.m. daily). There is also 24-7 water available from a spout near the separate restrooms.

Back on the trail, and just past red basalt outcrops of Miocene age, a PCT marker (220.3–2,610') leads you northeast across the Whitewater River's bouldery granite and marble bed to a narrow canyon peppered with boulders of basalt and gneiss, among junipers, catclaws, and bladderpods patrolled by collared lizards. Here the best track jogs northwest, paralleling the

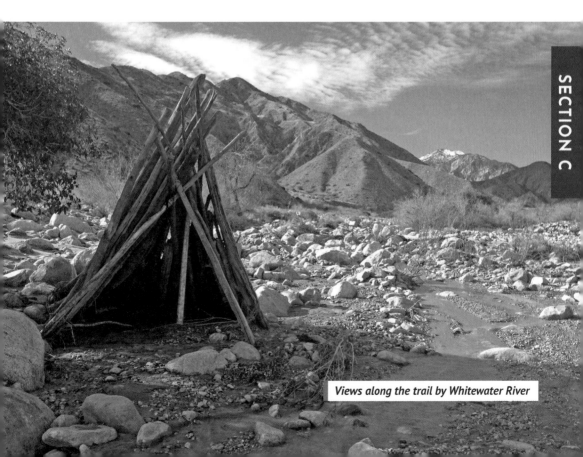

Views along the trail by Whitewater River

SECTION C

riverbed for a moment, to find a resumption of trail at a wood PCT signpost. From the post your path ascends moderately northeast in a terrain not unlike Death Valley, soon switchbacking to gain a ridgetop (221.1–3,166') in deeply incised gneiss and fanglomerate. Fiddleneck and foxtail brush against one's legs on the descent northeast from this saddle, and you soon reach and turn north beside West Fork Mission Creek Road. Minutes later the PCT veers north, away from this dirt road, in a dry, sandy wash. Look for wood posts, following them east into a side canyon, then up, arcing across the north side of the small valley and across its head, and then ascending its south wall to an east-ascending nose, eroded from Cenozoic sediments.

VIEWS Atop this ridge, views are panoramic and startling. The southern horizon is dominated by 10,804-foot San Jacinto Peak, often frosted with snow in winter and spring and contrasting markedly with the red, yellow, and gray hues of the desert's alluvial landscape, in the foreground. To the west, gneissic rocks support Kitching Peak, while the Whitewater River Canyon ascends as a rocky scar northwest to the Jumpoffs below barren San Gorgonio Peak. The gully just north of the ridge that you ascended, plus West Fork Mission Creek, Catclaw Flat, and Middle Fork Whitewater River, are all aligned with the north branch of the San Andreas Fault, which is partly responsible for this region's varied geology.

The PCT continues to wind northwest up the ridgetop dividing the East and West Forks of Mission Creek; then the ascent gives way to a moderate descent east of a chaparral nose to East Fork Mission Creek Road.

CAMPING Here you turn northwest upcanyon to cross usually flowing East Fork Mission Creek in about 0.5 mile (226.2–3,128'). Continue along its shadeless north bank to the end of the dirt road. From this point your hike up Mission Creek is often difficult, despite the installation of boulder bridges across each of the stream fords. There

are numerous primitive options for camping along the lower reaches of Mission Creek.

Mission Creek's narrow gorge, incised in tortured granite gneisses, leaves little room for a trail, so washouts are frequent and the path is often vague through alluvial boulder fields and jungles of baccharis (false willow), alder, willow, and cottonwood. Rattlesnakes—as well as garter snakes, racers, horned lizards, antelope ground squirrels, summer tanagers, and bobcats— inhabit the grassy stream margins, so keep an eye open while making any of the 20-plus fords of Mission Creek south of Forks Springs. Note, too, where prominent faults cross the canyon—at 3,400 feet, at 3,900 feet, and at 4,080 feet, where the Pinto Mountain Fault further tortures the banded gneisses.

PLANTS Chia, yerba santa, catclaw, baccharis, and bladderpod are the most frequent plants, but you also see notable specimens of Joshua tree, yucca, and cactus.

One species that hikers thankfully won't have to see as much anymore is cattle. Mission Creek Ranch, which once owned land traversed by the PCT, alternating in a checkerboard fashion with Bureau of Land Management–owned tracts, has now been purchased by the nonprofit Wildlands Conservancy. All cattle grazing has been eliminated from the area.

Mission Creek Preserve, also a Wildlands Conservancy property, is about 2 miles off the PCT but offers few amenities for PCT hikers. A historical stone house has a picnic table, toilets, and nonpotable water but is open only to group campers and requires a reservation. About 2 miles beyond the house is a parking area and four stone casitas with picnic tables. For more information, contact the ranger station at 760-369-7105 or visit wildlandsconservancy.org.

WATER ACCESS

Just below the confluence of the South and North Forks of Mission

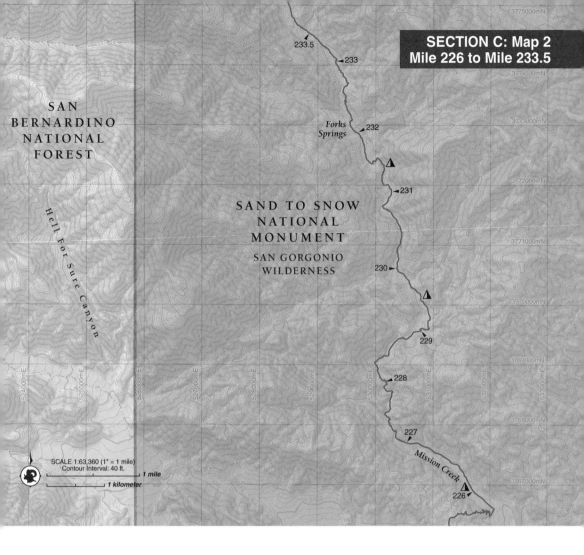

SAN
BERNARDINO
NATIONAL
FOREST

SAND TO SNOW
NATIONAL
MONUMENT

SAN GORGONIO
WILDERNESS

Hell For Sure Canyon

Forks
Springs

Mission Creek

SCALE 1:63,360 (1" = 1 mile)
Contour Interval: 40 ft.

1 mile

1 kilometer

Creek, you cross this major creek (232.1–4,834'), which is fed just upcanyon by Forks Springs. Water is generally available here year-round but may not be elsewhere in Mission Creek due to the porous sediments of its bed.

North of Forks Springs, the now discernible PCT keeps usually to northeastern banks in an ocean-spray chaparral. Near 5,200 feet the path crosses granitic bedrock emplaced at the same time as Sierran granites. Later, at 5,600 feet, the tread turns to sugar-white and yellowish Saragossa quartzite.

CAMPING Near 5,900 feet the PCT veers away from Mission Creek into a side canyon and quickly reaches a pleasant creekside camp (235.5–6,128') shaded by incense cedars, Jeffrey pines, and interior live oaks.

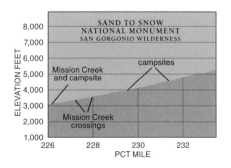

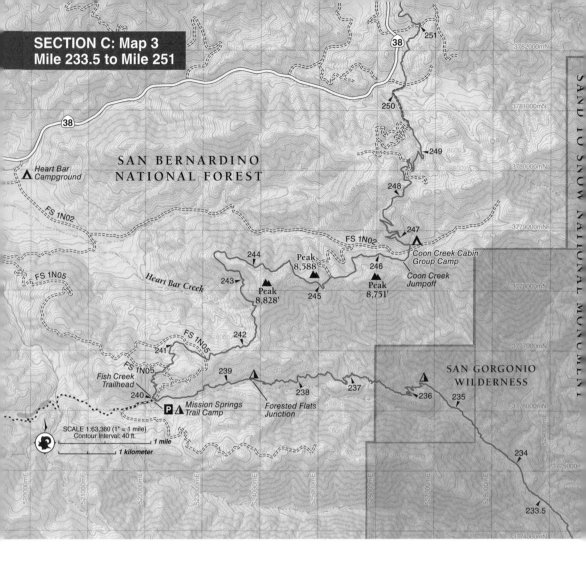

SAND TO SNOW NATIONAL MONUMENT

SAN BERNARDINO NATIONAL FOREST

Heart Bar Campground

FS 1N02

FS 1N05

Heart Bar Creek

FS 1N02

Coon Creek Cabin Group Camp

Coon Creek Jumpoff

Peak 8,588'

Peak 8,828'

Peak 8,751'

FS 1N05

FS 1N05

Fish Creek Trailhead

Mission Springs Trail Camp

Forested Flats Junction

SAN GORGONIO WILDERNESS

SCALE 1:63,360 (1" = 1 mile)
Contour Interval: 40 ft.
1 mile
1 kilometer

Eight switchbacks lead west from this spot, elevating you to a phyllite-and-quartzite promontory. The instability of the quartzite bedrock is demonstrated both by vegetational scarcity and by a massive landslide cutting across your path as you contour a steep slope shortly after gaining this ridge. Just past this slide, you leave BLM jurisdiction for San Bernardino National Forest.

WATER ACCESS

White firs and Jeffrey pines soon shade the PCT as it resumes its ascent close beside Mission Creek, which usually has flowing water near its headwaters. Tank up here,

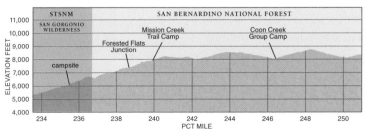

for there might not be water at Mission Springs Trail Camp.

CAMPING A rough jeep road, built to log the forested flats south of Mission Creek, is met at Forested Flats Junction (238.7–7,371'), which may still be marked by yellow paint daubs on nearby trees. The next water on-route, if Mission Springs Trail Camp is dry, is at Deer Spring in 17.5 miles.

CAMPING Follow the jeep road's overgrown tracks west up along creekside meadows to meet gravel Forest Service Road 1N93 (239.9–7,928') at a PCT marker. A sign here announces MISSION SPRINGS TRAIL CAMP, which is merely a pleasant flat spot with fire rings, south of North Fork Mission Creek.

FIRE The Lake Fire in 2015 burned 32,000 acres and led to the closure of the PCT between Mission Creek and Onyx Summit near Big Bear. San Bernardino National Forest officials reopened the trail in late 2016, but hikers should use caution throughout this area in years to come due to sustained hazards that may include loose soil and rocks, unstable terrain, and flash flooding. Check pcta.org or visit the San Bernardino National Forest website at fs.usda.gov/sbnf for updates.

PCT tread resumes here, starting north from FS 1N93 on a well-graded trail in an open stand of pines. The route rounds northeast, with some fine backward glimpses of subalpine Ten Thousand Foot Ridge in San Gorgonio Wilderness. Soon you reach a sandy gap and cross FS 1N05 (240.6–8,235'). Now you have some fine views northwest to rounded Sugarloaf Mountain and its smaller western sibling, Sugarlump. Next on your agenda is a level traverse, first north then southeast, in fire-ravaged

forest on the north side of the divide separating the Santa Ana River and the Whitewater River drainages. Eventually the trail dips easily to a post-marked crossing of FS 1N05 (241.4–8,118') at a saddle. Now, the easy route leads east under a forested summit, and you have panoramas northwest to Sugarloaf Mountain.

The PCT then heads north, contouring at first, then making a sustained moderate ascent through a patchy woodland of blackened needleless pines, mountain mahogany, foothigh manzanita, and scraggly white fir. Vistas gradually unfold southwest over to San Gorgonio Peak and Ten Thousand Foot Ridge and west down Heart Bar Creek to Big Meadows and the popular Barton Flats camp area. Bending northwest, the path soon levels out atop the long west ridge of Peak 8,828, and then it swings east into mixed conifer forest lying north of that summit.

PLANTS For a few minutes the PCT skirts across white, granular Furnace marble, and the surrounding vegetation also changes markedly: edaphic effects (see "Biology" in chapter 3, page 48) allow only hardy whitebark pines and junipers—the former normally found in higher, colder climes—to muster a scattered occupation of the crumbly slopes.

Rounding to the east of Peak 8,828, you descend gently to a ridgetop and join an unpaved road (244.7–8,490'), where you will enjoy good views southeast over North Fork Mission Creek to the San Jacinto Mountains and the Coachella Valley.

You continue east down the poor dirt road to a road junction located on the ridge east of Peak 8,588. From here the PCT continues east along the ridgeline. The route soon crosses onto north slopes, becomes a trail, and drops gently around Peak 8,751 to Coon Creek Jumpoff—a spectacular, steep granitic defile at the head of a tributary of North Fork Mission Creek.

GEOLOGY The steep wall here points to rapid erosion east of the

Jumpoff and illustrates the process of stream capture. The small stream draining the Tayles Hidden Acres basin to the northeast used to connect with Coon Creek, to the west, but accelerated headward erosion of Mission Creek at the Jumpoff has intercepted that stream. Its waters now flow southeast, eventually to the Salton Sea, rather than west to the Santa Ana River and the Pacific Ocean.

CAMPING From this thought-provoking overlook, the trail climbs easily for a moment to Coon Creek Road 1N02 (246.4–8,089'). Reservations-only Coon Creek Cabin Group Camp, with tent camping, parking, and toilets, but no water, is just to the east.

The way now attacks—via moderate switchbacks through scattered pines, firs, and montane chaparral—the south slopes of the ridge dividing Coon and Cienega Creeks.

VIEWS Extensive views compensate for the climb. Seasonally snowy Grinnell and San Gorgonio Mountains loom in the southwest, Mounts Baldy and Baden–Powell mark your upcoming travels west, and glimpses of the Santa Rosa Mountains and Palm Springs shimmer in the southeast.

Rounding north of a hillock covered with conifers and alive with mountain bluebirds, Clark's nutcrackers, white-headed woodpeckers, and dark-eyed juncos, you strike a trail that cuts perpendicularly across your route and meets a jeep road immediately east of your trail. The PCT continues ascending 0.3 mile, passing under small granitic cliffs before reaching a viewless, forested ridgetop. This 8,750-foot point is the highest spot your trail reaches in the San Bernardino Mountains.

Now the way drops sandily on a gentle gradient to cross a dirt road, then switchbacks down into a canyon, the path flanked by tall mountain-mahogany shrubs. At the mouth of a gully in the canyon bottom, you cross a jeep road, and then the PCT momentarily parallels its northward course before routing itself onto this road. Private land in this area prevents the U.S. Forest Service from constructing PCT tread, so you continue north on the jeep road. Soon the jeep road yields to a better dirt road (249.3–8,387'), which you trace north downcanyon to a five-way junction—four roads and a trail—located beside often-dry Cienega Creek. In another mile you will reach Predators in Action, a sort-of home for exotic animals trained to perform for movies and television. Hikers who have yet to come upon a wild cougar or bear during their trek may have a chance to see them here, though there will be comforting—if perhaps off-putting—chain-link cages separating them.

From the five-way junction, the PCT rises north, out of lodgepole pine into stands of juniper and mountain mahogany, then descends west along a dirt road 130 yards to a junction (251.0–8,395'). From here, the trail picks up again to contour the west slope of Onyx Peak over to a dirt road (252.1–8,531') that is just east of CA 38 and Onyx Summit.

The PCT crosses the road and climbs gently to moderately above FS 1N01, gaining increasingly good views of Baldwin Lake and Gold Mountain, in the northwest. Presently the path levels; crosses FS 1N01 (253.2–8,636'); and then descends, first north then west, below a ridge. Lower, the well-marked route crosses

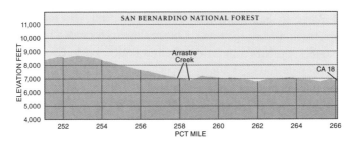

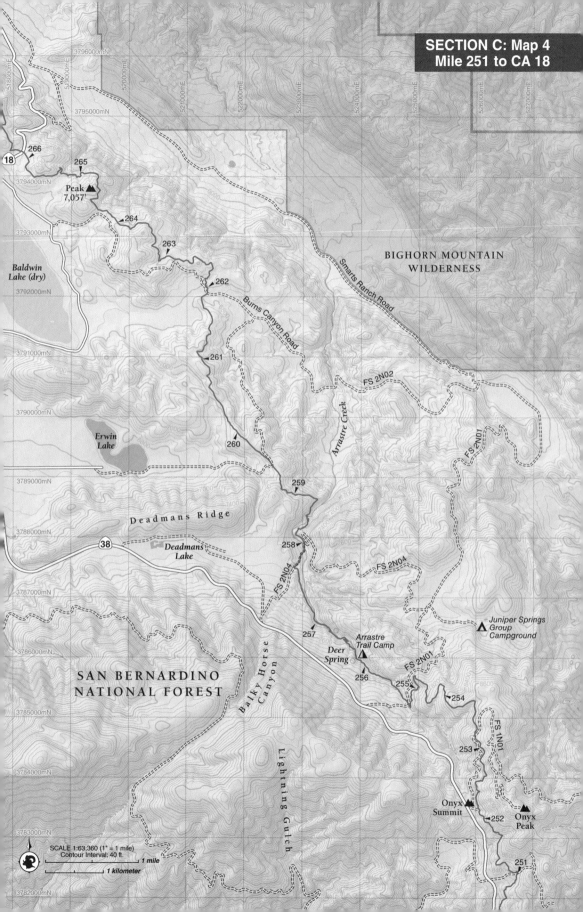

BIGHORN MOUNTAIN
WILDERNESS

Smarts Ranch Road

Burns Canyon Road

Arrastre Creek

FS 2N02

FS 2N01

Baldwin
Lake (dry)

266

18

265

Peak
7,057'

264

263

262

261

Erwin
Lake

260

259

258

Deadmans Ridge

38

Deadmans
Lake

FS 2N04

FS 2N04

FS 2N01

257

Deer
Spring

Arrastre
Trail Camp

256

255

254

Juniper Springs
Group
Campground

SAN BERNARDINO
NATIONAL FOREST

Balky Horse Canyon

Lightning Gulch

253

FS 1N01

Onyx
Summit

252

Onyx
Peak

251

SCALE 1:63,360 (1" = 1 mile)
Contour Interval; 40 ft.

1 mile

1 kilometer

a jeep road twice in quick succession before a switchback drops the trail to Broom Flat Road 2N01 (255.3–7,899'), a good dirt road running alongside shaded Arrastre Creek.

CAMPING Now you enter fragrant white fir groves to descend easily northwest along the seasonal creek and soon find Arrastre Trail Camp at Deer Spring (256.2–7,605'). This area has tent sites, a picnic table, log benches, and a faucet that has proven to be unreliable in recent years.

WATER ACCESS

Tank up at the spring 0.5 mile north of the camp (256.7–7,456'), if possible, as your next water source is 12 miles away at Doble Trail Camp.

Two minutes onward, you turn north at a junction with a jeep road (2N04) that leads to Balky Horse Canyon. The route continues down Arrastre Canyon to Balky Horse Canyon and crosses FS 2N04.

PLANTS The subtle changes in vegetation that have occurred on the descent into this region are influenced more by the Mojave Desert's parching winds than by moisture-laden ocean breezes.

Minutes later, you reach wooden berms that lead under Camp Oakes' rifle range, and then you climb gently across Saragossa quartzite in a true high-desert plant community: pinyon pines, buckwheat, and ephedra, a shiny yellow-green shrub with wiry stems called Mormon tea—after its use by Mormon pioneers. Atop a 7,240-foot shoulder, you gaze east and see gold mines near Tip Top Mountain's summit, as well as a high-desert woodland of Joshua trees and pinyon pines.

Now paralleling an expansive, desertlike ridge, the PCT crosses two jeep roads and first gives you views west over seasonal Erwin Lake and east to the Mojave, then later views

west to large, shallow, sometimes completely dry Baldwin Lake. Eventually the sandy path descends to cross FS 2N02 (261.9–6,782') amid pinyon pines, Joshua trees, and sagebrush. From that road the PCT climbs north, then contours northwest for alternating vistas of desert and mountain as it wanders among pinyon pines and crosses the Doble Fault just northeast of Peak 7,057.

GEOLOGY Here the rock underfoot abruptly changes from banded Precambrian gneiss to whitish Paleozoic quartzite. The Helendale Fault, stretching from north of Victorville southeast to Tip Top Mountain, runs parallel to Nelson Ridge, lying below you to the northeast.

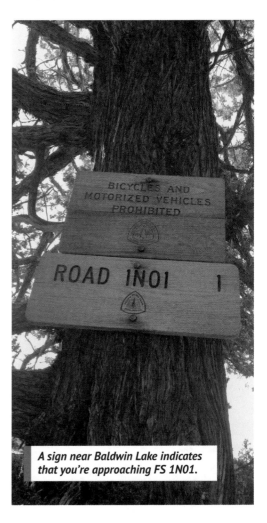

A sign near Baldwin Lake indicates that you're approaching FS 1N01.

Presently, with fleeting glimpses of Baldwin Lake, you descend to meet CA 18 (266.1–6,830') and a large dirt parking lot, just yards west of some interesting mining prospects.

RESUPPLY ACCESS

Head 5.4 miles southwest on CA 18 to reach Big Bear City, which has a small grocery store, restaurants, and motels.

North of the highway, find the trail angling left of a metal gate across a jeep road at the edge of a small pinyon forest, west of a bulldozed-bare slope. The PCT next switchbacks to cross the jeep road and then contours north of Nelson Ridge before angling west down through a dense stand of pinyon pines to meet paved Holcomb Valley Road just south of the county dump. West across Holcomb Valley Road the trail curves and contours south across three jeep tracks in sagebrush and rabbitbrush, affording good views of Baldwin Lake's playa surface beyond the ruins of Doble.

HISTORY Baldwin Lake is named for Elias J. "Lucky" Baldwin, owner of the prosperous Doble Gold Mine, located high on the slopes above you.

CAMPING The PCT contours low on Gold Mountain and soon reaches a short, indistinct, and unsigned spur trail (268.6–6,902') down to signed Doble Trail Camp. Look for the first lush patch of rushes and iris under scattered pinyons and junipers to mark the junction. The camp has a pit toilet, a corral, a horse trough, and two faucets of varying reliability.

On the PCT, you make a gentle ascent in scrubby vegetation, crossing two jeep roads and making three switchbacks to gain a saddle on the northeast ridge of Gold Mountain. Here you leave pinyon pines behind for incense cedars, Jeffrey pines, and junipers. A gentle traverse around Gold Mountain's northern flanks bisects a jeep road and offers vistas over Arrastre and Union Flats, scenes of the fevered Holcomb Valley mining excitement in the 1860s.

HISTORY This gold rush began when William F. Holcomb discovered flecks of placer gold at the head of Van Dusen Canyon, 1 mile west of Arrastre Flat. Hired by other prospectors for his ability with a rifle, Holcomb and a companion trailed a wounded grizzly bear north from Poligue Canyon. Holcomb's experience prospecting in the mines of the Sierra Nevada's mother lode paid off when his bear-tracking led to the alluvial flats on Caribou Creek. Soon the sagebrush- and pine-dotted basin swarmed with prospectors, and a camp named Belleville was erected.

History records that this settlement was one of the least law-abiding of the California gold camps—more than 40 men died by hanging or gun battles. Causes for argument included not only the usual charges of claim-jumping and theft but also political affiliations in the Civil War. Southern sympathizers were particularly numerous, as they had been forcibly ejected from many pro-Northern mining camps in the mother lode. Although the site of fevered and hectic activity for almost a decade, Holcomb Valley was relieved of most of its readily accessible placer gold by 1870, and its inhabitants moved on to greener pastures. Belleville was soon a ghost town. Interest in the region revived, however, when hard-rock mines opened to seek the local mother lode—the source of the Holcomb Valley placer gold. Soon shafts and their adjunct tailings dotted the land. Lucky Baldwin's Doble Mine was one of these, but, like the other hard-rock mines, it failed to locate the mother lode, and it is doubtful that Baldwin recouped his $6 million purchase price for the mine.

The PCT veers south along Gold Mountain's flanks to strike one jeep road, then a second (272.7–7,688'), which leads north 0.7 mile to Saragossa Spring. About 0.25 mile beyond the next small rise, you cross a better road, then

SECTION C

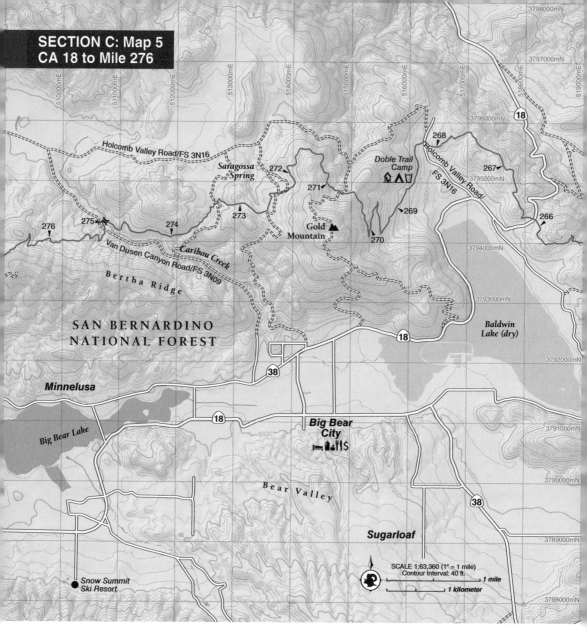

Holcomb Valley Road/FS 3N16

Saragossa Spring

272

Doble Trail Camp

268

267

266

271

269

273

Gold Mountain

270

275

274

276

Van Dusen Canyon Road/FS 3N09

Caribou Creek

Bertha Ridge

Holcomb Valley Road/ FS 3N16

Baldwin Lake (dry)

SAN BERNARDINO NATIONAL FOREST

18

38

Minnelusa

18

Big Bear City

Big Bear Lake

Bear Valley

38

Sugarloaf

Snow Summit Ski Resort

SCALE 1:63,360 (1" = 1 mile)
Contour Interval: 40 ft.

1 mile

1 kilometer

---

turn southwest down to a tributary of Caribou Creek, dotted with mining ruins.

WATER ACCESS

A mile-long contour then leads to Caribou Creek itself (274.9–7,257'), which rarely flows later than early June. The next water for northbound PCT hikers is not until Little Bear Spring Trail Camp, 10.7 miles away.

Just 0.1 mile beyond Caribou Creek the trail bisects Van Dusen Canyon Road 3N09 (275.1–7,264'), which leads southeast 2.8 miles to Big Bear City.

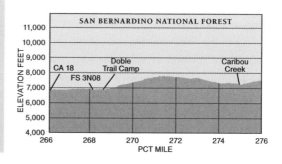

SAN BERNARDINO NATIONAL FOREST

ELEVATION FEET

11,000
10,000
9,000
8,000
7,000
6,000
5,000
4,000

CA 18

FS 3N08

Doble Trail Camp

Caribou Creek

266   268   270   272   274   276
PCT MILE

RESUPPLY ACCESS

Big Bear City, the best resupply town in this section, is closest from this point.

More mountain mahogany, Jeffrey pines, and junipers shade the PCT as you leave Van Dusen Canyon, crossing numerous jeep tracks as you make a gentle ascent west under Bertha Ridge. Finally, a switchback leads to a saddle north of Bertha Peak, where you cross a jeep road, then another, leading to the summit, in excellent exposures of marble. West of the second road, sweeping vistas open up to the south across dammed Big Bear Lake to Moonridge and to the high summits of the San Gorgonio Wilderness. Just beyond these vistas, the PCT meets the Cougar Crest Trail 1E22 (277.7–7,674').

RESUPPLY ACCESS

This enjoyable path starts west, then heads south 2.7 miles to CA 38, near the ranger-staffed Big Bear Discovery Center and Serrano Campground on the north shore of Big Bear Lake—a convenient place from which to hitchhike either west to Fawnskin, with its limited supplies, or east to Big Bear, with more complete provisions.

The PCT recrosses the last jeep road midway down to wide Polique Canyon Road 2N09 (278.6–7,550').

RESUPPLY ACCESS

From here travelers can head 3.7 miles to Fawnskin for supplies by first walking south along the dirt road, which descends Polique Canyon to reach CA 38 beside Big Bear Lake, then walking west along the highway.

From Polique Canyon Road the PCT continues its traverse of the San Bernardino Mountains' spine by continuing west, easily up along the south side of Delamar Mountain's east ridge.

SECTION C

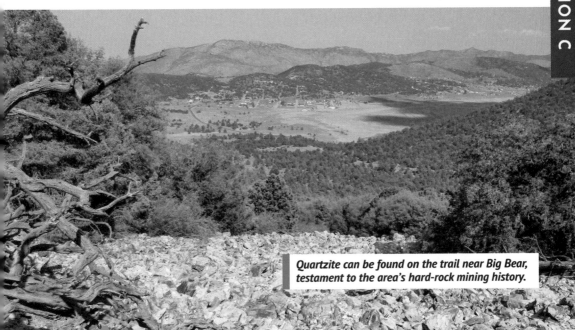

Quartzite can be found on the trail near Big Bear, testament to the area's hard-rock mining history.

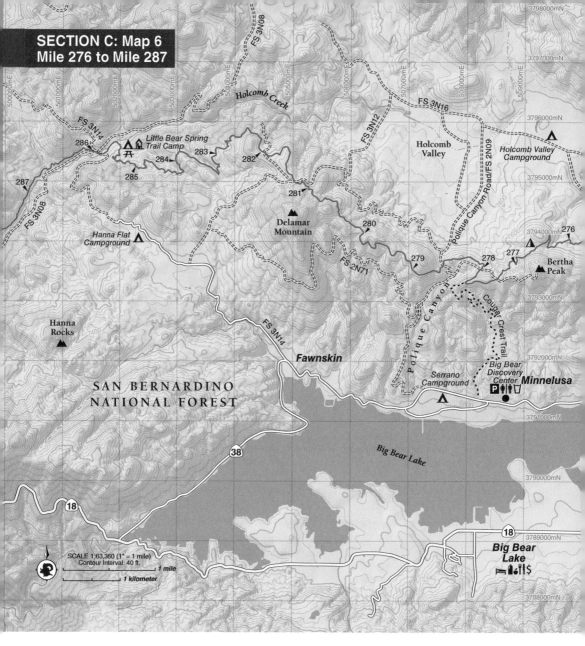

Holcomb Creek

FS 3N16

FS 3N14

286

Little Bear Spring
Trail Camp

283

284

282

285

287

FS 3N08

281

Holcomb
Valley

Holcomb Valley
Campground

280

Delamar
Mountain

Hanna Flat
Campground

FS 2N71

279

278

277

276

Bertha
Peak

Cougar Crest Trail

Hanna
Rocks

FS 3N14

Fawnskin

Big Bear
Discovery
Center

Minnelusa

Serrano
Campground

**SAN BERNARDINO
NATIONAL FOREST**

Big Bear Lake

38

18

18

**Big Bear
Lake**

SCALE 1:63,360 (1" = 1 mile)
Contour Interval: 40 ft.

1 mile

1 kilometer

Unfortunately, several wildfires have swept through here in recent years, and the damage is evident. Charred oaks and bare hillsides mark much of this stretch, which ends after a long mile when the route crosses to the shadier north side of the ridge to pass an east-ascending jeep track, then descends to FS 3N12, atop a saddle.

The PCT contours north from FS 3N12, then arcs west around a nose covered with mountain mahogany before crossing another good dirt road. Dropping gently, the trail rounds north on a steep hillside with vistas east over Holcomb Valley but soon turns southwest and eventually strikes a jeep road, which you follow downhill 35 yards before resuming trail tread. Another 0.3

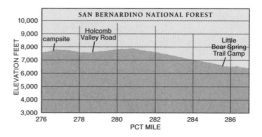

SAN BERNARDINO NATIONAL FOREST

campsite

Holcomb
Valley Road

Little
Bear Spring
Trail Camp

ELEVATION FEET

PCT MILE

mile of descent leads into a small canyon, then northwest along its south wall, then into another, similar canyon, now just below a dirt road.

CAMPING Later, near the bottom of Holcomb Creek's wide canyon, the route switchbacks, crosses one poor dirt road, then another, and immediately reaches Little Bear Spring Trail Camp (285.6–6,577').

WATER ACCESS

Little Bear Spring Trail Camp has a corral, an open-air outhouse (essentially a plastic toilet surrounded by a low wall), a table, and a spring-fed trough and faucet, though you may find it dry by midsummer. If it's available, southbound hikers should tank up here, as the next seasonal water is 10.7 miles away, at Caribou Creek in Van Dusen Canyon.

Most wilderness lovers will likely not spend the night at this poorly sited campground, which is a haven for buzzing motocross enthusiasts, though good camping can be found across the creek from the main camping area. Many PCT-ers prefer to sack out farther down Holcomb Creek, choosing a site at least 200 feet from the water and trail.

From the trail camp the PCT turns northwest down a creek's mouth to quickly reach the willow-lined, sagebrush-dotted banks of year-round Holcomb Creek. The trail follows its south bank, crossing a jeep road leading to the trail camp, then parallels the lower shoulder of Coxey Road 3N14 as it descends west a few yards to cross Holcomb Creek (285.9–6,502').

The PCT resumes above Holcomb Creek's north bank, 35 yards up Coxey Road, and proceeds gently downcanyon in an open ponderosa pine forest still recovering from wildfires,

staying just above canyon-bottom FS 3N93, a dirt road that is repeatedly drowned under beaver-dammed pools. The trail passes two dirt roads and a jeep track, and then about 0.5 mile later it turns west up a side canyon, climbing moderately to a saddle. From it a gentle descent southwest in warm groves of conifers and black oaks leads across a dirt road, beyond which the route follows a sunny, rock-dotted divide north of Holcomb Creek. Drier conditions prevail as the easy descent continues, eventually leading to a rock-hop crossing of the Cienega Larga fork of Holcomb Creek. From it the trail parallels some 50 feet above shaded, bouldery Holcomb Creek, soon passing some nice campsites and dropping to cross it via boulders. Moments later the streamside canopy of willows and cottonwoods opens where wide Crab Flats Road 3N16 (292.2–5,469') meets rough FS 3N93.

The PCT now continues on Holcomb Creek's south bank, via very rocky tread under white alders.

FIRE Wildfires have swept through this area several times in the last two decades, and the damage is still evident. Expect scarred hillsides and skeletal forests, interspersed with streamside vegetation and thorny brush encroachment. Be sure to check pcta.org or with the San Bernardino National Forest before proceeding.

CAMPING Pushing on, you soon enter a sandy flat with adequate campsites (293.2–5,331') and again cross Holcomb Creek.

The trail now winds northwest above it in a dry chaparral of mountain mahogany, buckwheat, and yellow, fleshy-petaled flannelbush. Turning more to the west, the way drops once again alongside Holcomb Creek, traverses the perimeter of a bouldery sand flat with a good camp, and then crosses the permanent Cienega Redonda fork of Holcomb Creek to find the north-branching Cienega Redonda equestrian trail.

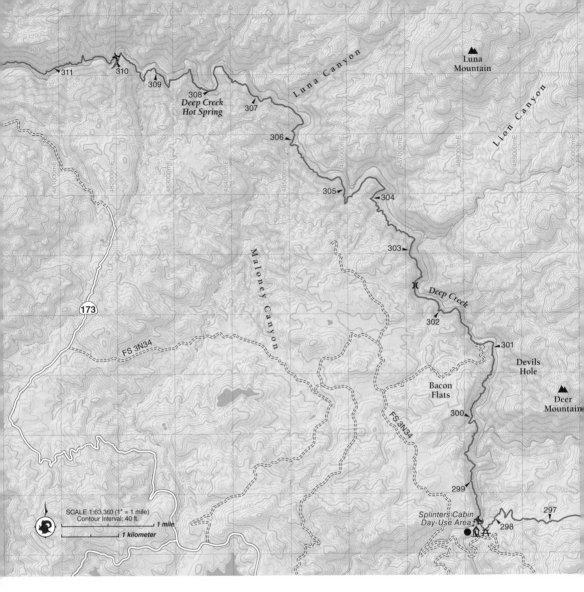

CAMPING Many horned lizards might appear as the trail continues its gentle descent west on rotting granitic rock along Holcomb Creek and soon enters a grassy flat to reach Holcomb Crossing Trail Camp (294.1–5,215'), with fire pits and several large Jeffrey pines.

Minutes later, on a sidehill traverse, you pass the enormously rutted Crab Flats Trail, which has been heavily abused by motocross riders.

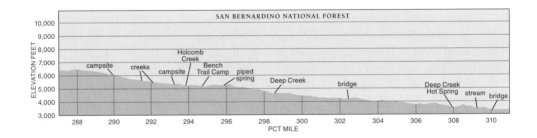

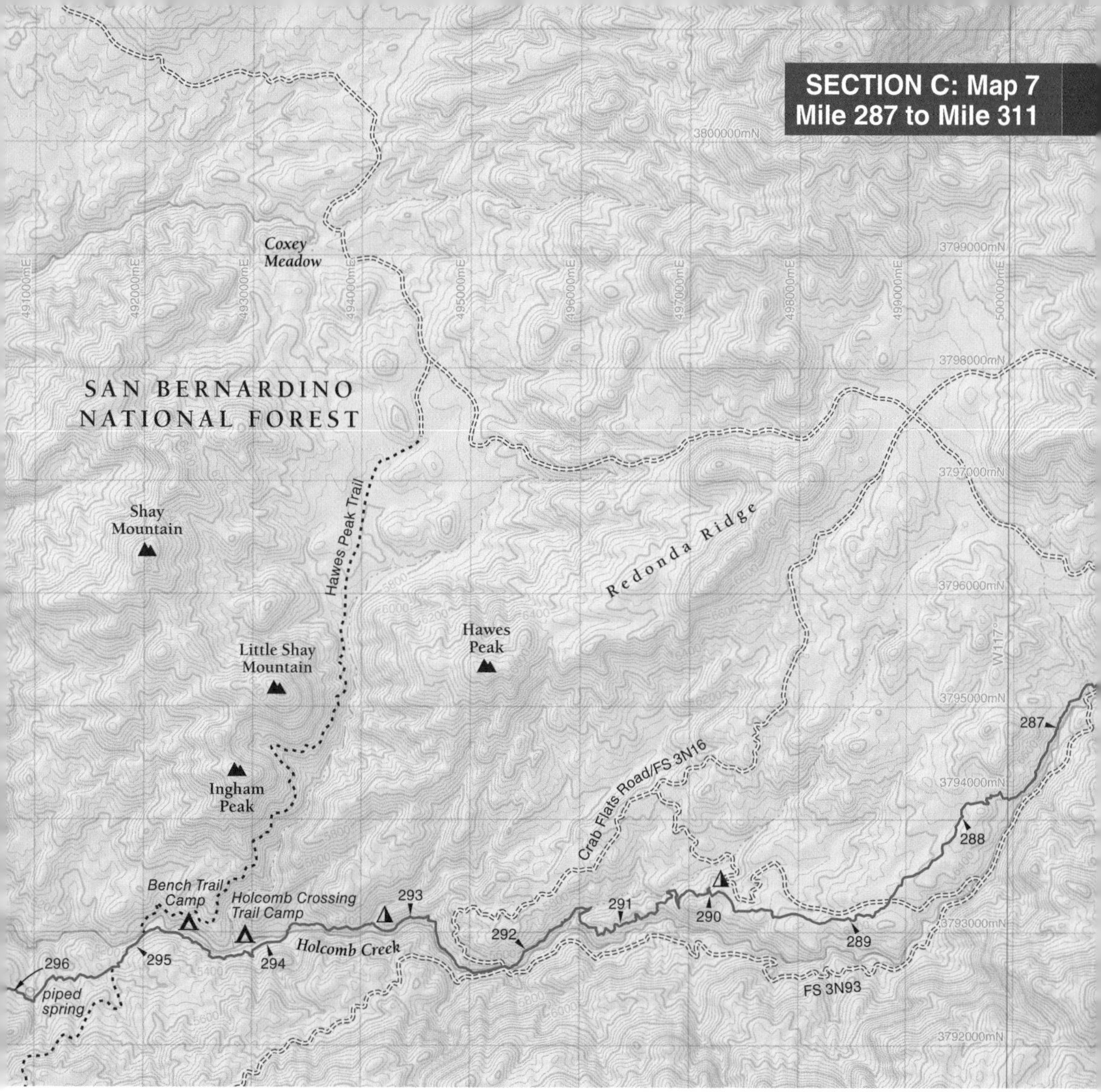

Coxey
Meadow

SAN BERNARDINO
NATIONAL FOREST

Shay
Mountain

Hawes Peak Trail

Redonda Ridge

Little Shay
Mountain

Hawes
Peak

Ingham
Peak

287

288

Crab Flats Road/FS 3N16

Bench Trail
Camp

Holcomb Crossing
Trail Camp

293

296   295   294

291   290

292

289

Holcomb Creek

FS 3N93

piped
spring

| CAMPING | Nearing the alder- and cedar-shaded banks of Holcomb Creek once again, you pass less appealing, signed Bench Trail Camp (294.7–5,185').

Soon after, you approach a junction with the Hawes Peak Trail (294.9–5,158'), just shy of the PCT's bouldery fourth ford of Holcomb Creek. The trail ascends onto hillsides still recovering from wildfires. In a mile the trail begins to descend and eventually heads northwest, dropping via four oak-shaded switchbacks to a beautiful 90-foot steel and wood bridge (298.5–4,581') spanning Deep Creek, where no camping is allowed. Here the stream drops between large granitic boulders and harbors a good population of rainbow trout. Note that all of Deep Creek is a Wild Trout Area (with a two-fish daily limit, minimum 8 inches each, no bait allowed, and barbless hooks required).

RESUPPLY ACCESS

Just beyond the bridge, a signed trail briefly strikes left and back upstream to cross diminutive Bear Creek and hit the end of dirt Hook Creek Road 3N34C.

The busy trailhead, called Splinters Cabin, has toilets, tables, and a shady ramada—a perfect lunch spot while waiting for a ride up to Lake Arrowhead. Hook Creek Road leads upcanyon (west) 0.5 mile to cross FS 3N34, then later becomes paved and designated 2N26Y, climbing 3.5 miles total past numerous homes and cabins to Lake Arrowhead. There you find the Cedar Glen Post Office and supermarkets just before meeting CA 173 near the lakeshore.

After crossing Deep Creek the PCT briefly climbs northeast, then contours under live oaks and near crumbling granitic parapets. After 0.5 mile the path descends gently, matching the gradient of Deep Creek, which is flanked by spruces and pines 140 feet below. The way presently becomes hot and exposed near ocean spray and hollyleaf cherry, and many will wonder why the trail wasn't routed lower, along the cool streamside. Soon you get your answer, in the form of steep bluffs, above which the PCT must skirt. Later, the route bends west and strikes unpaved Bacon Flats Road 3N20 (301.3–4,263'), just above the popular Devils Hole fishing area. It offers the last chance to head out to Lake Arrowhead to resupply.

Across Bacon Flats Road the PCT winds along the canyon walls, well above quietly flowing Deep Creek and its streamside willows, cottonwoods, and alders. Though sometimes shaded by steep, granitic bluffs, your route soon becomes more exposed to sun and seasonally stifling heat.

WILDLIFE Your proximity to the Mojave Desert is reflected in both the shimmering heat and in the flora and fauna. Coarse chamise chaparral, harboring flitting phainopeplas and somnolent horned lizards, lines your way, while scurrying insects and pursuant roadrunners share your sandy path. Rattlesnakes are also seen, although not in the heat of day—their cold-blooded metabolism cannot stand extreme ground temperatures, but they love to bask when shadows are long.

Soon after passing a streamside terrace, your undulating descent alters its northwestward course to a more westward one. Shortly thereafter, it passes a jeep road that rolls 0.5 mile east to Warm Spring, and then it drops 0.25 mile south to Deep Creek Hot Spring (307.9–3,522'), which is situated on a prominent northeast–southwest fault. The hot spring, with its bubbling water, high-diving rocks, and warm sunbathing, is a popular and crowded spot at almost any time of the year. Unfortunately, human waste, graffiti, and trash left by careless day-trippers have marred the area. You might be tempted to carry out some of the water bottles and beer cans.

TRAIL INFO Trail-dusty would-be swimmers should heed this caution: a very rare, microscopic amoeba living in the hot water has caused deadly amoebic meningoencephalitis by invading swimmers' bodies through their noses. Swimming may cut your hike short! Also be advised that camping is not allowed in this area, and rangers patrol the trail frequently.

Taking leave of the skinny-dippers, you eventually cross Deep Creek via an arched bridge (310.0–3,318') and then start a traverse west along the almost barren north wall of Deep Creek canyon, pocked with graffiti, tracing the route of an old aqueduct. This walk ends at the spillway of the Mojave Forks Dam (313.0–3,135').

HISTORY Standing in the maw of the spillway, you find a small exhibit that describes efforts to save the endangered arroyo southwestern toad. You are also in the vicinity of an old Mojave Indian village called Atongai. It was visited by Padre Garces, a member of Juan Bautista de Anza's expeditions, in 1776. A mission was built hereabouts in 1819.

The designated route from atop the dam actually drops southwest back to the foot of the dam, on flats beside Deep Creek, but an overgrowth of brush, fields of nettle and foxtails, and a welter of dirt-bike paths have essentially obliterated the way. Instead, cross the spillway, then turn up to the crest of the dam at a paved spur. Now proceed left, in a westward arc across the top of the boulder-faced dam, treading a one-lane paved road. The dam ends on the eastern shoulder of Hill 3,353 at a road junction, close beside a small concrete building with a tall radio mast.

ALTERNATE ROUTE AND RESUPPLY ACCESS

In wet years, the trail below the dam may flood, and crossing the creek can be difficult. In this case, hikers may opt to walk west on the paved road, swinging north around Hill 3,353 and then across the top of another dam segment, eventually reaching busy, two-lane, paved Arrowhead Lake Road.

To reach Hesperia and its amenities from this point, walk north about 6 miles. Hesperia Lake Park is found on the right in just 2.8 miles, offering cool, shady camping beside a small lake, with showers and a small convenience store. For more information, visit hesperiaparks.com/hesperia-lake -park or call 760-244-5951.

To return to the trail, turn left (south) and follow Arrowhead Lake Road to CA 173. Turn left again, follow the highway briefly to its paved end, and look for metal PCT signs marking the trail on either side of the road.

From the western end of Mojave Forks Dam, the PCT turns left (southeast) from atop the dam's paved road, dropping moderately down a gravel road that traces the edge of the dam's face. Paralleling the gravel road is a row of 4- to 5-foot-high posts that mark theoretical depths of the reservoir, should it experience a flood of biblical proportions. At the base of the dam, a 10-foot-tall, white-metal depth marker indicates the point where the now more visible original PCT route joins levelly from the left (east). Turn right (southwest) on the sandy trail, and in just a moment plunge through a phalanx of willows to a usually shallow but wide and rocky ford to the south side of Deep Creek. Now scramble up a sandy bank to a low alluvial terrace, just west of the mouth of a small, rocky canyon. Here the trail—an old jeep track—becomes more distinct. Trace it west above a fringe of baccharis and willows before dropping again to the creekside. Here, Deep Creek is sucked north through the dam, down a massive, iron-gated outlet tunnel.

From here, you're back on a trail that winds west in a thicket of willows and cottonwoods that show evidence of beaver cuttings. These trees are just south of another sandy arroyo, this one draining ephemeral West Fork Mojave River. Presently you cross the base of a narrow ravine, where your trail begins to trace the grade of an abandoned, torn-up paved road. This is followed moderately uphill, and soon you level out on a terrace to strike a wide turnout on a curve of CA 173 (314.3–3,127').

Across CA 173, pick up the signed PCT and follow it almost levelly south across a swath of land that may still show signs of damage from the 2016 Pilot Fire, which burned more than 8,000 acres between Deep Creek and Silverwood Lake State Recreation Area. After a bit, the path

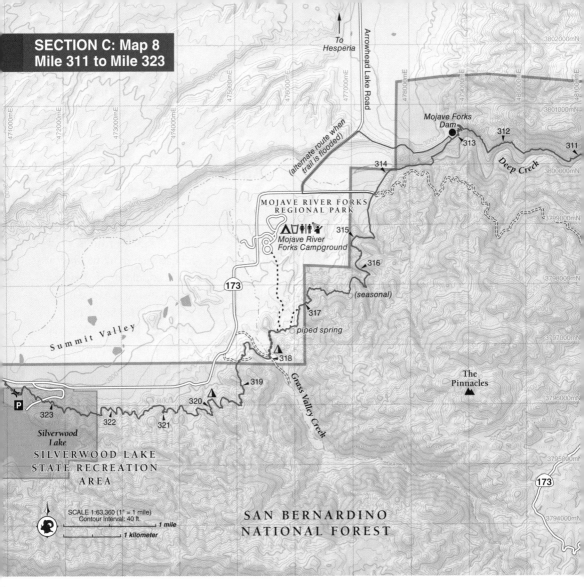

begins an easy, sandy ascent, soon striking the end of a little-used jeep road. Follow the signed PCT marker south along the boulder-lined path past a seasonal rock-framed waterfall, as the path climbs briefly south into a small canyon, then ascends around several ridges on a winding course to the south, soon leveling in the process to undulate at about 3,500 feet.

Just after heading around a north-dropping ridge, you reach a small canyon that spawns a trailside spring (316.6–3,482'), which sometimes offers water in early spring but cannot be relied upon and has been choked by poison oak in recent years.

CAMPING Just past the spring is a turnoff for Mojave River Forks Regional Park (317.6–3,371'), which sits 0.75 mile off the trail and has campsites, bathrooms, and hot showers. Information: 17891 CA 173, Hesperia, CA 92345; 760-389-2322; parks.sbcounty .gov/park/mojave-river-forks-regional-park.

Turning more to the west, the route travels hillsides ravaged by fire but clothed intermittently with low chaparral of chamise, buckwheat,

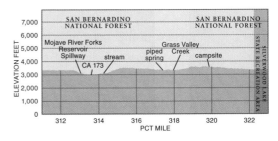

and flannelbush, with panoramas northwest over the expanse of Summit Valley to the aberrant alluvial scarp forming its northern limit.

GEOLOGY This long, steep-faced ridge is actually the upslope edge of an early Pleistocene alluvial fan, whose sediments originally came from canyons of the San Gabriel Mountains, seen far to the west. However, subsequent right-lateral movement along the San Andreas Fault displaced the range northwest, thereby cutting off the source of the sediments. Continuing lateral and vertical movement along the San Andreas Fault and associated parallel faults not only altered the landscape but also brought about drastic changes in the stream-drainage pattern.

The PCT drops slightly as it winds south into a broad valley, then climbs to a ridgetop saddle where it joins a jeep road (317.7–3,411') serving a power line.

WATER ACCESS

CAMPING This jeep road travels south to an easy ford of Grass Valley Creek (318.0–3,331'), which flows most summers but is often dry by fall. Camping is nearby.

The trail resumes just across the stream, on the jeep road's left (east) side and momentarily crosses a second, poor jeep track before climbing northwest. Around a nose, the trail hairpins south across another steep jeep road, then undulates interminably west in and out of gullies and ravines in shadeless chaparral. About halfway to Silverwood Lake, you come to a flat area where an ascending jeep road from CA 173 seems to terminate upon reaching the PCT (321.3–3,474').

You continue winding almost levelly west. Eventually the way strikes FS 2N33, a paved road ascending west to the nearby east end of Cedar Springs Dam. Walking a few minutes up to that end will give you vistas over giant Silverwood Lake, which is part of the California Aqueduct system. From FS 2N33 the PCT descends steeply, then turns south around a sharp ridge and joins a west-branching dirt road close under the base of 249-foot-high, rock-filled Cedar Springs Dam.

TRAIL INFO PCT travelers lacking a fast mode of transportation might

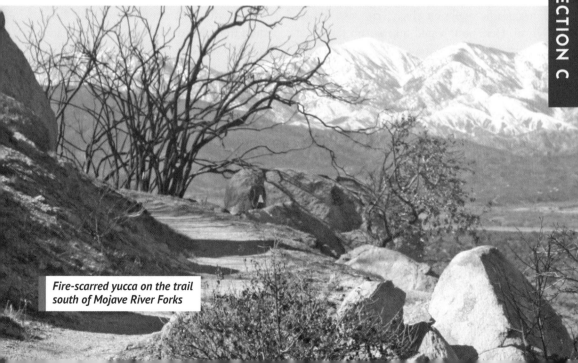

Fire-scarred yucca on the trail south of Mojave River Forks

SECTION C

be less than enthused to learn that the active Cleghorn Mountain Fault lies not far south of the dam site: the reservoir's northern east–west arms lie along the fault.

Now, possibly with a brisker stride, you turn west down the dirt road a few yards to the end of a poorly paved road that bridges the canyon bottom and continues northwest to some dam-maintenance facilities. Follow the poor road left, gently up onto a sandy flat, to a paved road just east of the large maintenance sheds. Turn right (north) along that short road's west shoulder, through a hurricane fence and out to two-lane paved CA 173 (323.8–3,166') at a line of junipers. Now walk left (west) on the highway shoulder, crossing a bridge that straddles the concrete spillway flume of Cedar Springs Dam. In a pinch, water can be had from the algae-ridden pools below the dam, but filtering is strongly advised. Pass dirt Las Flores Ranch Road and an access road to the Mojave Siphon Power Plant to reach a dirt road angling southwest (324.4–3,201'), up the brushy hillside. Here the PCT's trail tread resumes, climbing parallel to the dirt road, which is immediately above it.

Entering Silverwood Lake State Recreation Area, the PCT continues below the road for a bit, then crosses it and switchbacks southeast to a nearby saddle, on which it crosses a similar road. Here northbound hikers gain their first vistas over windy Silverwood Lake. The warm water will likely prove irresistible to most, as the PCT route traverses near the reservoir's western shoreline. Twice you follow jeep roads 60 yards as the route winds through sparse chaparral, crossing many gullies. North of the westernmost arm of northern Silverwood Lake,

a meager spring wets the trail, and then the path meanders south before climbing moderately east above the Chamise Boat-In Picnic Area, which has covered picnic tables but lacks running water. Now 200 feet above the reservoir, you pass onto a hillside, and the trail bends south to an unsigned spur trail that drops south to another trail and to Garces Overlook—an octagonal hilltop gazebo—which makes a fine, albeit waterless, picnic spot.

TRAIL INFO Water-quality levels at Silverwood Lake vary throughout the year. If quality is poor, swimming is prohibited and warning signs are usually posted around the lake, but hikers are advised to check with rangers or visit parks.ca.gov for updated information. The park's main phone number is 760-389-2281.

Back on the PCT, you descend easily west across a jeep road and eventually come to a paved, two-lane bike path (328.7–3,392') next to a paved road leading east to unremarkable Cleghorn Picnic Area, which has water, tables, and bathrooms. This junction is not signed but is easy to spot, coming southbound on the PCT, if you look carefully: it is 80 yards east of where the infant, usually dry West Fork Mojave River passes under the bike path via a cattle grate. The trail leaves from a curve in the path that is farthest from the paved road to the picnic area. Heading toward Oregon on the PCT, walk southwest across the Mojave River's wash and slightly up to a signed junction with another paved bike path that leads west, toward the group-camp complex. Follow the path up to the paved entrance road of Silverwood Lake State Recreation Area (329.0–3,397').

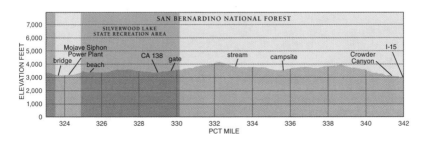

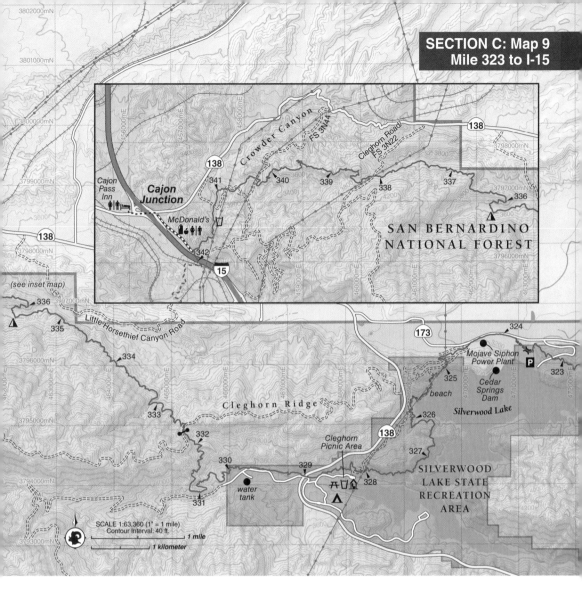

RESUPPLY ACCESS

This road may be traced south to the entrance station and then 1.7 miles east beyond it for camping, water, showers, telephones, and a small store and café at the reservoir's marina. PCT campers may stay in the Hike and Bike section for a reasonable $5 per night.

WATER ACCESS

Northbound hikers should note that the next certain water lies in lower Crowder Canyon, 12.6 miles west of the state recreation area, while, except for the reservoir, the next water for those southbound flows in Grass Valley Creek, 10.9 miles east.

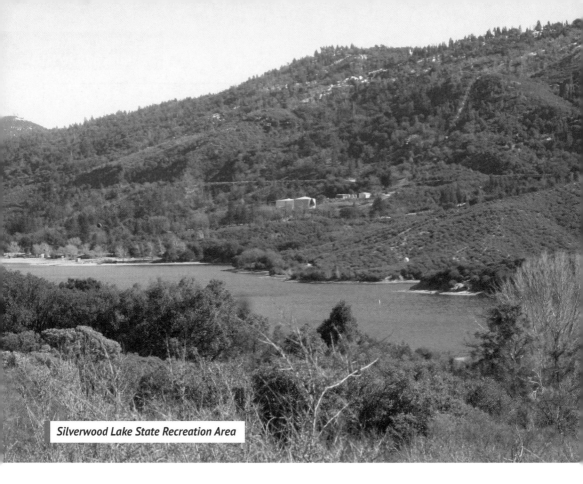

Silverwood Lake State Recreation Area

Continuing on the PCT route from the SRA entrance, you first walk west under the CA 138 overpass to its off-ramp. From here you may hitchhike southeast to Crestline for supplies at its post office and stores. Here, too, the trail resumes at the off-ramp's junction with the SRA's entrance road. PCT posts lead northwest from a concrete culvert across a small grassy field to five sycamores clustered against the northern hillside. Here tread becomes more distinct. The PCT leads gently upcanyon and then dips into West Fork Mojave River's sandy wash for a moment before crossing a dirt road that serves a small, seemingly abandoned picnic area (329.5–3,468'). From it the route continues up along the base of a canyon wall cloaked in chamise, buckwheat, and pungent yerba santa. The trail's tread is interrupted as you follow the paved group-camp access road 25 yards; then it resumes to strike a narrow paved road that climbs steeply to a water tank (with no access). Several group camps, including one equestrian group camp, lie just down this road, in Silverwood Lake State Recreation Area.

Now you leave the SRA and begin climbing in earnest, winding southwest up numerous dry gulches, then around an east-jutting nose, and finally turning north to join a jeep road (331.9–4,023') at a small promontory. Here the PCT turns west, following the track, which climbs moderately 0.3 mile to its junction with a road atop scenic Cleghorn Ridge.

GEOLOGY To the east you can see the Lake Arrowhead region, Miller Canyon, Silverwood Lake, and West Fork Mojave River, the last three aligned along the east–west Cleghorn Fault, which separates Mesozoic granitic rocks, found here, north of the fault, from older Precambrian metamorphic rocks south of the fault.

Resuming your trek, you follow the ridge road north 100 yards down to where the trail's tread resumes. The way descends moderately northwest across hillside gullies, presently reaching a deeper canyon with a small stream (333.1–3,829'), which usually flows through late spring. No camping is possible, however. The next leg winds northwest across numerous similar ravines while it contours above ranches in Little Horsethief Canyon.

HISTORY This canyon and Horsethief Canyon to its north commemorate Captain Gabriel Moraga's pursuit of an American Indian band whom he suspected of horse thievery in 1819. The first known crossing by Europeans of nearby Cajon Pass occurred in 1772, and this key pass was heavily used by the Mormon Battalion and Death Valley borax teams, the legendary Old West wagon trains that hauled borax between Death Valley and railheads to the south in the late 1800s.

Eventually the route drops into the canyon's head, where PCT posts show the way through a grassy flat. Your trail turns north across Little Horsethief Canyon's dry creekbed (335.6–3,587'), ignoring a use trail that continues upcanyon and then climbs again to a narrow ridgecrest, which you traverse in low, bedraggled chamise chaparral—an impoverished indicator of your proximity to the Mojave Desert. The Blue Cut Fire of 2016 charred and severely altered the landscape along the trail between here and Wrightwood. Be prepared for little shade.

The PCT then proceeds west up into another draw, and near its head strikes a road under a huge power-transmission line. You walk across Cleghorn Road 3N22, then west along a spur beneath a mammoth power pylon. Trail tread continues west from here, vaguely at first along a gravelly wash, then more obviously as it climbs to an overlook of spectacularly eroded badlands above Cajon Canyon.

GEOLOGY The Pliocene sediments here were eroded from the infant San Gabriel Mountains, then were shifted east, relatively speaking, along the San Andreas Fault, which now cuts through Cajon Canyon below. Because these sediments have been removed from their source, stream flow has easily carved their once gently sloping surfaces into a dramatic series of razorback ridges.

The path climbs to top the most spectacular of these ridges, then winds tortuously down, west, along it, giving you superb vistas of the San Gabriel Mountains' crown, Mount San Antonio, and Lytle Creek Ridge, which you will climb on the PCT in the next section. Presently you cross FS 3N44 (340.4–3,350'), and minutes later you pass through a burned gate on a saddle and then descend easily southwest. You quickly cross another road, from which well-marked trail tread resumes to lead west, momentarily passing under a power-transmission pylon to strike the previous descending dirt road (341.0–3,165'). Here the PCT turns left, south, down the road as it drops steeply into quiet Crowder Canyon.

There, just shy of a hop-across ford of sandy, always-flowing-a-little Crowder Canyon Creek, you end the descent at a post-marked merger with a better dirt road (341.3–3,150'), which goes briefly downcanyon to another power pylon.

A cluster of cottonwoods and baccharis, teeming with birds, at this three-way junction, once made this an ideal place to set up camp. Fire again lamentably altered the landscape in 2016, and there is little shade until you reach the rock walls of Crowder Canyon. This area still makes the best camp since Silverwood Lake, though there is little protection from the area's notorious winds. From the junction, you follow the PCT, which proceeds right (northwest), directly across the cress-decked creekbed, then leads 90 yards uphill across a buried gas pipeline to a PCT post, which marks the resumption of trail heading left (south) onto an alluvial bench.

WATER ACCESS

This still-pleasant path winds along the narrow, shady gorge of lower Crowder Canyon, where, on occasion, pools and trickles of water afford the last on-route water most likely until Lamel Spring, a long 33.7 miles away.

The trail ends abruptly at six-lane I-15 (342.0–2,995') in Cajon Canyon, just south of a road-end memorial to Santa Fe Trail pioneers.

RESUPPLY ACCESS

Just 0.5 mile northwest up the access road to the trail's terminus, 0.1 mile before the CA 138 cloverleaf, is a Chevron gas station with a large convenience market and a McDonald's restaurant. If no potable water is available in lower Crowder Canyon, this restaurant is a recommended detour. Just west of the cloverleaf are two more gas stations, another minimart, a Del Taco restaurant, and the Cajon Pass Inn (described in the "Resupply Access" section on page 132).

SECTION C

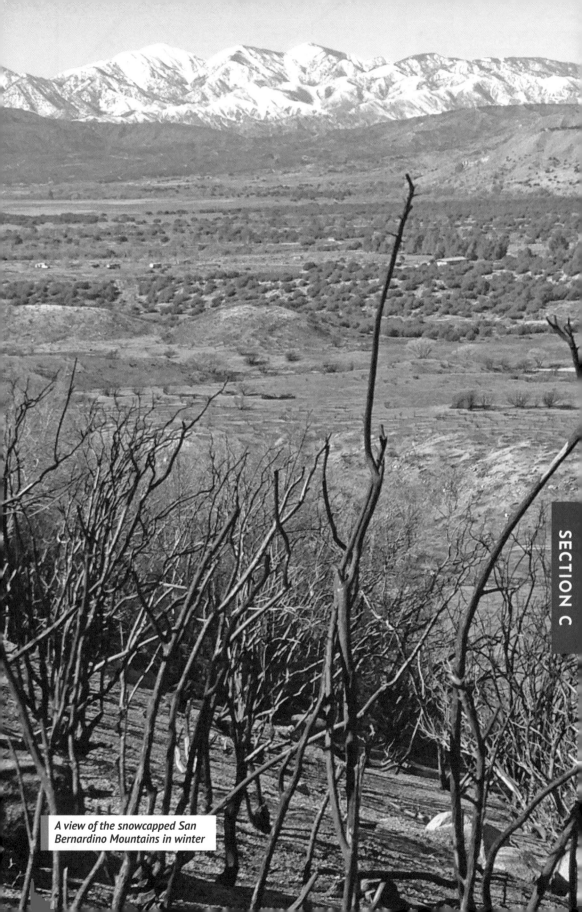

A view of the snowcapped San Bernardino Mountains in winter

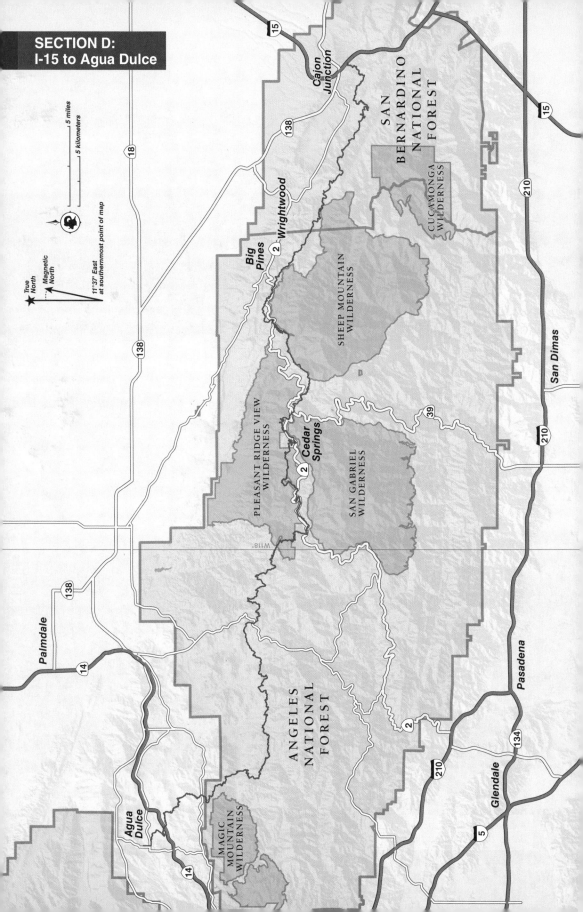

5 miles

5 kilometers

11°37' East
at southernmost point of map

True
North

Magnetic
North

18

15

138

Cajon
Junction

138

SAN
BERNARDINO
NATIONAL
FOREST

15

210

Wrightwood

2

Big
Pines

CUCAMONGA
WILDERNESS

SHEEP
MOUNTAIN
WILDERNESS

San Dimas

39

Cedar
Springs

2

PLEASANT RIDGE VIEW
WILDERNESS

SAN GABRIEL
WILDERNESS

210

W118°

138

Palmdale

14

ANGELES
NATIONAL
FOREST

2

Pasadena

134

210

Glendale

Agua
Dulce

MAGIC
MOUNTAIN
WILDERNESS

5

14

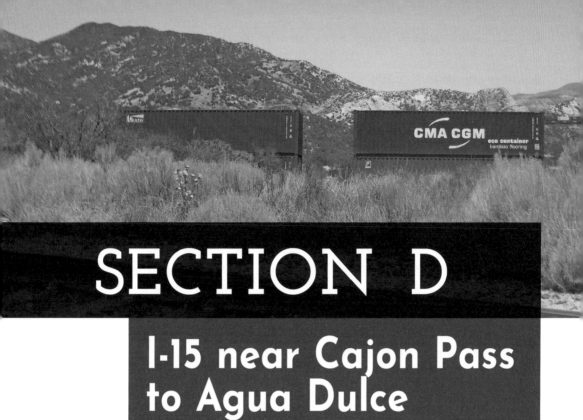

SECTION D

I-15 near Cajon Pass to Agua Dulce

TRUE TO ITS NAME, the Pacific Crest Trail (PCT) through the San Gabriel Mountains remains on or close to the watershed dividing streams that flow into the Pacific Ocean from those that run north, losing themselves in the sand or evaporating from muddy playas in the Mojave Desert. The PCT climbs quickly from smoggy, arid Cajon Canyon to the subalpine reaches of the San Gabriel Mountains and soon ascends its Southern California apex— wind-torn, 9,399-foot Mount Baden-Powell. Most of the PCT's winding route lies between these two extremes, treaded in pine-needle duff under groves of shading, hospitable Transition Zone forest trees: Jeffrey pine, incense cedar, black oak, sugar pine, white fir, and water-loving white alder.

Except for frequent roads and resorts that the PCT skirts, much of the trail route traverses country unchanged, at first glance, by the encroachment of modern civilization. But on closer inspection, you see that the San

Above: Trainspotting from the PCT, west of the Cajon Pass

Gabriels are no longer the wild and remote range that moved legendary mountaineer John Muir to call them "more rigidly inaccessible than any other I ever attempted to penetrate." Man has tamed the San Gabriels' clawing chaparral and steep-walled gorges with miles of highway and has prevented once-devastating floods with dams and catchment basins. Bears and bighorn sheep, which once roamed the range, have been driven by thousands of hikers, skiers, picnickers, hunters, and loggers into the most remote and forbidding canyons. The forests, however, show the most insidious and far-reaching effects of California's burgeoning population. Though Los Angeles's infamous smog is much less prevalent than it used to be, at times it rises well into the surrounding mountains. Drought, bark beetles, tree disease, and other factors also contribute, but the damage is evident in the yellowed needles on thousands of acres of dying pines and firs.

A part of the Transverse Ranges geologic province, the San Gabriels are thought to be rather young, at least in their present stature. Despite their relative youth, geologists state that some of California's oldest rocks lie in the San Gabriels. Both Precambrian anorthosite (a light-colored, plutonic rock composed almost entirely of plagioclase feldspar and high in aluminum content) and gabbro estimated to be 1.22 billion years old line the PCT route in the vicinity of Mount Gleason. These rocks are much older than most of the rocks along the San Gabriel Mountains segment of the PCT. Most of the trail tread lies in familiar granitic rocks of Mesozoic age; these were intruded at the same time as similar rocks in the Sierra, San Bernardino, and San Jacinto Mountains and in Baja California. Other rocks, such as the Pelona schist, which you first encounter on Upper Lytle Creek Ridge as you enter the San Gabriels, are metamorphic rocks, once volcanic and ocean-bottom sediments, which may have been altered by the intruding granites.

The present-day San Gabriels are a complex range, cut by and rising along numerous faults that occur along their every side. The major San

Andreas Fault is the most famous, and it bounds the San Gabriels on their northern and eastern margins. This great fault stretches from near Cape Mendocino southeast about 1,000 miles into the Gulf of California. Geologists now know that hundreds of miles of horizontal shift along the fault (with the western side moving north) have occurred in the last 30 million years, since about the time the fault first formed. Where the San Andreas Fault slashes through Cajon Canyon, at the start of this section, you can see an example of long-term motion along the fault: the bizarre Mormon Rocks and Rock Candy Mountains, all sedimentary rocks, lie northeast of the fault about 25 miles east of related rocks at the Devil's Punchbowl, on the fault's southwest side. The Punchbowl and the trace of the San Andreas Fault can be seen easily atop Mount Williamson, a short side hike from the PCT.

DECLINATION 11°37'E

USGS MAPS

Cajon	Valyermo	Pacifico Mountain
Telegraph Peak	Crystal Lake	Acton
Mount San Antonio	Waterman Mountain	Agua Dulce
Mescal Creek	Chilao Flat	

POINTS ON THE TRAIL, SOUTH TO NORTH

	Mile	Elevation in feet	Latitude/Longitude
I-15 near Cajon Pass	342.0	2,995	N34° 18' 16.680" W117° 27' 54.720"
Swarthout Canyon Road	347.3	3,568	N34° 17' 46.980" W117° 30' 25.130"
Acorn Trail to Wrightwood	363.4	8,247	N34° 20' 11.940" W117° 38' 30.420"
Inspiration Point/CA 2 to Wrightwood	369.4	7,372	N34° 22' 21.120" W117° 42' 37.740"
Vincent Gap/CA 2/Mount Baden-Powell	374.0	6,582	N34° 22' 23.760" W117° 45' 08.640"
Little Jimmy Spring	383.7	7,435	N34° 20' 43.500" W117° 49' 46.200"
Islip Saddle	386.0	6,666	N34° 21' 25.320" W117° 51' 01.980"
Eagles Roost (endangered-frog detour)	390.2	6,654	N34° 21' 15.480" W117° 52' 41.040"
Camp Glenwood Boy Scout Camp	400.6	6,252	N34° 21' 07.740" W117° 57' 28.320"
Three Points Trailhead	403.1	5,928	N34° 20' 36.050" W117° 58' 59.270"
Fountainhead Spring	411.0	6,436	N34° 22' 50.610" W118° 01' 37.920"
Mill Creek Summit/Angeles Forest Highway	418.6	4,979	N34° 23' 23.880" W118° 04' 51.420"
North Fork Saddle Ranger Station	436.1	4,185	N34° 23' 17.041" W118° 15' 11.779"

SECTION D

continued on next page

POINTS ON THE TRAIL, SOUTH TO NORTH *(continued)*

	Mile	Elevation in feet	Latitude/Longitude
Soledad Canyon Road to Acton	444.2	2,245	N34° 26' 15.420" W118° 16' 20.400"
Vasquez Rocks Natural Area	452.9	2,482	N34° 29' 06.350" W118° 18' 42.780"
Agua Dulce	454.5	2,537	N34° 29' 46.260" W118° 19' 34.920"

CAMPSITES AND BIVY SITES

Mile	Elevation in feet	Latitude/ Longitude	Number of tents	Feature	Notes
361.7	8,135	N34° 19' 48.900" W117° 37' 32.280"	>5	Near Mount Baldy turnoff	
364.4	8,251	N34° 20' 27.960" W117° 39' 17.040"	>10	Guffy Campground	Seasonal water, picnic table, fire ring, pit toilet
367.3	7,894	N34° 21' 33.480" W117° 41' 16.260"	>10	Blue Ridge Campground	Pit toilet, no water
377.0	8,638	N34° 21' 51.360" W117° 45' 38.640"	>5	Baden-Powell spur	
383.9	7,479	N34° 20' 50.220" W117° 49' 49.860"	16	Little Jimmy Campground	Pit toilets, fire rings, spring nearby
395.2	6,235	N34° 21' 40.140" W117° 55' 15.660"	6	Cooper Canyon Trail Camp	Pit toilet, picnic tables, stream nearby
406.6	5,270	N34° 22' 02.273" W117° 59' 17.660"	6	Sulphur Springs Trail Camp	Pit toilets, picnic tables
411.7	6,682	N34° 23' 20.640" W118° 01' 42.780"	5	Below Pacifico Mountain	Some shade
415.1	6,219	N34° 23' 49.980" W118° 03' 14.700"	5	Scenic desert views	Flat, wind-prone
430.4	5,886	N34° 22' 52.380" W118° 11' 24.060"	10	Messenger Flats Campground	Fire-damaged but accessible, flat campsites; no water; views
444.3	2,226	N34° 26' 18.120" W118° 16' 19.620"	Dozens	Soledad Canyon Road/KOA	Large campground 0.4 mile off trail with PCT hiker area, food, showers, swimming pool
453.6	2,482	N34° 29' 17.280" W118° 19' 16.560"	>15	Vasquez Rocks Nature Center	Campsites behind building, water

WEATHER TO GO

Mount Baden-Powell and the other San Gabriel crest peaks usually maintain a heavy snowpack until mid-May. But May through summer and fall are otherwise the nicest times to traverse this section. During winter, expect most of the trail to be snowbound. By June, the trail's lower reaches, at either end of the section, can be oppressively warm.

SUPPLIES

At the Start of Section D, minimal supplies can be purchased at either of two convenience stores at the freeway overpass 0.6 mile north of the section's beginning. A complete selection of needed items may be purchased in San Bernardino, 17 miles south on I-15. Be sure to restock on water before leaving Cajon Canyon; sources like the spring at Guffy Campground are no longer reliable. Wrightwood, a ski-resort community with a post office, stores, restaurants, and motels, is the next possible supply point. There is a PCT register, along with maps, supplies, and trail angel information, at Mountain Hardware Store (mtnhardware.com). This community hub also lets hikers wash up and air out their packs on its back patio. Camp Wrightwood, a Methodist church camp, sometimes offers bunks, showers, and laundry facilities to hikers; they post availability on a sign at their driveway entrance, but it's best to call ahead if possible: 760-249-3453. Wrightwood is a 4.4-mile round-trip detour down from the PCT via the Acorn Trail, 21 miles from I-15. Alternatively, reach it by hitchhiking east on busy Angeles Crest Highway (CA 2) at Inspiration Point, 27.4 miles from the start of this section. From Wrightwood, inexpensive public buses leave four times daily to Victorville. This large, sprawling Mojave Desert community has neither Wrightwood's charm nor cool temperatures, but it does afford more conveniences.

Acton, a small town with a post office, grocery stores, and a motel, lies 5.8 miles east off the PCT route in Soledad Canyon, about 100 miles from I-15. Santa Clarita, a larger city with complete amenities, lies west of the PCT some 12.5 miles from the same point in Soledad Canyon. Agua Dulce, at the end of Section D, is the most logical resupply point, and a long carry from Wrightwood. The village of Agua Dulce has several good restaurants, a hardware store, a feed store, and a hair salon. The closest post office is in Acton.

WATER

While generally well watered, the San Gabriel Mountains nonetheless pose a challenge to the hiker in search of regular water sources. This is especially true at either end of the mountain chain, where lower elevations and the proximity to the fiery Mojave Desert create an arid chaparral, with few permanent springs or streams. Carry plenty of water for the long, hard uphill day at the start of this section. Check pctwater.org before you begin, as hikers have found the once-reliable spring at Guffy Campground to be dry and the pipe in disrepair in recent years. After Wrightwood, you should encounter water a few times a day, from natural sources or campgrounds. By summertime, however, don't count on stream-flowing water in most creeks. West of North Fork Saddle Ranger Station, the pickings again become slim—don't count on water, except at man-made facilities.

PERMITS

No wilderness permits are required for overnight PCT campers, though section hikers are encouraged to obtain them when possible in the event of an emergency. A California campfire permit is required to use portable stoves containing gas, jellied fuel, or pressurized liquid fuel outside of campfire use sites. Permits may be obtained online at readyforwildfire.org/permits/campfire-permit.

SPECIAL CONCERNS

Refer to page 36 for information about poodle-dog bush. For information about poison oak, see page 35.

Due to the extreme fire danger, open fires are *not allowed* at any site outside of a designated campground in the Angeles National Forest—even with a campfire permit. This is a compelling reason for all hikers to carry a gas stove throughout their trip.

ON OCTOBER 10, 2014, President Barack Obama designated 342,177 acres of the Angeles National Forest and 4,002 acres of the San Bernardino National Forest as the San Gabriel Mountains National Monument. The 87 miles of the PCT that traverse this monument include Mount Baden-Powell, the northern ridgeline of the Sheep Mountain Wilderness, and Pleasant View Ridge Wilderness. Rich in biodiversity and unique geology, the San Gabriels include the San Andreas Fault and provide critical habitats for threatened or endangered species, such as the California condor, mountain yellow-legged frog, and Nelson's bighorn sheep.

The Omnibus Public Land Management Act of 2009 added 2 million acres of wilderness, including 26,757 acres that comprise Pleasant View Ridge Wilderness; thousands of miles of National Wild and Scenic Rivers; and other additions to federally protected public lands.

I-15 NEAR CAJON PASS TO AGUA DULCE

>>>THE ROUTE

Reach the beginning of Section D by taking I-15 north 17 miles from San Bernardino to the CA 138/Silverwood Lake exit. Atop the off-ramp, turn right and head 12 yards east along CA 138 to paved Wagon Train Road, the frontage road that branches south. Paralleling I-15, take this road down past a gas station, minimart, and McDonald's 0.6 mile to its end beside the Santa Fe–Salt Lake Trail monument, a stone tribute to the pioneers who made their way by caravan across the rocky gorges and canyons surrounding you. This spot is just short of narrow Crowder Canyon, the PCT's route. Just south of the monument, the PCT curves south under the freeway (342.0–2,995') via a boxed culvert, emerging on the other side in a thicket of dry brush. The route becomes a sandy-muddy jeep track paralleling the freeway. Moments later, you pass under a wooden railroad trestle and then turn right to follow a jeep road west, just below the tracks. Just north of a fenced private home, PCT tread resumes, branching obliquely left (west–southwest) from the jeep trail. The path winds levelly through desert chaparral, then swings south, up and over a sandy ridge on a well-signed route, and dips to a rough dirt road that heads west to Sullivan's Curve, a historical railroad grade. Cross this road, then walk down a short trailless wash to a culvert under another railroad track (342.9–2,969'). Now walk right (southwest) up a faint path that parallels the rails to find the PCT climbing south once again via two small, overgrown switchbacks.

Soon the trail crosses more railroad tracks (343.1–3,013') and swings right along a dirt access road 30 yards before bending southwest to wind among the hills and sandstone-conglomerate outcrops of the Mormon Rocks, a badland of Miocene alluvium. At one point you amble south along a jeep road (keeping right where the road forks) 100 yards before trail tread resumes on the right side of the road.

HISTORY The Mormon Rocks commemorate Mormon pioneers who were among the first Caucasians to use Cajon Pass and who settled San Bernardino Valley. Pedro Fages, who on one trip discovered the Colorado Desert and the San Jacinto Mountains, crossed the mountains in this vicinity when he tired of leading a contingent to capture Army deserters, and an urge to explore captured him. The forces of Juan Bautista de Anza and Father Francisco Garcés passed near here four years after Fages, in 1776, on their way north from Sonora, Mexico. By 1813 the Cajon Pass route, part of the Santa Fe Trail, was seeing frequent use by American trapper-trader Ewing Young and others. The Mormon Battalion used this route both coming from and going to the Great Salt Lake, and borax teams from Death Valley Railroad also crossed here.

Pushing on, you cross first one power line road, FS 3N49, and then in 0.25 mile cross another (344.3–3,335') amid bush sunflower, chamise, and scattered cacti. Upon reaching the second power line road, ascend south up the road 150 yards before resuming trail tread on the right side of the road. Next the PCT ascends to a sandy ridge dominating lower Lone Pine Canyon, eroded along the San Andreas Fault. The path traverses this ridge, which presents some striking blue clays, then cuts across sandy washes under the south face of Ralston Peak to dirt Swarthout Canyon Road 3N28 (347.3–3,568'). Just before the road, trail angels have built a simple wooden kiosk housing a trail register and water cache for hikers about to make the steep ascent to Wrightwood (see page 16 for more about water caches).

From Swarthout Canyon Road, the PCT route strikes invisibly west from the road, marked by 4-by-4-inch posts in the cobbly

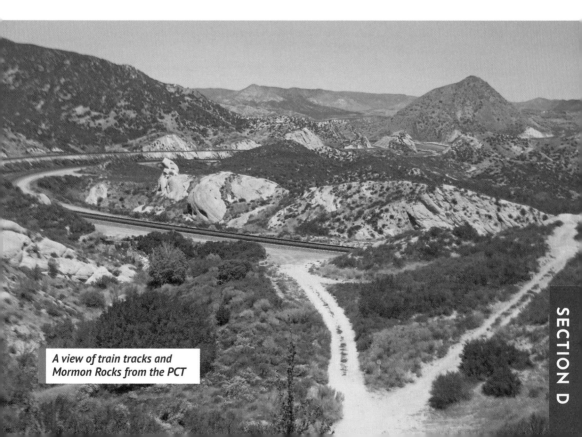

A view of train tracks and Mormon Rocks from the PCT

SECTION D

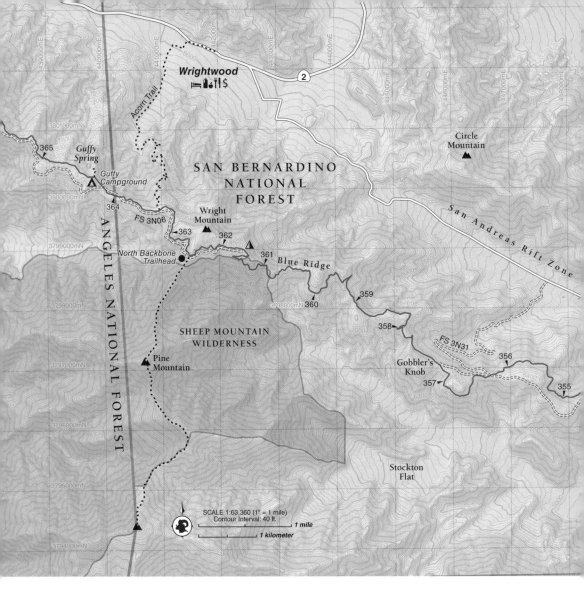

alluvium, then turns south across a bouldery wash to a jeep road (347.7–3,685'). Two concrete tubs at Bike Spring are found just yards north, but they have been dry more often than not in recent years. Even when water is running, its heavily polluted nature relegates it to emergency use only. Four white PVC pipes have been driven here in the dry wash, with the seeming intention of building a well.

Attacking the fire-scarred eastern flanks of Upper Lytle Creek Ridge, the trail swings into a canyon, then switchbacks north, up across three canyons, to finally strike dirt Sharpless Ranch Road 3N29 (351.8–5,195') near the ridgecrest. Now you round a nose and amble more or less levelly west on the cooler northern slopes, just yards below ridgetop Sheep Creek Truck Road 3N31. At the next gap in the ridge, you find remains of the old south-side PCT tread and might choose to walk up to the ridgetop to gain cooling vistas of the snow-dappled Mount San Antonio massif and the rugged Cucamonga Wilderness, to the west and southwest, above North Fork Lytle Creek.

HISTORY In the 1890s Lytle Creek was the setting for a spirited but short-lived gold rush.

Your path ascends gently, keeping to the ridge's steep north side, where you parallel arid Lone Pine Canyon from a slightly cooler

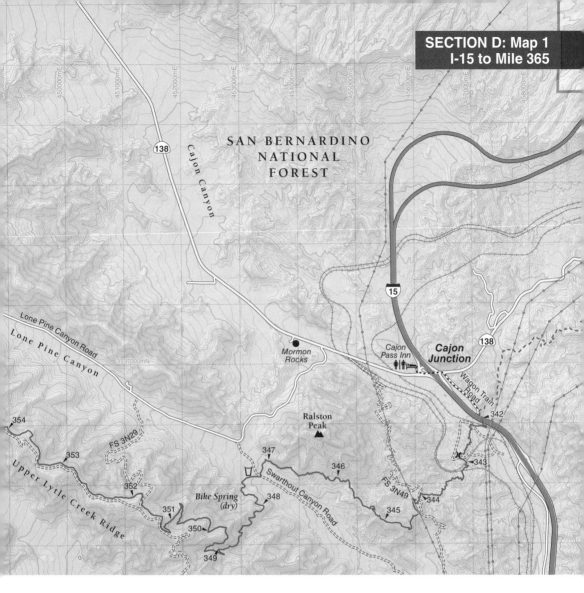

SAN BERNARDINO
NATIONAL
FOREST

vantage. Eventually, you cross dirt Sheep Creek Truck Road 3N31 (356.2–6,293') at an intersection where it turns northwest to drop into Lone Pine Canyon.

Now your chia-lined path crosses to the south side of the ridge and in a few minutes finds a small, scenic ridgetop flat and a cluster of shady big-cone spruce.

Beyond it, you wind south around a prominence to a road-end just east of Gobbler's Knob.

FIRE   The massive Blue Cut Fire swept through this area of the San Bernardino National Forest in 2016. Its path impacted 20 miles of the PCT. Its damage to surrounding hillsides once rich with groves of juniper, big-cone spruce, and mountain mahogany

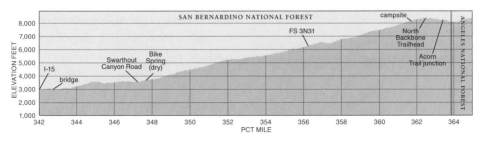

will be evident for years to come. Hikers should exercise caution in this area and be sure to stay on the trail. As the route swings under Blue Ridge, both Devils Backbone and Dawson Peak dominate the southern horizon, thrusting ridges of platy brown Pelona schist above treeline. These points mark the eastern boundary of Angeles National Forest's new Sheep Mountain Wilderness, a 43,600-acre preserve that protects the rugged San Gabriel River drainage, just west of Mount San Antonio.

CAMPING Look for black-granular phyllite and outcrops of white quartz and fibrous green, shiny actinolite, a close relative of asbestos, in the schist before the PCT switchbacks east up to a jeep road (361.7–8,135') atop Blue Ridge, where wind-prone camping may be found.

This road climbs northwest to a posted trailhead (362.5–8,312') to Mount Baldy just north of the jeep road's intersection with FS 3N06. Here you can gaze north down to Wrightwood, across the north face of Wright Mountain, where cycles of mudflows, triggered by the melting of winter snows, have cut a spectacular, barren swath. The PCT contours south around Jeffrey pine–forested Wright Mountain, staying just above dirt FS 3N06.

VIEWS Prairie Fork San Gabriel River comes into view, incised along the San Jacinto Fault. Mount Baden-Powell dominates the western horizon, while San Gabriel Valley smog is partly screened by the Pine Mountain Ridge to the south.

West of Wright Mountain you meet the Acorn Trail (363.4–8,247'). Just before the junction, a memorial stone at the base of two large trees honors the memory of two hikers who died nearby while attempting to thru-hike the PCT in winter 1983.

RESUPPLY ACCESS

This path descends 2 miles north past quaint mountain homes to a road that drops 1.5 miles to the western edge of Wrightwood. Hikers may also opt to hitch a ride to Wrightwood from Inspiration Point, another 6 miles away. The next possibilities for provisions on the route lie in either Acton, 80.9 miles away, or Agua Dulce, 91.1 miles away.

CAMPING The PCT continues west up Blue Ridge, sometimes on FS 3N06 but often to its north on short trail segments. It enters Angeles National Forest and arrives at Guffy Campground (364.4–8,251').

WATER ACCESS

CAMPING Guffy Campground, the first logical campsite west of I-15, sometimes has water in April and May at a spring reached by a side trail down Flume Canyon to the north. It is not dependable, especially in late spring and summer of drought years. A better strategy for thru-hikers is to detour to Wrightwood and avoid the uncertainty.

The trail, often sited on old, narrow dirt roads, continues mostly north of Blue Ridge's crest, offering vistas north over Swarthout Valley and the San Andreas Fault Zone to pinyon-cloaked ridges abutting the Mojave Desert. You descend easily in fine mixed-conifer forest around Blue Ridge's high point, eventually reaching a dirt road (366.6–8,130') beside an artificial lake enclosed by a high fence. This is one of two reservoirs serving the snowmaking operations of the Mountain High Ski Area, which has ski-lift terminals that you will pass in

ANGELES
NATIONAL FOREST

Big Pines Highway/N4

Jackson
Lake

372

Jackson Flat
Group Campground

371

373

Jackson Flat Road/FS 3N26

2

Table Mountain

Big Pines

Inspiration
Point
Trailhead

370

Mountain High
Ski Resort

2

Swarthout Valley

375   374

Grassy Hollow
Visitor Center

369

E. Blue Ridge Road/
FS 3N06

Vincent Gap

376

368

Lamel Spring

377

378

SHEEP MOUNTAIN
WILDERNESS

Blue Ridge
Campground

367

Mount-
den-Powell

Blue Ridge

366

SCALE 1:63,360 (1" = 1 mile)
Contour Interval: 40 ft.

1 mile

Prairie Fork

365

1 kilometer

---

the next mile. Turn left (south) briefly up over the ridgecrest, through a large, white pipe gate to FS 3N06, which you follow right (west) for a minute to access a resumption of PCT pathway on the west side of the reservoir. This leads back up to the ridgetop, from which you wind down in nice fir forest, beside a ski run, to again strike East Blue Ridge Road (367.1–7,937').

CAMPING As indicated by white metal PCT posts, you cross the road and descend a few feet to traverse the western perimeter of pleasant but waterless Blue Ridge Campground (367.3–7,894').

Beyond the campground, you parallel the boundary of Sheep Mountain

Wilderness, the rugged chaos of mostly trailless ridges and gorges to the southwest.

Atop the second hill along your way, you find the second artificial lakelet and more ski lifts, and the path is forced directly onto the brink of Bear Gulch's steep headwall. Beyond, you cross or swing next to now-paved FS 3N06 several more times. Black oaks and white firs join the

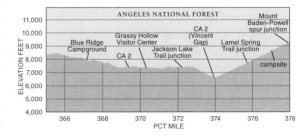

ecosystem as you near Angeles Crest Highway (CA 2) (369.4–7,372') just east of Inspiration Point, a sweeping overlook with picnic tables, of the East Fork San Gabriel River basin.

Carefully cross the highway to a paved parking area, which has bathrooms but no water. Here a metal PCT post marks your route, branching left (west). Ascend easily past a returning loop of the nature trail, then drop west through flats of whitethorn and bitter cherry to reach forested Grassy Hollow Visitor Center (370.3–7,310'), which usually has water, as well as toilets, a large interpretive center, and a part-time ranger station. The center is open only on weekends, but PCT hikers may use the pit toilets in the day-use area.

About 0.5 mile northwest of the center, the PCT route goes along Jackson Flat Road 3N26 for 100 yards before returning to trail tread on the north side of Blue Ridge. Next on the itinerary is a short spur to walk-in Jackson Flat Group Campground, in shading pines and firs. It's closed November–late April. It usually has piped water and toilets throughout summer, but it can't be relied upon. After passing north of Jackson Flat, the PCT drops south across FS 3N26, then switchbacks moderately down past interior live oaks and ocean spray to Angeles Crest Highway at Vincent Gap (374.0–6,582').

South of the highway, beside a parking area and a trail east to the interesting Bighorn Mine, is the Mount Baden-Powell Trail—a popular pilgrimage for Southern California Boy Scouts. You take this trail, which starts southwest before switchbacking gently to moderately up in Jeffrey pine–white fir groves on crunchy Pelona schist tread. After a number of switchbacks you reach a side trail (375.7–7,768') that contours 100 yards south to Lamel Spring. This marks a good rest stop.

Above, the switchbacks become tighter, the air grows crisper, and firs give way to lodgepole pines, which yield in turn, above 8,800 feet, to sweeping-branched, wind-loving limber pines. Some botanists believe that these hunched,

gnarled conifers along the Mount Baden-Powell Spur Trail are 2,000 years old (377.9–9,245'). The Wally Waldron tree, an especially grizzled and striking specimen, stands at the junction of the PCT and Mount Baden-Powell Trail. It is named after a local Scout leader and makes a fine place to stop and admire the ridgetop views.

SIDE TRIP Take this side hike to the 9,399-foot summit for superlative views north across desert to the southern Sierra; west to Mount Gleason; south down Iron Fork San Gabriel River (in Sheep Mountain Wilderness) to the Santa Ana Mountains; and east to Mounts San Antonio, San Gorgonio,

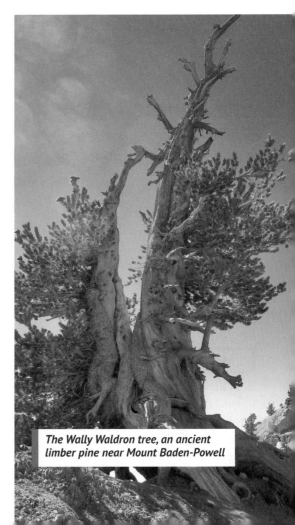

The Wally Waldron tree, an ancient limber pine near Mount Baden-Powell

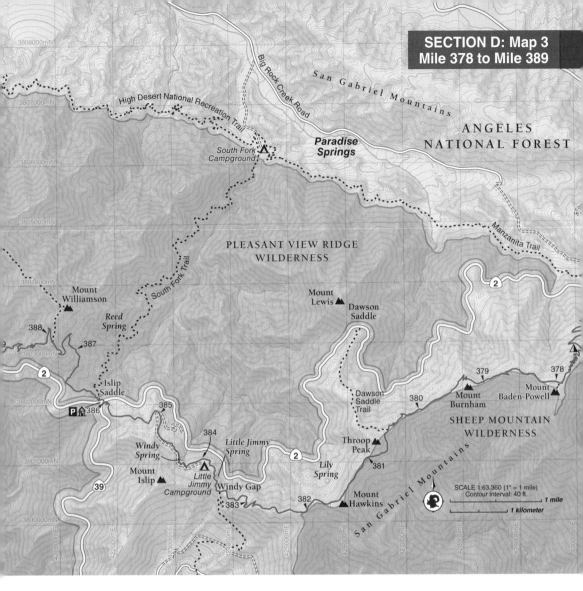

San Gabriel Mountains

Big Rock Creek Road

High Desert National Recreation Trail

Paradise Springs

ANGELES NATIONAL FOREST

South Fork Campground

Manzanita Trail

PLEASANT VIEW RIDGE WILDERNESS

South Fork Trail

Mount Williamson

Reed Spring

388

387

Mount Lewis

Dawson Saddle

2

379

378

Mount Baden-Powell

2

Islip Saddle

385

Dawson Saddle Trail

380

Mount Burnham

SHEEP MOUNTAIN WILDERNESS

P 386

384

Little Jimmy Spring

2

Throop Peak

381

Windy Spring

Mount Islip

Little Jimmy Campground

Windy Gap

Lily Spring

San Gabriel Mountains

39

383

382

Mount Hawkins

SCALE 1:63,360 (1" = 1 mile)
Contour Interval: 40 ft.

1 mile

1 kilometer

San Gabriel Mountains

and San Jacinto. On the clearest days, Mount Whitney, still three to four weeks north, and Telescope Peak, overlooking Death Valley, can be seen. A concrete monument here is a tribute to Lord Baden-Powell, founder of the Boy Scout movement. This summit marks the terminus of the Silver Moccasin Trail, Scouting's 53-mile challenge through the San Gabriel Mountains, which is congruent with the PCT until Three Points, about 25 miles away.

Back on the PCT, you bear west, descending the steep ridge under Mount Burnham.

Later, ascend two small switchbacks and pass a signed spur trail that heads north down the shoulder of Throop Peak to Dawson Saddle (380.5–8,856'). You climb briefly in open pine and fir forest, with an understory of manzanita,

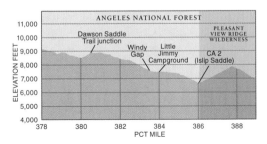

ANGELES NATIONAL FOREST

PLEASANT VIEW RIDGE WILDERNESS

Dawson Saddle Trail junction

Windy Gap

Little Jimmy Campground

CA 2 (Islip Saddle)

ELEVATION FEET

11,000
10,000
9,000
8,000
7,000
6,000
5,000
4,000

378   380   382   384   386   388

PCT MILE

whitethorn, and sagebrush, to navigate Throop Peak's east and south slopes, where you briefly enter the Sheep Mountain Wilderness. More descent follows, past a lateral trail to the summit of Mount Hawkins. Then, on the sparsely conifered ridge west of that peak, you pass a lateral that drops 0.3 mile north to Lily Spring. Just a bit later, you pass another lateral trail, this one south to South Mount Hawkins, before an aggressive descent ensues, bringing you to aptly named Windy Gap (383.5–7,576'), from which a trail drops south to campgrounds in the Crystal Lake Recreation Area.

WATER ACCESS

From here the PCT descends north off the ridge to Little Jimmy Spring (383.7–7,435'), which lies just below the trail.

CAMPING   Little Jimmy Campground (383.9–7,479') is just a couple of minutes farther, with toilets, tables, and fire pits. Bears can be common visitors in summer,

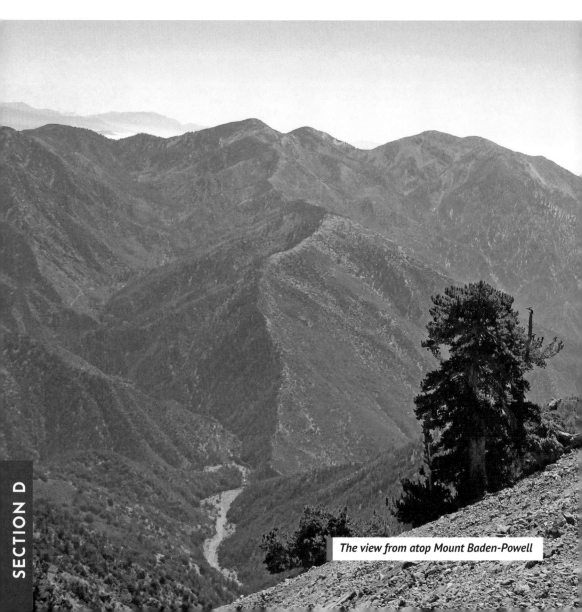

The view from atop Mount Baden-Powell

so be sure to secure your food in provided bear-proof boxes or bring your own bear canister.

Beyond the campground you curve west on a trail that soon passes above Windy Spring. Now your route parallels dirt FS 9W03, keeping some distance below it. Presently, the road hairpins across the trail, where you should find a sign identifying the PCT route. The trail heads west moderately down to Angeles Crest Highway (386.0–6,666'), reaching it just east of its Islip Saddle intersection with closed-to-cars CA 39.

Just west of the parking area and restrooms on Islip Saddle, turn right on Mount Williamson Trail 9W02, and ascend moderately northwest past white firs and whitethorn ceanothus to the Mount Williamson Summit Trail (387.9–7,774'), which climbs 0.4 mile north to views of fault-churned Devil's Punchbowl. While you switchback west down from your ridgetop, you can look south down deep ravines in the tonalite to the San Gabriel Wilderness, which is a Southern California refuge of mountain bighorn sheep. Ending the descent, the route merges with a jeep road for 200 yards, and then crosses Angeles Crest Highway (389.3–6,700').

The trail resumes about 50 yards west to ascend Kratka Ridge in a heterogeneous forest of white fir, sugar and ponderosa pines, interior live oak, and mountain mahogany. Soon you descend back to Angeles Crest Highway, where you walk along the southern road shoulder, past a large tan-metal highway-maintenance shed, 180 yards to waterless Eagles Roost Picnic Area (390.2–6,654').

DETOUR This detour is a complex and ever-changing issue. Check with the U.S. Forest Service for the latest updates; the PCTA also offers up-to-date information on its website.

The mountain yellow-legged frog once held court as the most abundant amphibian in the Sierra Nevada and Southern California mountain ranges.

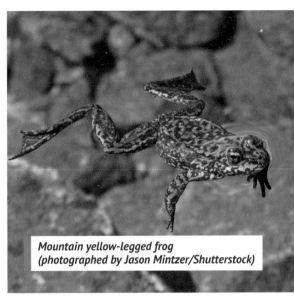

Mountain yellow-legged frog (photographed by Jason Mintzer/Shutterstock)

Today, it is an endangered species, threatened and decimated over the years by the introduction of nonnative trout to lakes and streams, human encroachment on habitat, and a fungal disease epidemic that hindered breeding. In an effort to protect a known frog habitat in the San Gabriels, rangers closed a stretch of the PCT between Eagles Roost (mile 390.2) and the Burkhart Trail junction (mile 394.0), but the U.S. Forest Service announced in 2018 that attempts to breed the endangered frog are going well, and plans are in the works that may lead to the reopening of the segment.

For years, most hikers have opted to road walk nearly 3 miles along busy Angeles Crest Highway between Eagles Roost and the Burkhart Trailhead, then follow the Burkhart Trail 2 miles to resume hiking the PCT. The curvy mountain highway is often buzzing with motorists, especially on weekends, so use extreme caution.

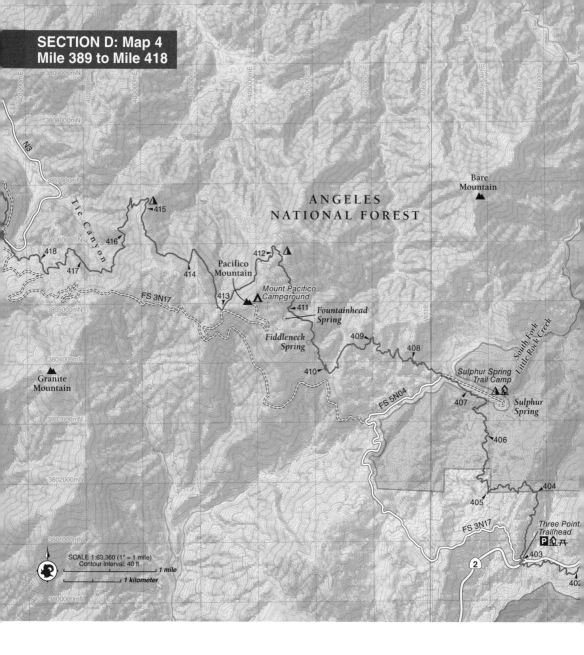

If the route has reopened, at the entrance to Eagles Roost Picnic Area just west of the highway, turn west down a rocky, unsigned, and unused dirt road, and descend to its end at Rattlesnake Trail (391.4–6,165') in a shady gully. This little-used path drops north, under the stone gaze of the cliff now known to rock climbers as Williamson Rock, and crosses melodious Little Rock Creek (391.7–6,080') in cedar-lined Rattlesnake Canyon (a proposed bridge would lead hikers above the creek instead of beside it). The PCT continues, contouring to Rattlesnake Spring and another spring a mile later. Past the second spring, the PCT merges with Burkhart Trail 10W02 (393.8–5,675') and turns south across the stream to ascend southwest into Cooper Canyon.

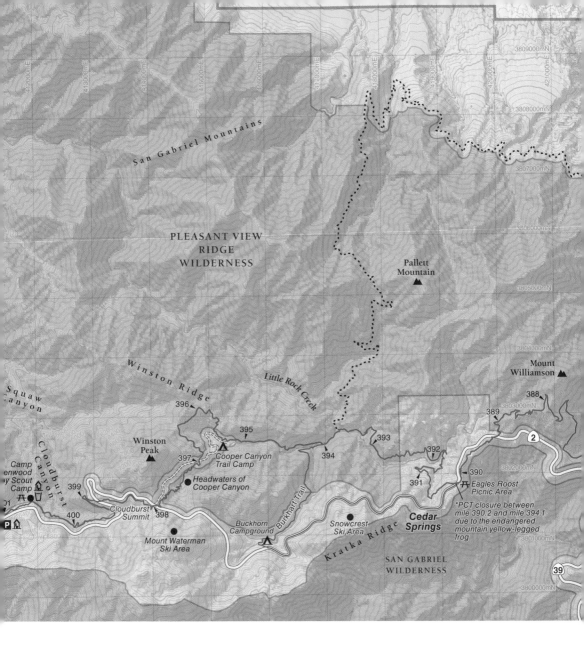

PLEASANT VIEW
RIDGE
WILDERNESS

San Gabriel Mountains

Pallett
Mountain ▲

Mount
Williamson ▲

Winston Ridge

Little Rock Creek

388

Squaw
Canyon

389

Cloudburst Canyon

396

395

393

392

Winston
Peak ▲

397

Cooper Canyon
Trail Camp

394

390

Camp
enwood
y Scout
Camp

399

Headwaters of
Cooper Canyon

391

Eagles Roost
Picnic Area

2

*PCT closure between
mile 390.2 and mile 394.1
due to the endangered
mountain yellow-legged
frog

Cloudburst
Summit

398

Burkhart Trail

Cedar
Springs

400

Buckhorn
Campground

Snowcrest
Ski Area

Kratka Ridge

Mount Waterman
Ski Area

SAN GABRIEL
WILDERNESS

39

Whether you took the detour or the official route has reopened, continue past a pristine waterfall and the south-branching Burkhart Trail (394.0–5,721'), which climbs 1.5 miles to popular Buckhorn Campground (38 campsites, pit toilets, and piped water). The PCT route becomes an often steep jeep road, FS 3N02.

CAMPING You ascend this road to pleasantly shaded Cooper Canyon Trail Camp (395.2–6,235'), which has reliable water, picnic tables, and an outhouse.

Here the PCT tread branches right (northwest) from the still-climbing road, briefly

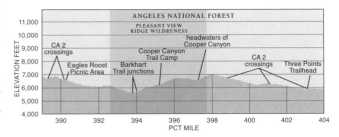

ANGELES NATIONAL FOREST

PLEASANT VIEW
RIDGE WILDRENESS

headwaters of
Cooper Canyon

CA 2
crossings

Cooper Canyon
Trail Camp

CA 2
crossings

Three Points
Trailhead

Eagles Roost
Picnic Area

Burkhart
Trail junctions

ELEVATION FEET

11,000
10,000
9,000
8,000
7,000
6,000
5,000
4,000

390   392   394   396   398   400   402   404
PCT MILE

paralleling it before turning north up a ravine. In a sunny open forest of Jeffrey pine amid tufts of silvery-leaved, multi-hued lupine, the way winds up and across a hillside, merges subtly with a disused jeep road, and winds to a ridge-top gap at the head of Winston Ridge. Here you can look west down brushy Squaw Canyon to the Sulphur Springs vicinity. Now the jeep road–cum–trail ambles gently up over the eastern shoulder of Winston Peak, then drops momentarily to cross the better dirt road (396.9–6,645') that returns to Cooper Canyon Trail Camp.

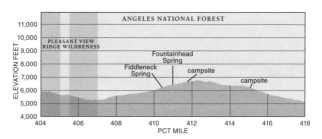

Below that road, your way traverses south-west back into Cooper Canyon, where a tier of sandy flats, shaded by pine, fir, and cedar, lie next to the permanent, trickling headwaters of Cooper Canyon Creek.

Now, via small, steep switchbacks, the PCT tackles the final slopes to gain the better dirt road just below its end at Cloudburst Summit (398.0–7,032'). Here, you cross the Angeles Crest Highway again.

On the west side of this forested gap, the path drops to contour just south of the high-way in open forest then crosses the highway (398.8–6,733'), again below a hairpin turn. Now you follow another gated jeep road, 10W15, which makes a switchback down into the head of Cloudburst Canyon, where you find a road junction with a dirt spur leading west down to Camp Pajarito. Here brown plastic PCT posts point your way straight ahead, contouring southwest across the dry creekbed and below two water tanks as you cross the Pleasant View Ridge Wilderness boundary.

An easy, shaded descent carries you below the highway to soon reach a small saddle atop which sits Camp Glenwood Boy Scout Camp (400.6–6,252'). Water is usually available here May–November. Two minutes west of the camp's lodge, treading on the dirt access road, you pass a 14-foot-high, narrow steel water tank. Here the PCT drifts right (west–southwest), away

from the road, onto a poor dirt road indicated by plastic posts. In a moment, you dip across a culverted gully and walk up to a slightly better dirt road, which strikes left (south) just a few yards to reach CA 2 (401.1–6,268'). Now turn right (west) on the highway shoulder 80 yards to a saddle with a large parking pullout. Here you cross south to briefly ascend a dwindling dirt road (still 10W15). After a few minutes, the gentle descent resumes, this time above the highway, to emerge from big-cone spruce at Three Points Trailhead (403.1–5,928') on the Angeles Crest Highway.

RESUPPLY ACCESS

Three Points Trailhead at Santa Clara Divide Road marks the closest major access point from the PCT to Pasadena and downtown Los Angeles. It's also 1.3 miles via the Angeles Crest Highway to Newcomb's Ranch, a historical roadhouse frequented by motor-cyclists and weekend adventurers. Cold drinks, burgers, salads, and adventure-fueled camaraderie can be found here. Check the website for hours and weather-forced closures: newcombsranch.com.

FIRE   In 2009 the Station Fire, the largest wildfire ever recorded in Los Angeles County, burned 160,000 acres—nearly one-quarter—of the Angeles National

Forest. Its unprecedented and fast-moving fury affected the PCT between Three Points and Messenger Flats Campground, and recovery of the surrounding forest and hillsides will take decades. The trail itself has reopened, but the fire's impact is still sadly evident. The Sand Fire of 2016 covered less territory but also damaged parts of Section D, most notably between Mill Creek Summit and just south of CA 14. Check the PCTA's trail closures section, or call the U.S. Forest Service for updated conditions: 818-899-1900.

The Chilao Flat/Waterman Mountain Trail here continues southwest, but the PCT goes north across the highway. In a moment it reaches Horse Flat Road 3N17 and a trailhead parking area with restrooms and two picnic tables. This is just beyond the left-branching Silver Moccasin Trail, which continues west to Bandido Campground and Chilao Flat. Across gravel Horse Flat Road, the PCT, indicated by a signpost, continues north, climbing slightly onto a granite-sand hillside shaded by interior live oaks. A northward contour on this slope soon ends as the PCT swings west through a gap, then drops gently west under big-cone spruces to an unused dirt road. Turn left along this track, descending to reach, in 200 yards, a continuation of the trail, which branches right from the track. This short leg drops to another dirt road that, like the one before it, leads left to a group camp. The PCT here follows the gently descending dirt road north just 130 yards down to a resumption of trail where the road ends.

Winding in and out of small, sandy ravines, the trail leaves Pleasant View Ridge Wilderness and descends easily out onto a chaparralled ridge on a more or less northward tack. This descent ends at a usually dry streambed, where the trail climbs for a moment to terminate on an old jeep road. Turn right (east) down the ravine for a moment to find a signed trail junction. Here the hiker-only PCT branches left (northwest), while the signed equestrian PCT heads right (northeast) down to a dirt road-end.

This used to be the equestrian section of Sulphur Springs Trail Camp (406.6–5,270'), but it has since closed.

WATER ACCESS

CAMPING Stream water, usually lasting until summer, is available in the main part of Sulphur Springs Trail Camp, 0.2 mile east down the access road.

The PCT leaves the environs of the campground via two different routes. From the trail junction southwest of the former equestrian camp, the foot trail contours northwest on the shaded hillside above South Fork Little Rock Creek, then gently descends to step across that spring-fed rivulet. A minute later, you merge with the signed equestrian trail. The horse route leaves the campground at its western entrance via its previously paved access road 5N40H. This ambles northwest, just north of South Fork Little Rock Creek, to a resumption of trail tread, which drops left (southwest) away from the road a few yards to merge with the foot trail. Now you wind upcanyon (generally west–northwest) through sagebrush and scattered pines to clamber to the shoulder of dirt Little Rock Creek Road 5N04 (407.4–5,315'), just a moment west of its junction with the road to Sulphur Springs Trail Camp. Across the road, the tread steeply ascends a brushy ravine, then circles northwest. Continuing, you seamlessly merge with old trail alignment and gently but relentlessly proceed up the brushy hillside.

Soon your path starts to zigzag in and out of numerous small ravines, sometimes shaded at the bottom by interior live oaks but usually a sunny mixture of ocean spray, hoary-leaved ceanothus, yellow-blossomed flannelbush, and pungent yerba santa. Eventually the PCT winds through a gap and turns southwest at the head of Bare Mountain Canyon, but not before you

SECTION D

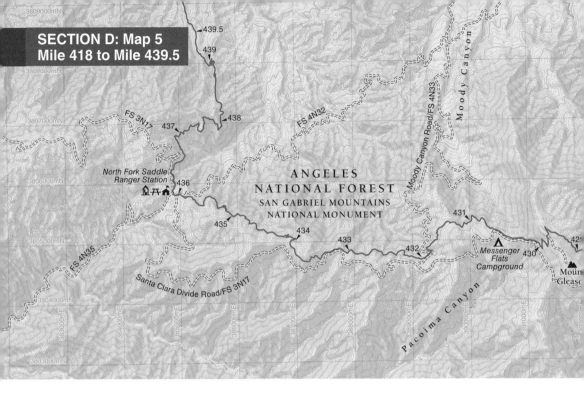

notice how easily the orange-rust-stained, rotting granite is quickly eroded by torrential rains into a badland of sharp-crested, barren ravines.

Just below the level of a saddle at the head of Bare Mountain Canyon, the route turns northwest, switchbacks briefly south, and then ascends easily northwest to a grassy flat just shy of shaded, seeping Fiddleneck Spring (410.4–6,232'), which emerges from the side of Pacifico Mountain.

Leaving the spring, your path climbs north to a notched ridge and then swings west to a chaparral-and-boulder-choked canyon dampened by Fountainhead Spring (411.0–6,436'), 140 feet above you. Like the previous spring, it may be waterless by early summer in dry years. No camping is afforded here.

Next your trail leads into and out of many small gulches clothed in 10-foot-high greenbark ceanothus but soon leaves these behind for a gentle amble up through an open forest of Jeffrey pine floored with rabbitbrush. After gaining Pacifico Mountain's north ridge, the trail swings southwest to a bare ridgetop vista point, giving panoramas north down Santiago Canyon to Little Rock Reservoir, Soledad Pass,

and the environs of Lancaster and Palmdale in the Antelope Valley.

From here the PCT begins a gentle descent southwest on steep, sparsely shaded slopes, passing above Sheep Camp Spring. Where the trail turns north in a shady gap (413.0–6,650'), trekkers may leave the PCT and walk south a few yards to a dirt road that can be ascended east to Mount Pacifico Campground for outstanding sunrise views. There is no water here, and it closes to campers for the season, typically mid-November–mid-May.

CAMPING Returning to the PCT, you descend gently northwest then west under interior live oaks and bigcone spruces to a jeep road, which you follow north down to its end and a resumption of trail. Now the path gently descends the head of spruce-mottled Tie Canyon, named for the railroad ties that were lumbered here in the late 1800s. Several nice, if wind-prone, campsites can be found before the descent.

Lower, you swing west through a U.S. Forest Service tree nursery and under the first of a pair of high-tension power lines, where you find a signed spur trail (418.5–4,980'). It climbs left,

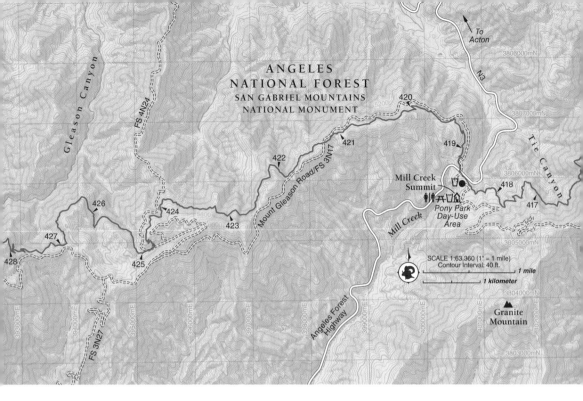

south, just a few feet to Pony Park Day-Use Area, with a parking area, toilets, a picnic table, and a spigot (filtering is strongly recommended).

WATER ACCESS

If the water is turned off, walk northwest down the paved road for just a minute to the Mill Creek Fire Station for water. Be sure to tank up here, as the next likely water on the northbound PCT is at North Fork Saddle, 17.5 miles away.

The PCT itself rounds down below the ranger station and a highway-maintenance yard,

soon making tiny switchbacks to reach Angeles Forest Highway at Mill Creek Summit, a small picnic area with a pit toilet that has been left shadeless by the Station Fire (418.6–4,979').

HISTORY Cut by the Mill Creek Fault, the cause of this saddle, the Mill Creek–Big Tujunga Wash area was the scene of a considerable mining rush in the 1880s, as men searched for the legendary Los Padres gold mines.

The PCTA Southern California Trail Gorillas have worked hard to clear the trail of overgrowth and poodle-dog bush in recent years, but hikers should use caution, stay on the trail at all times, and heed the camping restrictions. Hazards might include loose soil and rocks, unstable trees and terrain, flash flooding, and debris flows.

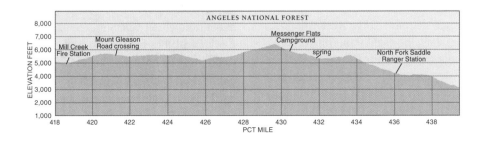

North across Angeles Forest Highway, the PCT begins to climb close alongside paved Mount Gleason Road 3N17, then leaves yerba santa scrub as it turns west, just north of the ridgetop, in shading interior live oak stands. Frequent glimpses north include the shimmering Antelope Valley and the barren Sierra Pelona (Spanish for "bald range"). The PCT dips to cross Mount Gleason Road (421.2–5,595'), then keeps north of and below that road. An undulating traverse at about 5,600 feet eventually turns south across the nose of a ridge. There it finds a short side trail that leads to a couple of small, shrub-protected campsites. The PCT continues south and soon switchbacks down to a narrow dirt road in a small northeast-trending canyon. Your route follows this track 0.1 mile southwest gently down to dirt FS 4N24 (424.8–5,521'). Across the road, trail resumes amid a skeletal collection of interior live oaks, ponderosa and Coulter pines, and brodiaea still recovering from wildfires.

Here, in a ravine, a flat (425.8–5,195') just below the trail contains water that is typically available only in earliest spring. Beyond the flat, the way begins to climb easily, first north around a ridge, then south and west.

HISTORY Nearby lie the remains of a Los Angeles County prison camp, which also served as one of a dozen Project Nike antiaircraft-missile installations in the Los Angeles area in the 1950s. Gutted by the unprecedented 2009 Station Fire, Camp 16, as it was known, housed more than 100 inmates who were trained to work on firefighting crews. Two crew members died in the line of duty.

Later, the PCT switchbacks up to a junction with a south-branching trail. Ignoring a north-branching trail, which was part of an earlier, now defunct PCT route down to Acton, you start along the south trail, which climbs for a moment to top Mount Gleason's north ridge and cross a narrow dirt road. You could ascend southeast about 300 yards along this road to Mount Gleason's scenic 6,502-foot summit.

The PCT, however, crosses the road and abruptly turns downhill into the head of Pacoima Canyon. Soon you are switchbacking down on poorly maintained, heavily eroded tread in a charred woodland of oak and manzanita.

CAMPING The trail then quickly makes a traverse just above Santa Clara Divide Road, but after a short while you leave the burned brush behind and, at the entrance to Messenger Flats Campground (430.4–5,886'), come to within a few feet of that road.

VIEWS With no water and shuttered toilets, it is no longer the bucolic pine-shaded spot it once was, but its expansive flat area and excellent views draw many hikers to rest or nap here after the semi-arduous climb from Mill Creek.

The next certain water is at North Fork Saddle Ranger Station, in 5.7 miles. Water is sometimes found in early spring just before the

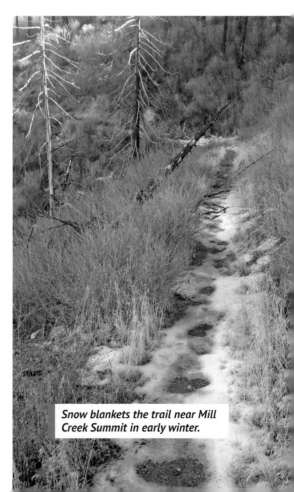

Snow blankets the trail near Mill Creek Summit in early winter.

PCT crosses Moody Canyon Road—1.5 miles from Messenger Flats Campground.

Leaving the campground, the PCT descends northwest momentarily, staying on the road's northern shoulder. This gentle descent soon becomes moderate to steep, however, as the trail veers from the roadside to traverse under the north rim of the Santa Clara Divide. This 1980s trail segment is narrower and more tortuous than you have become used to, though volunteers have worked hard in recent years to improve it. It was built by U.S. Forest Service crews, local Boy Scouts, and service clubs after it had become apparent that the original PCT route, northward through Acton, had to be abandoned due to private-property considerations.

Initially you are shaded by the now familiar, often fire-scarred trio of big-cone spruce, live oak, and ponderosa pine, but as the route drops, low, chamise chaparral supervenes. The otherwise monotonous scrub does, however, allow excellent, if smog-shrouded, vistas north over Soledad Canyon and Acton and northwest to ranks of low, seasonally green mountains, over which the PCT will pass on its way to the High Sierra. Soon you dip into a small ravine to strike Moody Canyon Road (431.9–5,375'). Seasonal water is sometimes available here, from the headwaters of Mill Canyon.

The PCT crosses west below Moody Canyon Road and adopts a fairly level route, once again under open oak-and-spruce shade. This course eventually leads you to intersect a ridgeline gap and its Santa Clara Divide Road. Here the PCT and the road coincide, descending gently west for just a moment to the next gap on the ridge, where PCT tread resumes. Climbing west, initially beside a poor jeep road, the trail now keeps on the sunnier south side of the divide, in low, dry chaparral. Beware of ticks residing on the brush hereabouts, and check your legs for them often. Presently, an easy ascent yields to a gentle descent; then the PCT reaches a firebreak atop the main divide and descends from its steeply west-descending jeep track.

After an initial descent northeast, the PCT turns northwest to descend moderately across the forested head of Mill Canyon. A few short switchbacks lead to a more earnest descent on often rocky tread. You get frequent glimpses down into Soledad Canyon, and later, as the tree cover thins, you can look northwest to the fantastic red Vasquez Rocks, the next major point of interest on your northward agenda.

Another set of small switchbacks presently deposits you at North Fork Saddle, where you find BPL Road 4N32 (436.1–4,185') under a crackling high-tension power line. On the north side of the saddle is the U.S. Forest Service's North Fork Saddle Ranger Station.

WATER ACCESS

There is a picnic table, shade, and a sometime water cache maintained by rangers here (see page 16 for more about water caches). Northbound trekkers will find their next certain water in Soledad Canyon, 8 miles away, while southbound trekkers are advised to carry water all the way to Mill Creek Summit, a long 17.5 miles away.

Bound for Soledad Canyon, the PCT descends north from the BPL road, initially just under Santa Clara Divide Road but soon far below it, on a diagonal descent on steep, rocky hillsides above Mill Canyon. Soon you are clambering steeply up and down across narrow ravines. Later, the PCT drops at a gentler angle, but as it rounds the east side of point 4,173, the path virtually plummets north into the head of Mattox Canyon. For the most part, your PCT stretch steeply traces a ridgetop firebreak, but in one place switchbacks do relieve the strain of your aching thigh muscles. When you can afford not to watch your footing, views east reveal a tree plantation in Mill Canyon.

PLANTS Beside the trail in springtime, yerba santa bears fragrant blue blossoms, and chia and fiddleneck show small purple and white flowers, respectively.

Eventually, you encounter a second set of switchbacks, which deposit you at a step-across ford of Mattox Canyon Creek (440.2–2,685′). This small stream usually flows into May but should not be relied on for water. Water access may be more certain a short way back upcanyon.

Pushing on, you ascend moderately west and north through dry chaparral to gain a 3,000-foot ridgecrest. A short drop from its north end leads to a contouring traverse above Fryer Canyon. From here, you can identify the PCT route, under some large pink cliffs, climbing the north slopes of Soledad Canyon. About 1 mile later, your path starts a swoop down to a nearby saddle, just feet above Indian Canyon Road 4N37.

GEOLOGY This pass is formed by the Magic Mountain Fault, one of a series of southwest-to-northeast-trending faults that transect the PCT in the next few miles. Notice how the Precambrian feldspar-rich granitic rocks have been crushed to a fine white powder by the fault's action.

Now the PCT makes a steep initial climb, paralleling Indian Canyon Road 4N37 and staying just above it. In a few minutes you reach a pass and dip to cross this dirt road (443.1–2,619′), which switchbacks steeply north down into Soledad Canyon. The PCT instead continues west, traversing gently down above the mouth of Indian Canyon before rounding back east to terminate on Indian Canyon Road at a point just 35 yards above that road's signed junction with two-lane, paved Soledad Canyon Road (444.2–2,245′).

RESUPPLY ACCESS

Congratulations are in order at this time, for you have now finished walking the length of the San Gabriel Mountains! Acton, with a post office, a market, restaurants, and a PCT register, lies 5.8 miles east up Soledad Canyon Road. Santa Clarita, a larger city with complete facilities, is 12.5 miles west down the road. The Acton KOA Campground on Soledad Canyon Road has water and welcomes hikers with discounted rates, showers, a small store, and a pool. They also accept resupply boxes for hikers.

WATER ACCESS

Northbound, the next certain water is in Agua Dulce, 10.3 miles ahead. Southbound trekkers will next get water up at North Fork Saddle, a usually hot 8-mile ascent into the San Gabriel Mountains.

It can be difficult to navigate the chaotic route of the northbound PCT across the Santa Clara River on the floor of Soledad Canyon. To succeed, simply keep in mind that you want to attain the railroad tracks running along the north side of the canyon, and respect private property as you go.

From Indian Canyon Road 4N37, northbound PCT travelers amble east along the shoulder of Soledad Canyon Road about 50 yards to a short, poor dirt-road spur that drops left (downcanyon) toward the riverside. Trail tread resumes from the eastern verge of this spur, marked by a brown metal PCT post.

CAMPING Two tiny switchbacks drop 20 feet to the alluvial flat (444.3–2,226′). Here you can walk east 3 minutes to KOA Campground.

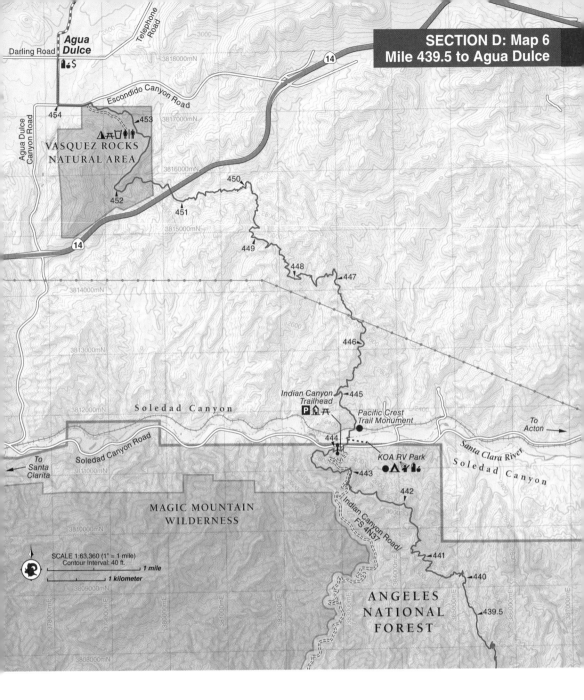

Agua
Dulce

Darling Road

Telephone Road

Escondido Canyon Road

454
453

Agua Dulce Canyon Road

VASQUEZ ROCKS
NATURAL AREA

452

451

450

449

448

447

446

445

Indian Canyon
Trailhead

Pacific Crest
Trail Monument

444

Soledad Canyon

KOA RV Park

443

Santa Clara River

Soledad Canyon

To Acton

Soledad Canyon Road

To Santa Clarita

442

MAGIC MOUNTAIN
WILDERNESS

Indian Canyon Road
FS 4N37

441

440

SCALE 1:63,360 (1" = 1 mile)
Contour Interval: 40 ft.

1 mile

1 kilometer

ANGELES
NATIONAL
FOREST

439.5

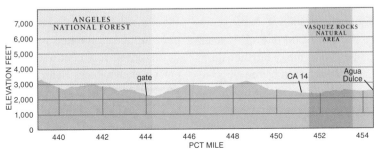

ANGELES
NATIONAL FOREST

VASQUEZ ROCKS
NATURAL
AREA

gate

CA 14

Agua
Dulce

7,000
6,000
5,000
4,000
3,000
2,000
1,000
0

ELEVATION FEET

440   442   444   446   448   450   452   454

PCT MILE

You pass a stand of Fremont cottonwoods to reach a ford of the Santa Clara River.

Don't dismay if you lose the route as you emerge on the extensively bulldozed north banks of the river. Trail tread is washed away by every spring's floods, so the way is often confusing. Your indistinct path empties onto a flat alluvial maze of dirt roads, debris piles, and other assorted rubble. Head north toward the far valley wall via the easiest route. Find a dirt road adjacent to a barbed wire fence, just south of railroad tracks. Now follow the road a short distance right (east) to a break in the fence marked with PCT emblems. It ushers you left (north) across another dirt road tracing the southern shoulder of the railroad tracks. You step north, up to a stop sign marking your crossing of railroad tracks (444.5–2,256'). A 3-foot-high cobble-and-concrete obelisk stands to the left of the trail, with a brass plaque commemorating PCT completion ceremonies, held here on June 5, 1993.

Leaving the shady canyon bottom to climb briskly back onto a fire-scarred hillside, the trail quickly gains a saddle but hardly pauses before continuing up. Soon you pass beneath strange, pinkish cliffs—our first encounter with the Vasquez Formation, which is a conglomerate of igneous and metamorphic cobbles set in fine-grained pink siltstone. The sometimes steep ascent finally abates as the trail rounds the east side of a summit to cross Young Canyon Road, which serves a trio of parallel, humming, high-voltage transmission lines. Across the good dirt road the way swings northwest, descending gently to moderately below the road, soon to cross a gap near the head of Bobcat Canyon. Around here you see, to the southwest, a spectacular formation of pink Vasquez outcrops. Next the PCT climbs a bit, then drops into Bobcat Canyon's dry wash before climbing in earnest to cross a jeep road on the divide separating Soledad and Agua Dulce Canyons.

As you catch your breath, you gain vistas south, east to Mount Gleason, and north to the Sierra Pelona; then you descend west, quickly recrossing the jeep road once and then again at a saddle, from which the trail leaves the ridgetop. The trail north from this saddle wastes no time—nor does it spare your knees—in a willy-nilly, steep descent north to a narrow branch of Escondido Canyon. After a bone-jarring 0.5 mile, the incline abates as the route hops to the ravine's west side, then levels out to turn west along a terrace above Escondido Canyon's seasonal creek. White-trunked sycamores in the canyon bottom contrast starkly with the surrounding red, rocky bluffs, dappled by yellow lichens, while yerba santa and white-flowered buckwheat dot the ruddy hillside.

VIEWS Across the canyon to the north is an even greater contrast—four-lane Antelope Valley Freeway (CA 14) climbing toward Palmdale.

A gradual descent carries you down to the level of the streambed at a side canyon and a use trail from the south. Now Escondido Canyon's trickling springtime stream, lined with watercress, bends more northward, and the PCT follows it, to abruptly enter a lengthy, graffiti-covered 10-foot-high tunnel under Antelope Valley Freeway (451.1–2,379').

PLANTS Emerging from the north end of the 500-foot passage, you find an abrupt change of scenery. Here the creekside is lined by thickets of willows and baccharis shrubs, while lush groves of squaw-bush, flannelbush, and poison oak stand just back from the creek's edge. The air is noticeably cooler, and myriad birds call from the underbrush.

Your route proceeds directly down the shallow, sandy streambed a few yards and then picks up a well-traveled path near the creek's north edge. You continue downcanyon and enter Vasquez Rocks Natural Area.

GEOLOGY In the park, note how the canyon's south wall begins to steepen into pink and red cliffs of sandstone and conglomerate. These rocks are layered sediments of Oligocene and Miocene age, having a nonmarine origin.

Your path soon crosses to the canyon's south side and then ascends slightly under a fantastic precipice of multilayered overhangs. Rounding north of this cliff, the route then drops to cross once again to the north bank.

Here, at a major side canyon from the north, the southern cliff bulges into a huge, cobbled overhang. Just downstream, the northern canyon wall is also overhung by cliffs. The PCT continues to head southwest (downstream) between the purple walls of rock. You will cross the creek six more times, where it seasonally pools and trickles over a sandy bottom. Look for tadpoles, and beware of poison oak and nettles. For a lunch stop, find a delightfully cool cave under an overhang of the tallest southern cliff, or pick the shade of a checkerboard-barked sycamore tree.

Next, you climb easily northwest away from the streamside, up and over the southwest end of a low ridge. A few yards later, find a three-way signed junction with an equestrian trail, which takes off to the left (southwest). Follow the PCT right, heading northeast up a steep section of trail. This deposits you on a little-used dirt road on the north rim of Escondido Canyon, surrounded by a springtime profusion of Whipple's yucca and a sign memorializing a July 2007 wildfire that burned the surrounding hillsides. Once on the canyon's rim, you find a different world, an almost flat upland dotted with low buckwheat, sagebrush shrubs, and head-high junipers. Lying in the northwest are the spectacular Vasquez Rocks, the 1850s hideout of famed bandit Tiburcio Vásquez.

Now begin a gentle ascent northeast as you parallel the western rim of the major tributary of Escondido Canyon, ignoring a north-branching track. Soon, across the canyon from some ridgetop homes, the route strikes a junction with another poor dirt road, descending west. This junction is marked by a sign, and on the road you follow a succession of similar posts west down past a cluster of picnic tables

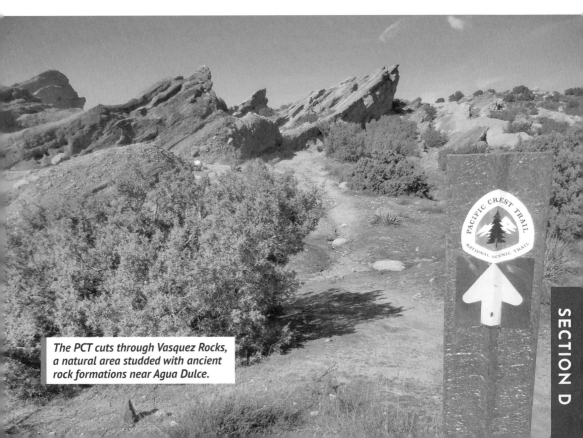

The PCT cuts through Vasquez Rocks, a natural area studded with ancient rock formations near Agua Dulce.

SECTION D

and across a large grassland to a gate (452.9–2,482') at a large parking area.

Just before this gate is a horse hitching post and the delightful shade of a large Brazilian pepper tree—a perfect lunch spot.

From the gate, the treadless PCT veers right, north, a few yards and then, developing a discernible tread, heads northwest, just north of a 20- to 30-foot-high, overhanging, cobbly cliff band. Walking here may give you a sense of déjà vu—and appropriately so, as these spectacular rock outcrops have been made famous by dozens of cowboy movies and TV ads.

From a rocky gap below the summit of these rocks, you descend easily west. The path now serves dual duty as a nature trail, and signs teach you the names of many chaparral species that you encounter throughout the park. Soon you wind near a number of homes just outside the park's north boundary, then amble northwest, around a half-dozen clifflets, to strike Escondido Canyon Road (453.6–2,482') at the signed entrance to Vasquez Rocks Natural Area.

CAMPING The ranger station and a modern nature center, where you can find information concerning camping and water, are just a minute's walk south down the entrance road. A large group camping area is just behind the nature center.

For the next 2 miles, the PCT is sited along the shoulder of busy paved roads. For the time being, though, here you turn left (west) along Escondido Canyon Road, soon coming to a stop sign at Agua Dulce Canyon Road.

RESUPPLY ACCESS

Turn right, north, onto it, and head into the village of Agua Dulce. Passing a café, you soon reach "downtown" Agua Dulce at Darling Road (454.5–2,537'). Restaurants are nearby, as is a feed-and-supply store for equestrians.

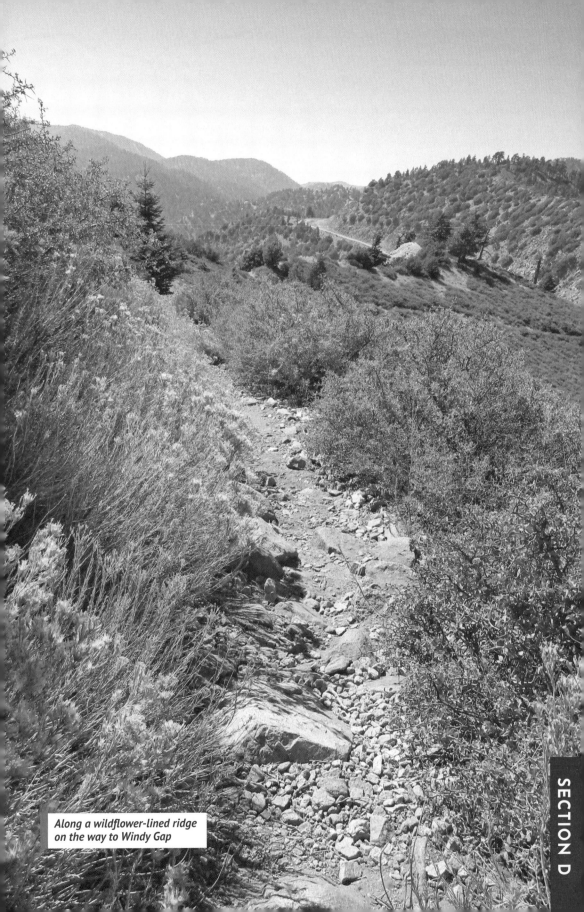

Along a wildflower-lined ridge on the way to Windy Gap

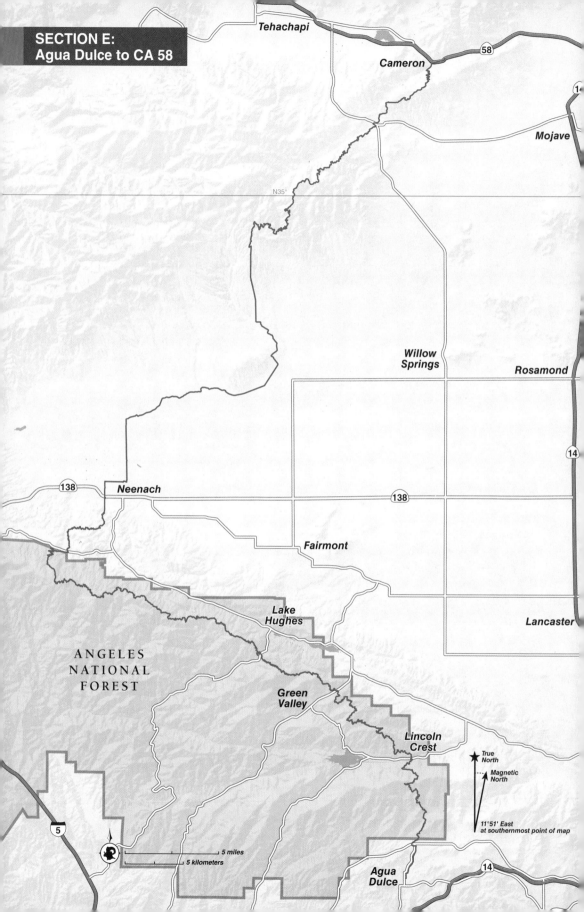

SECTION E:
Agua Dulce to CA 58

Tehachapi

Cameron

58

1

Mojave

N35°

Willow
Springs

Rosamond

138

14

Neenach

138

Fairmont

Lake
Hughes

Lancaster

ANGELES
NATIONAL
FOREST

Green
Valley

Lincoln
Crest

★ True
North

Magnetic
North

11°51' East
at southernmost point of map

5

5 miles

5 kilometers

Agua
Dulce

14

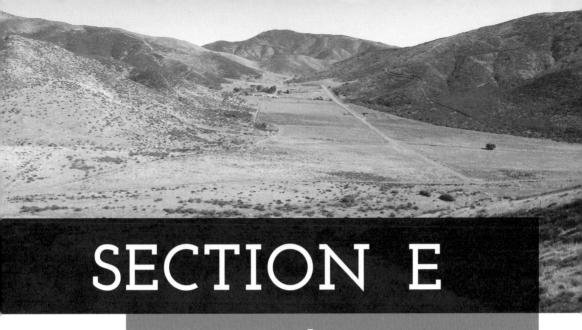

SECTION E

Agua Dulce to CA 58 near Mojave

THE MOJAVE DESERT is the arid setting for this short, often onerous segment of the Pacific Crest Trail (PCT). Some of the route is not even really trail, but rather it follows dusty dirt roads along the Los Angeles Aqueduct. Congress's original intent was to align the PCT atop the ridge of Liebre Mountain, going all the way west to the vicinity of Quail Lake. At the time of trail construction, the U.S. Forest Service (USFS) could not secure right-of-way easements over the necessary private lands and had to route the trail along the desert floor instead. Currently the USFS is working with the Tejon Ranch Corporation, Tejon Ranch Conservancy, and Pacific Crest Trail Association (PCTA) to negotiate a trail right-of-way easement that would relocate the PCT across private land along the crest of the Tehachapi Mountains, the start of the Sierran chain. This route would relocate the trail to the original location

Above: Views of arid terrain on the trail above Agua Dulce

envisioned by Congress, thereby enhancing the scenic nature of the PCT with mountain vistas, cool black oak and pine forests, and numerous springs.

For the time being, the PCT climbs slopes covered in chaparral on Grass Mountain, skirts Lake Hughes, and then attacks Sawmill Mountain's east flank before dropping north from Liebre Mountain, abandoning any pretense of being a crest route, and strikes north across the heart of the Antelope Valley, which is the western arm of the immense Mojave Desert. The pronghorn antelopes seen by John C. Frémont in 1844, when he forced passage through Tejon Pass via this valley, are gone, exterminated by hunters and later by encroaching alfalfa fields, but Antelope Valley's desert flavor remains.

Even in early spring, temperatures can soar over 100°F, and swirling dust devils can send unwary hikers sprawling or ducking for cover behind a Joshua tree. The route strikes due north across the shrub-dotted desert, and then, at the alluvial stoop of the Tehachapi Mountains—a southern extension of the Sierra Nevada—you turn east beside the underground Los Angeles Aqueduct, then continue up into the Tehachapis across several ravines, past dirt-bike trails, and through welcoming stands of junipers and piñon pines with vistas of the Antelope Valley.

Beginning in the Owens Valley, on the east side of the Sierra, the Los Angeles Aqueduct was the brainchild of William Mulholland, a former Los Angeles County water superintendent. It was constructed in 1913 and later extended north to the Mono Lake basin. Bitter disputes, court battles, and even shooting wars raged when Owens Valley farmers realized that the water needs of a growing Los Angeles would turn their well-watered agricultural region into a dust bowl. But Mulholland is a hero to some Angelenos, for millions of Southern Californians drink Owens Valley water, and without this project Los Angeles might have remained a sleepy patchwork of orange groves.

DECLINATION 11°51'E

USGS MAPS

Agua Dulce	Lake Hughes	Fairmont Butte
Sleepy Valley	Burnt Peak	Tylerhorse Canyon
Green Valley	Liebre Mountain	Tehachapi South
Del Sur	La Liebre Ranch	Monolith

POINTS ON THE TRAIL, SOUTH TO NORTH

	Mile	Elevation in feet	Latitude/Longitude
Agua Dulce	454.5	2,537	N34° 29' 46.680" W118° 19' 33.420"
Bear Spring	463.2	4,331	N34° 34' 13.958" W118° 18' 56.552"
Bouquet Canyon Road	465.5	3,334	N34° 34' 58.380" W118° 19' 21.180"
Spunky Edison Road 6N09	471.5	3,747	N34° 36' 34.360" W118° 21' 47.460"
San Francisquito Canyon Road/ Green Valley Ranger Station	478.2	3,392	N34° 38' 04.080" W118° 23' 23.940"
Lake Hughes Road to town (amenities)	485.7	3,058	N34° 39' 34.860" W118° 27' 37.560"
Liebre Mountain Truck Trail (guzzler nearby)	504.6	5,554	N34° 42' 49.500" W118° 38' 07.680"
Pine Canyon Road	510.9	3,839	N34° 44' 09.780" W118° 38' 33.000"
CA 138	517.6	3,052	N34° 46' 33.180" W118° 36' 20.520"
Los Angeles Aqueduct faucet	520.9	2,889	N34° 48' 10.760" W118° 35' 13.380"
Cottonwood Creek bridge	534.9	3,086	N34° 53' 51.420" W118° 27' 19.980"
Tehachapi Willow Springs Road to Tehachapi	558.5	4,145	N35° 03' 08.100" W118° 21' 30.420"
CA 58/to Mojave or Tehachapi	566.4	3,825	N35° 05' 57.840" W118° 17' 34.440"

CAMPSITES AND BIVY SITES

Mile	Elevation in feet	Latitude/ Longitude	Number of tents	Feature	Notes
465.9	3,453	N34° 35' 15.540" W118° 19' 18.540"	2	Small campsite	
468.2	3,976	N34° 35' 49.680" W118° 20' 17.760"	2	Campsite	
471.3	3,665	N34° 36' 32.520" W118° 21' 41.460"	2	Campsite	
493.0	4,643	N34° 41' 16.440" W118° 31' 18.000"	10	Maxwell Trail Camp	Guzzler; flat, semishaded tent sites; more sites near old road
498.2	5,188	N34° 42' 12.300" W118° 34' 34.140"	8–10	Sawmill Campground	Spring
504.4	5,400	N34° 42' 45.547" W118° 37' 56.812"	7	Bear Campground	Guzzler nearby
508.1	4,858	N34° 43' 53.160" W118° 39' 37.860"	5	Horse Camp	Picnic table, seasonal spring nearby
541.6	4,843	N34° 58' 45.960" W118° 28' 06.840"	>5	Tylerhorse Canyon	Seasonal creek

WEATHER TO GO

The second half of this section, north of the California Aqueduct, skirts the summer-sun-baked Mojave Desert. Ideally, you'd walk here in fall or early spring, after winter's incessant frosty winds and at the peak of wildflower displays but before the 100+°F days of June. Because most thru-hikers will come here in May, expect hot, sunny days with temperatures of up to 100°F, tempered by cool evenings and pleasant spring conditions in the higher elevations.

SUPPLIES

The village of Agua Dulce has several eateries and a small, well-regarded market but no post office (the closest is in Acton). It also has a hardware store, a feed store, and a hair salon. Hiker Heaven, a trail-angel property known far and wide for its hiker-friendly amenities, sadly closed its doors in 2019, as did another long-standing trail-angel property, Casa de Luna. Hiker Heaven may become an Airbnb-type rental; check hikerheaven.com for the latest information.

Later, the settlement of Green Valley is a short detour from the PCT where it drops into San Francisquito Canyon, 23.7 miles from Agua Dulce. Reach it by walking southwest 1.7 miles down San Francisquito Canyon Road to Spunky Canyon Road in quiet Green Valley, then heading southeast 0.9 mile to an intersection with a minimart and café.

A 2.2-mile detour to Lake Hughes, 31.2 miles into your journey, offers a post office, a restaurant with a few rooms to let, and a small store.

Lancaster might seem an improbable choice for resupply: it lies in the middle of sweltering Antelope Valley, fully 30 miles east of the PCT's crossing of CA 138, some 63.1 miles into this section. However, access is surprisingly easy, as CA 138 is very busy and hitchhiking should not pose a problem. Also, Lancaster is the largest town in this section, and it boasts a complete array of amenities for the PCT traveler, though its sprawl deters most hikers from seeking it out.

At the intersection of CA 138 and 269th Street, visible from the trail, sits Hikertown, an informal Old West–themed complex that has served as a trail-angel property in recent years with water, showers, and beds. Its future was uncertain at press time, however, and it's not recommended as an overnight stop.

A couple of cafés several miles east of Hikertown on CA 138 serve up burgers, burritos, and all kinds of hiker-friendly packaged goods.

Avangrid Renewables, also known as the Manzana Wind Project, offers 24-7 water via a 100-gallon tank (treating is advised) and accepts FedEx and UPS packages for hikers. Indicate ETA on package: Avangrid Renewables, 17890 Champagne Ave., Rosamond, CA 93560. From mile 536.9, walk east 1.3 miles across the wind farm property to a low-rise office building. Offices are open Monday–Friday, but hours may vary. Call ahead to confirm it is still accepting packages: 661-256-2220, ext. 4321.

Tehachapi lies 9.2 miles west of the PCT route at the end of this section. It is more easily reached, as described later, by Tehachapi Willow Springs Road, at the 558.5-mile mark, 7.9 miles before busy CA 58. Many hikers will exit here to minimize the need to carry heavy loads across the hot, dry Mojave Desert and Tehachapi Mountains segments. Tehachapi is a large and growing community, with many stores (including a Kmart), restaurants, motels, and laundromats, as well as a post office. Additionally, there are limited sporting goods available, as well as bus service and a small airport. Tehachapi has PCT host families who will help with travel to and from the trailhead.

Mojave is a desert town, also 9 miles from the PCT at the end of this section, reached via Tehachapi Willow Springs Road or east along CA 58. It is a fair-size community, with services similar to Tehachapi, and now sports a large shopping center with fast food, a pharmacy, groceries, and some chain motels that sit right at the junction of CA 58 and CA 14. This makes a visit to Mojave quite convenient. Mojave's two Motel 6 properties are popular with hikers.

How to choose between Tehachapi and Mojave for resupply? Tehachapi is much cooler, prettier, and quieter and has a somewhat greater depth of, though not a lot better, resources. For some, it will be a little harder to reach than Mojave. Mojave tends to be less expensive for lodging and meals and has a more compact town plan—it is easier for walkers. For the ravenous, it has a superior mix of fast-food restaurants. On the minus side, it is usually blisteringly hot, unattractive, and constantly barraged by the noise of a stream of auto traffic and passing trains—the antithesis of your ideal PCT experience.

WATER AND DESERT SURVIVAL

The Mojave Desert was a formidable barrier to early travelers, causing much hardship and greatly slowing Southern California's growth. That part of the Mojave traversed by the PCT is now tamed by crisscrossing roads and dotted with homes and ranches, eliminating past risks—as imagined by the uninformed—of dying like French Legionnaires, with parched throats and water-filled dreams. Still, the Mojave Desert stretch of the PCT can broil your mind, blister your feet, and turn your

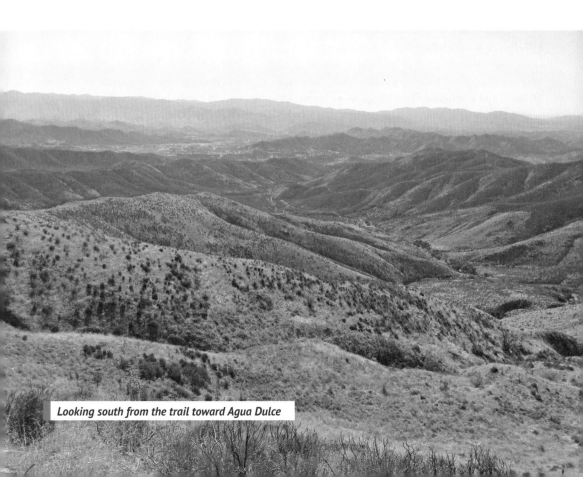

Looking south from the trail toward Agua Dulce

mouth to dust—in all, an unpleasant experience—if you are not adequately prepared. With a little forethought, enough water, and the right equipment, this hike can be a tolerable variation from the PCT's usual crest line surroundings.

Water is the key to all life, and enough of it will make yours more enjoyable. While planning your nightly stops or possible side hikes to water sources, you might consider the following government figures, arrived at by subjects operating under optimal experimental conditions (they weren't carrying heavy packs). Without water you can survive only two days at 120°F if you stay in one spot, five days at 100°F, and nine days at 80°F. If you walk during the day, you will survive only one-third as long. If you rest during the day and hike at night, then these figures become one, three, and seven days, with 12, 33, and 110 miles being covered. At 100°F, the midfigure, you would be able to hike 20 miles for every gallon of water you carried, though you would become hopelessly dehydrated and eventually incapacitated. Actual hiking conditions require at least 2 gallons a day while hiking in 100°F heat with a backpack, and most people will function better with 2.5 gallons.

Be aware that humans are the only mammals that do not drink automatically to replace the body's lost water stores, when water is available. Even when water is plentiful, exercising humans tend to become dehydrated, since most people drink only enough to keep their mouths and throats wet. Unfortunately, however, even a small degree of dehydration will exact a considerable toll on performance and endurance, and possibly result in health problems. Therefore, you must force yourself to drink enough water while exercising and to drink at frequent intervals. It is much better to drink a cup of water every 15 minutes or so than to stop every few hours and force down 2 quarts. When drinking, pick the most palatable liquid. The addition of a small amount of flavoring helps the chore of forced hydration, and some salts and a bit of sugar may actually help absorption of water from the stomach.

Hikers who drink plenty of water but fail to replace electrolytes after hours of grueling, hot-weather hiking can suffer from low blood sodium. Symptoms include nausea, muscle weakness, fatigue, and confusion. Including an electrolyte supplement in your daily routine—dozens of which are now available commercially—can also help keep the body's sodium balance intact, keep nausea and dizziness at bay, and often increase energy. Be aware, though, that most instant drink mixes, including many specialty athletic drinks, contain enough sugar and salts to actually delay stomach absorption and may lead to nausea during heavy exercise. Diluting commercial drinks to twice their volume usually prevents this problem. If you're not experiencing symptoms of hyponatremia, all that's necessary to make sure that vital body electrolytes are replaced during prolonged exertion is to eat a balanced diet and drink plain water. Most hiking foods contain more than enough salts to maintain body stores.

The best way to conserve water is to hike at night, and night hiking has added bonuses in the Mojave Desert: astounding star-filled skies, fewer passing cars, and the chance to observe some little-seen desert wildlife—inquisitive kit foxes sometimes play tag with hikers. Yucca night lizards, which spend their days under fallen Joshua trees, also scurry about at night. But use a flashlight, even on moonlit nights, because rattlesnakes like to lie on the warm roads.

If you prefer to hike in daylight, start early, before sunrise, say at 5 in the morning during spring. Hike about 4 hours, perhaps getting in 12 miles, rest until evening, and then hike about another 2 hours. By day, walkers should ignore their desire to shed sweaty shirts or pants, as clothing not only prevents excessive moisture loss and overheating but also forestalls an excruciating high-desert sunburn.

It is no secret that water is a critical issue throughout arid Section E, and especially so in drought years. After about May 1, don't count on water at any sites away from human improvement. Even before then, most streams are small seasonal trickles and likely to be polluted.

This should not overly inconvenience PCT travelers, since the (untreated) streams and springs that supply the campgrounds are still as accessible as ever. Treat all water with iodine, or use a filter before drinking water from any natural sources. In an emergency, you may be forced to try to obtain water from springs or creekbeds that are barely flowing.

Heat-related illnesses, most notably heat cramping, heat exhaustion, and heat stroke, can also be an issue in this section. Heat cramping occurs when you become dehydrated and experience leg or abdomen cramps and sweat more heavily than normal. Heat exhaustion can occur after you've been exposed to high temperatures for several days. Symptoms include heavy sweating, weakness, dizziness, dark-colored urine, fainting, fatigue, muscle cramps, and nausea. Heat stroke can be fatal and requires immediate hospital treatment. Signs include a throbbing headache, confusion, nausea, dizziness, shallow breathing, and unconsciousness.

PERMITS

No wilderness permits are required for overnight PCT campers, though section hikers are encouraged to obtain them when possible in case there is an emergency.

SPECIAL CONCERNS

No campfires of any kind are allowed in Angeles National Forest, outside of designated campgrounds. A California campfire permit is required to use portable stoves containing gas, jellied fuel, or pressurized liquid fuel outside of campfire use sites. Permits may be obtained online at readyforwildfire.org/permits/campfire-permit.

AGUA DULCE TO CA 58 NEAR MOJAVE

>>>THE ROUTE

Reach Agua Dulce (454.5–2,537') via CA 14, 18 miles east of its junction with I-5 in Sylmar or 21 miles south of Palmdale. Take CA 14's Agua Dulce Canyon Road exit, then head north 2.5 miles up that road to east–west Darling Road, in Agua Dulce. Your first chance for water north of town is at Bear Spring, 8.7 miles away. However, in recent drought years, Bear Spring has been quite unreliable, so plan to carry water until the next certain water, at San Francisquito

Canyon Road and Green Valley Ranger Station, 23.7 miles away.

Leave Agua Dulce by walking north on Agua Dulce Canyon Road very gently up grassy Sierra Pelona Valley. You pass numerous homes and side roads, a few businesses, an airfield, and finally a church before your road ends at wide, paved Sierra Highway. Turn left and go west along its north shoulder just a bit to paved Mint Canyon Road. Follow that road up and right (west) shortly to a low gap where paved Petersen Road branches north. Turn right on Petersen Road and descend gently to the southern edge of a ranch-dotted bench in Mint Canyon. Here a dirt road (456.7–2,755') servicing a line of high-tension electric wires branches right.

The PCT begins by climbing momentarily northeast up this road, ignoring a spur branching right, then descends for a short while. The road then ascends moderately again, on exposed slopes of withered chamise on the east flank of Mint Canyon. Pass a second right-branching spur. Walk up past a chain-link fence and reenter Angeles National Forest, where you resume trail tread some 50 yards beyond a large steel electrical tower. Follow the tread left (north) as it contours around a nose, then makes a long, easily descending traverse to the shadeless southeast banks of Mint Canyon's infrequently flowing stream. At a step-across ford of the creek, you pass a horse trail that continues upcanyon. The PCT, however, clambers west up onto a low bench with an equestrian trail register. Beyond, you walk straight uphill on an old jeep road, passing another that runs downcanyon. Where a jeep road climbs left along an old barbed wire fence, you follow the obvious PCT right, ascending north. You soon reach a promontory overlooking the valley and private ranches, and then the path climbs moderately northwest to survey more blackened chaparral on the headwall of Mint Canyon. By walking a few minutes more, you reach an unmarked trail astride a saddle.

Leaving the saddle, the PCT starts a traverse to the left of the ridge, gaining elevation gradually at first, on cobbly schist tread. You climb more rapidly as the path drifts northwest, presenting excellent over-the-shoulder vistas south to the bizarre Vasquez Rocks, purported refuge of bandit Tiburcio Vásquez, and farther east to Mounts Gleason, Williamson, and Baden-Powell. You now switchback steeply up almost to the ridge, where you switchback again, back north. When the climb moderates, you soon reach Martindale Ridge Road (462.3–4,500'). Now turn right (east) and walk gently up to a low saddle. Here, atop Sierra Pelona Ridge, wind gusts have been measured in excess of 100 miles per hour. Now PCT posts lead your way northeast via a disused jeep road, through a white pipe gate, then steeply down the hillside at the head of Martindale Canyon. The path soon crisscrosses the even more steeply descending jeep track multiple times and is easily lost on sloping hillside meadows of foxtails and grasses.

Presently, you circle just above the levelest such flat, grown waist-high in yellow mustard.

WATER ACCESS

Hidden in a tangle of wild grapevines is mosquito-infested Bear Spring (463.2–4,331'). The spring's pipe is about 35 feet uphill from the trail, while a metal trough is just below the trail. This water hole often runs late into spring but should not be relied upon.

Continuing down with vistas north across Antelope Valley to Owens Peak in the southern Sierra, you circle the upper reaches of fault-aligned Martindale Canyon, soon reaching a

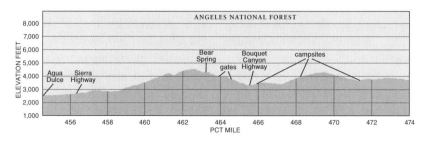

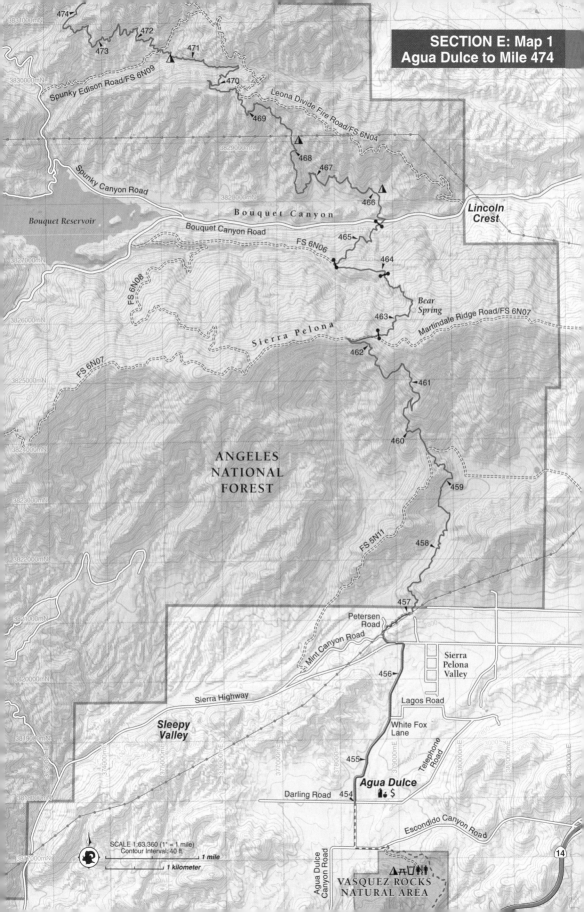

474

473

472

471

470

469

Spunky Edison Road/FS 6N09

Leona Divide Fire Road/FS 6N04

Spunky Canyon Road

468

467

466

Bouquet Canyon

Lincoln Crest

465

Bouquet Canyon Road

Bouquet Reservoir

FS 6N06

FS 6N08

464

Bear Spring

463

Martindale Ridge Road/FS 6N07

462

Sierra Pelona

FS 6N07

461

460

ANGELES NATIONAL FOREST

459

458

FS 5N11

457

Petersen Road

Sierra Pelona Valley

456

Mint Canyon Road

Lagos Road

Sierra Highway

White Fox Lane

Sleepy Valley

455

Agua Dulce

Telephone Road

Darling Road

454

Escondido Canyon Road

Agua Dulce Canyon Road

SCALE 1:63,360 (1" = 1 mile)
Contour Interval: 40 ft.

1 mile

1 kilometer

VASQUEZ ROCKS NATURAL AREA

14

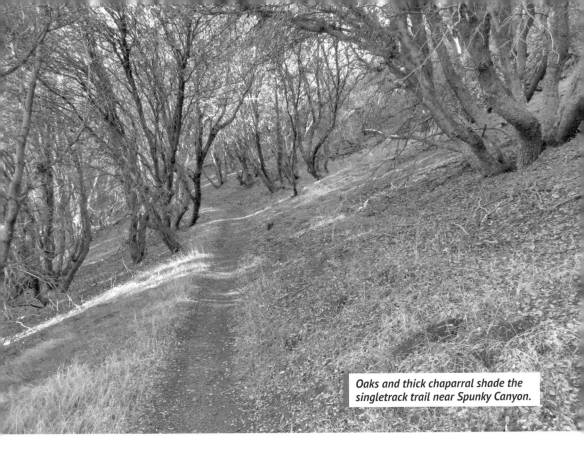

Oaks and thick chaparral shade the singletrack trail near Spunky Canyon.

ridgetop-firebreak jeep trail. This you descend, continuing west, to a junction with the old PCT alignment, which formerly climbed south to Big Oak Spring. Now you turn right for a more gradual descent on chaparral-choked trail, leading northeast to paved Bouquet Canyon Road 6N05 (465.5–3,334').

FIRE Tripped power lines started the 2013 Powerhouse Fire, which burned 30,000 acres of northern Los Angeles County, including the PCT between San Francisquito Canyon Road (mile 478.2) and mile 492. A fierce rainstorm in 2015 caused more destruction on the fragile hillsides and left a large swath of the trail impassable due to mudslides. For several years, hikers opted to detour via Elizabeth Lake Road through the town of Lake Hughes. The stretch reopened in 2017, thanks in part to the admirable efforts of the PCTA Southern California Trail Gorillas, a volunteer crew dedicated to maintaining and repairing the PCT between Campo and Kennedy Meadows. Due to the magnitude of the damage, the USFS and the PCTA repaired the trail employing an approach less commonly used on the PCT, using both hand crews and a trail-building machine that removed large amounts of dirt covering the trail and reestablished the actual path along the hillsides, while humans followed behind and smoothed it all out with shovels and hard labor. It was an amazing feat and a testament to this group's hard work and dedication to the trail.

GEOLOGY Merging under Bouquet Reservoir, 2.5 miles west, the San Francisquito and Clearwater Faults run Bouquet Canyon's length and separate southern Pelona schists from granites on the canyon's north wall.

The PCT drops across the dry wash draining Bouquet Canyon, then arcs easily up, northwest, to cross a jeep road near a water tank in a small canyon. Now the trail ascends moderately on coarse granitic sand to just north of a power

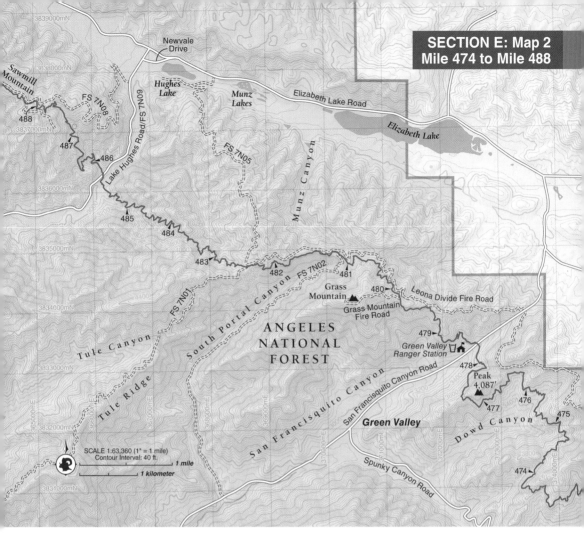

line, where the PCT branches northwest from the old California Riding and Hiking Trail, which continues north up to Leona Divide Fire Road 6N04.

The PCT climbs along the steep south-facing slope through sickly, low chamise; crosses a descending firebreak; and then veers more northward, just under the Leona Divide Fire Road, to gain a pass with another firebreak, which tops a ridge dividing Spunky and Bouquet Canyons. A gentle switchback in now-denser chaparral and occasional shading oaks drops you to the head of Spunky Canyon, where you turn downcanyon (west), then climb slightly to strike Spunky Edison Road 6N09 (471.5–3,747').

RESUPPLY ACCESS

If you're thirsty or need supplies, first walk west 1.7 miles down this dirt road to paved Spunky Canyon Road 6N11. On it, wind northwest about 2 miles to Green Valley, with a minimart, gas station, and café.

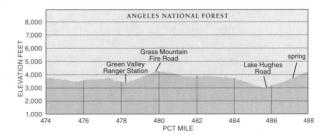

The PCT climbs gently away from FS 6N09, winding in and out of small ravines on a westward bearing. Eventually the path tops a small ridge, again with a firebreak, and then the trail angles northeast, through a gap, and down into the upper end of Dowd Canyon. Seen from here, Jupiter Mountain looms impressively across the valley. You reach a low point of 3,475 feet in Dowd Canyon, in a gully where native bunchgrasses grow; then you amble north–northwest before heading southwest around Peak 4,087 over to a ridgetop separating Dowd and San Francisquito Canyons.

From here a final northeastward swoop under shady interior live oaks brings the PCT to paved San Francisquito Canyon Road (478.2– 3,392'). Green Valley Ranger Station, with water, is 250 yards southwest; treat this water before drinking. About 1.7 miles southwest down San Francisquito Canyon Road is Green Valley, which has a minimart, gas station, and café, as well as phones and a fire station.

Across San Francisquito Canyon Road, the PCT begins its climb of Grass Mountain by ascending northwest into a nearby side canyon, above which it strikes a dirt road serving two power lines. The trail follows the road north momentarily, then switchbacks west and progresses unremittingly up chaparralled slopes to Grass Mountain Fire Road (479.8–4,270'), striking this dirt road just above its junction with Leona Divide Fire Road.

VIEWS Panoramas unfold northward over Elizabeth Lake—a sag pond on the San Andreas Fault—to distant Antelope Valley and the Tehachapi Mountains. If you are enjoying a smogless spring day, Owens Peak in the southern Sierra Nevada may be seen.

You enjoy this scenery as the path contours then descends the north slopes of Grass Mountain to a saddle (481.2–3,899'), where four dirt roads converge at the head of South Portal and Munz Canyons.

Keeping on a steep hillside south of the ridge, the PCT contours from this gap over to another saddle, where it crosses dirt Tule Canyon Road 7N01 by its junction with Lake Hughes Truck Trail 7N05. Onward the route rolls across dry ravines in dense chaparral, switchbacks once to pass through a gap, and then descends

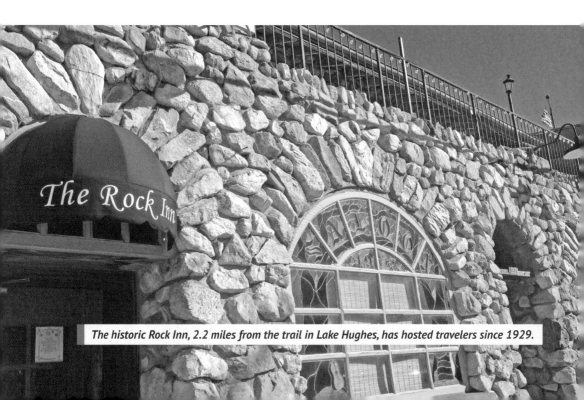

The historic Rock Inn, 2.2 miles from the trail in Lake Hughes, has hosted travelers since 1929.

unhesitatingly toward Elizabeth Lake Canyon by crossing an interminable array of narrow, rocky gulches. At the bottom of this segment, your path bursts from brush cover to traverse the broad, sandy wash of Elizabeth Lake Canyon. Northbound hikers head for nearby, paved Lake Hughes Road 7N09 (485.7–3,058').

WATER ACCESS

Water sources along this stretch between Lake Hughes Road and CA 38 can be unreliable and unsanitary. Be sure to verify which sources are truly available before heading out, and plan accordingly. Maxwell Trail Camp, a 0.6-mile detour that leaves the PCT in 7.3 miles, is typically a reliable source along this stretch.

RESUPPLY ACCESS

If you need water or supplies, you should detour 1.5 miles upcanyon (north) along Lake Hughes Road to Newvale Drive, which is on the west side of the small resort community of Lake Hughes. There you will find The Rock Inn (661-724-1855, historicrockinn.com), a historic café-bar with several upstairs rooms to let, plus a small convenience store. Reach these by following Newvale Drive east 0.3 mile to Elizabeth Lake Road, then walking 0.4 mile farther east along Elizabeth Lake Road. The Lake Hughes post office is another 0.5 mile east along the highway. The next chance to resupply on the northbound PCT is at a small market-café on CA 138 or in Tehachapi, which lies west of the PCT at the end of Section E.

PLANTS You will also see diminishing stands of Joshua trees. At one time Joshua trees, or tree yuccas, were more widely distributed, as evidenced by fossils of an extinct, giant, yucca-feeding ground sloth, found in southern Nevada where you no longer find Joshua trees. These giant members of the lily family, with their unusually branched, sometimes humanlike form, were likened by Mormon pioneers to the figure of Joshua, pointing the route to the Great Salt Lake.

Botanists now know that Joshua trees will not branch at all unless their trunk-tip flowers are damaged by wind or boring beetles. Each time a Joshua tree blossoms—an event determined by rainfall or temperature—it sprouts a footlong panicle of densely clustered, greenish-white blooms that produce football-shaped fruits later in the year.

Like that of other yuccas, Joshua tree pollen is too heavy to reach another plant, even in strong desert winds. Because they cannot pollinate themselves, they rely on a symbiotic relationship with the little, white yucca moth, also called the pronuba moth. Unlike other insects, which might unwittingly carry pollen from one plant to another, the moth makes a separate trip to carry pollen, which it stuffs deep into a Joshua tree blossom. It then drills a hole in the base of the flower, where it lays an egg. When the moth grub hatches, it has fruit to feed upon. Another animal that apparently can't live without Joshua trees or other yuccas is the small, mottled night lizard, which hides under fallen Joshua trees, feeding on termites, spiders, and ants.

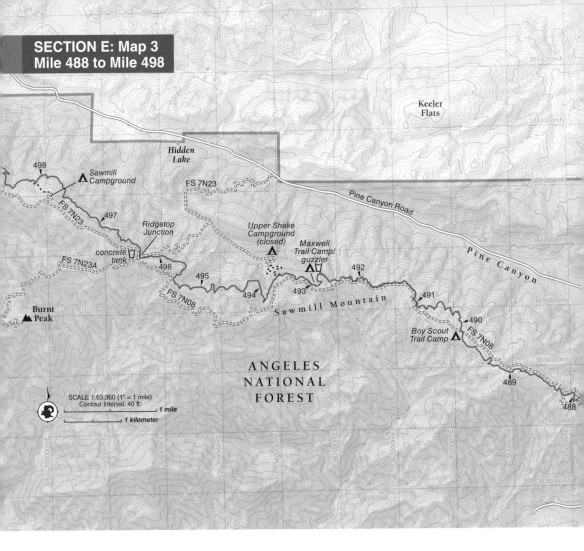

GEOLOGY Halfway across Antelope Valley, you're walking on sediments eroded from the Tehachapi and San Gabriel Mountains that geologists estimate are up to 5,000 feet thick.

PLANTS Note how evenly spaced the glossy-leaved creosote shrubs are. They secrete a toxin, washed to the ground by rain, that poisons nearby plant growth and provides the shrubs root space to collect sufficient water. Observant walkers may note some of the creosote bushes growing in clustered rings, up to a few yards apart. Botanists have discovered that root-crown branching by those shrubs results in rings of plants, each one a genetic clone of the colonizing plant. By radiocarbon dating and growth-rate measurements, scientists have

dated some creosote bush clonal rings in the Mojave Desert back an estimated 11,000 years—far older than the bristlecone pine.

Across Lake Hughes Road 7N09, the PCT attacks Sawmill Mountain's east flank. The trail climbs quickly northwest into a small valley with a sycamore-shaded flat. Soon the route, now back in chamise-and-oak chaparral, passes the mouth of an old graphite mine tunnel, then switchbacks

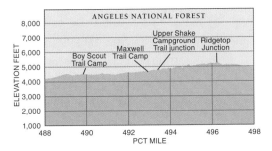

to climb more steeply southwest past two more tunnels. After reaching a ridge, the trail again swings northwest to ascend moderately through yerba santa and chamise back into the canyon. Here you find some shade in the form of interior live oaks and a cluster of disheveled big-cone spruces surrounding a trailside wet-season spring (487.1–3,734'). No camping is possible on the steep slope here. Continuing, the path leads up the now-narrow ravine, then veers southwest at its head to reach a scenic intersection with the Sawmill-Liebre Firebreak, just above a wide dirt road, Maxwell Truck Trail 7N08.

Now-familiar vistas north over the western part of Antelope Valley to the Tehachapi Mountains are presented here and accompany you as the PCT adopts a leisurely, traversing ascent of Sawmill Mountain's spine, always keeping just a stone's throw south of Maxwell Truck Trail. Repeated crossings of the ridge and its firebreak in a mix of chaparral eventually lead you to Maxwell Truck Trail 7N08 (489.9–4,530') in an open glade of black oaks.

You walk 35 yards northwest along the road to where trail tread resumes. The PCT drops slightly, then assumes an undulating traverse in and out of gullies on the north slope of Sawmill Mountain. After a short while the PCT becomes situated just below moderately ascending Maxwell Truck Trail and maintains that arrangement through chaparral sprinkled with Coulter pines. Eventually the PCT turns south into a larger ravine to cross two dirt roads in quick succession.

WATER ACCESS

CAMPING These access roads mark the site of a small plantation of trees, whose Coulter pines and incense cedars shade pleasant Maxwell Trail Camp (493.0–4,643'), which is just 100 feet north, down the first road. It has a unique guzzler self-filling water tank, where green algae–stained water is available to wildlife and hikers alike, though filtering is strongly recommended.

Pushing on, you ascend a shadier hillside and soon reach a trail intersection.

WATER ACCESS

The poorer branch climbs steeply southeast to Maxwell Truck Trail, while a good branch, descending northwest, drops via switchbacks 0.6 mile to permanently closed Upper Shake Campground. A small, usually flowing stream can be found in Shake Canyon, just north of the campground. In a pinch, hikers looking to leave the trail can descend 2 miles on an unpaved fire road to reach Pine Canyon Road, which turns into Elizabeth Lake Road to the east with access to the town of Lake Hughes.

The northbound PCT heads southwest gently up from the Upper Shake Campground trail junction, traversing the hillside first under shady oaks and big-cone spruces as it ducks into and then heads out of a small canyon. This pleasant segment crosses an abandoned jeep road that drops into the head of Shake Canyon, then continues to a ridgetop road junction. From here, Maxwell Truck Trail 7N08 starts south on a generally eastward traverse, Burnt Peak Road 7N23A traverses west, and Liebre Mountain Truck Trail 7N23 traverses northwest and descends northeast to Pine Canyon Road.

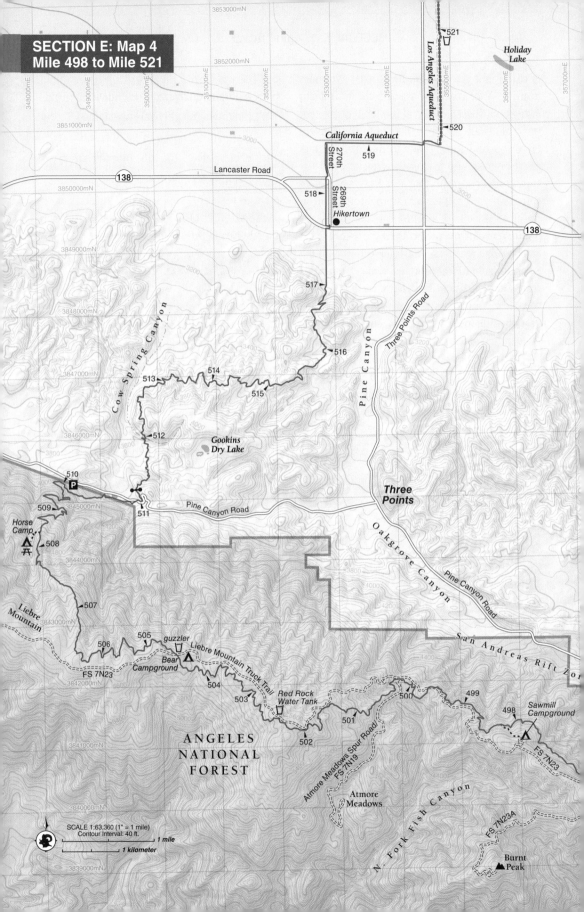

3853000mN

Los Angeles Aqueduct

521

Holiday Lake

3852000mN

520

California Aqueduct

519

270th Street

Lancaster Road

138

3850000mN

518

269th Street

Hikertown

138

3851000mN

3849000mN

517

Pine Canyon

Three Points Road

3848000mN

516

Cow Spring Canyon

514

513

515

3847000mN

512

Gookins Dry Lake

3846000mN

510

P

Three Points

509

511

Pine Canyon Road

Horse Camp.

508

Oakgrove Canyon

Pine Canyon Road

3845000mN

3844000mN

Liebre Mountain

507

San Andreas Rift Zone

506

505

guzzler

Liebre Mountain Truck Trail

3843000mN

Bear Campground

FS 7N23

504

503

Red Rock Water Tank

500

499

498

Sawmill Campground

FS 7N23

501

502

ANGELES NATIONAL FOREST

Atmore Meadows Spur Road

FS 7N19

Atmore Meadows

FS 7N23A

3841000mN

3840000mN

N. Fork Fish Canyon

Burnt Peak

SCALE 1:63,360 (1" = 1 mile)
Contour Interval: 40 ft.

1 mile

1 kilometer

3839000mN

CAMPING The PCT descends gently north under the upper branch of Sawmill Mountain Truck Trail, now in even shadier mixed forest and chaparral. Next a long descent leads across a broad black oak–clothed ridge nose to a junction (498.2–5,000'). From here a spur trail ascends southeast 0.2 mile to small Sawmill Campground. A wildlife guzzler often has water in the spring; it's about a mile from the campground up a fire road near a cluster of pine trees on a cleared slope.

You first contour and then switchback twice to resume a position just north of and below Liebre Mountain Truck Trail. Presently, you cross that road (499.4–4,792') at a large turnout. Across the road, your trail drops southwest, through a corridor of Coulter pines, then winds west around the head of wild, rugged North Fork Fish Canyon. Soon you reach a saddle junction of Liebre Mountain Truck Trail and Atmore Meadows Spur Road 7N19. The PCT follows the latter road southwest 80 yards to a resumption of trail tread in a steep ravine.

Next on the PCT's agenda of chaparral-cloaked summits is Liebre Mountain, and the steep, seasonally hot trail that climbs from Atmore Meadows Spur Road quickly dispels any thoughts of a sedate ascent. After an effort, you are high on brushy slopes, panting toward a grassy saddle (502.4–5,616'), which marks an end to the unpleasant grind. Step across a jeep road that crosses the saddle, then descend easily northwest, still just under the truck trail.

Now descending easily, zigzags lead northwest first close to Liebre Mountain Truck Trail, then into and out of interminable dry washes that alternate with brushy ridgelets. Sometimes you have good views south to the wildlands of deep Cienega Canyon.

CAMPING Eventually, the undulating descent ceases and the grade becomes a moderate ascent. Moments later, you encounter a junction with a spur trail that climbs north a few yards to waterless Bear Campground (504.4–5,400'). An additional 3 minutes' climb along the PCT leads to a crossing of Liebre Mountain Truck Trail 7N23 (504.6–5,554').

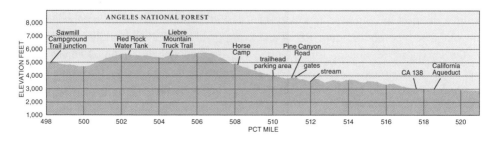

WATER ACCESS

A wildlife guzzler can be reached from this point. Walk back right (east) 100 yards down the road. Then look north down a shallow gully, under an open grove of black oaks, where a fiberglass water tank for the use of wildlife and hikers lies under a low, corrugated aluminum roof.

Now on the cooler north slopes of Liebre Mountain, your way becomes much nicer, winding almost level along hillsides shaded by open groves of black oaks. In spring the grassy turf underfoot is a green sea dotted with brodiaea, baby blue eyes, and miner's lettuce. Soon you cross a north-descending dirt road on a ridge nose as the PCT winds west close to the gentle summit of Liebre Mountain. You wind over two more small, delightfully oak-clothed ridgetops, then merge with a poor jeep track, still traversing more or less levelly, for just a minute to reach another jeep road (506.5–5,754') on the crest of a broad, open ridge. Here the PCT branches right (northwest) down the ridgetop on the jeep road briefly before striking a fair dirt road.

VIEWS Here, take a few minutes' detour, and walk left (south) back up to the top of Liebre Mountain's ridge for its expansive vistas south to the Santa Monica Mountains, the Pacific Ocean, and the highrises of Hollywood looming over the white roller coasters of Six Flags Magic Mountain. Possibly more interesting is an eastward inventory of terrain conquered: beyond Vasquez Rocks and across the San Gabriel Mountains, from Mounts Wilson and Gleason on the west to towering Mount Baden-Powell and Mount Baldy on the east, are all there for inspection.

The PCT heads downhill (north) on this closed ridgetop road, passing through a plantation of young black oaks and their older in-laws. Soon the downgrade steepens and sagebrush replaces much of the understory. Windswept panoramas over the westernmost corner of Antelope Valley remind you that you have now ended a sweeping, nearly 300-mile skirting of the southwestern border of the Mojave Desert, which has led you west from Whitewater along the summits of the San Bernardinos, the San Gabriels, and Sawmill and Liebre Mountains—a job well done!

Continuing your descent, you lose these views as you reenter big-cone spruce, pine, and oak cover below 5,200 feet in elevation. Soon thereafter, the road, which has diminished to a rough jeep track, ends.

CAMPING Switchbacks lower you gently from just beyond this point into a saddle—with a good but dry camp known as Horse Camp (508.1–4,858')—just short of a conifer-clad 4,923-foot knob. If you choose to camp here in early season, you may find water 100–200 feet down a steep gully to the east, though beware it may be infested with nettles and insects.

Beyond, the enjoyable trail enters thick chaparral, descends moderately via switchbacks, and presently levels out at a dirt road spur (510.0–4,003') atop a minor pass just south of paved Pine Canyon Road.

This trail segment heads right (south), away from the road spur, descending easily in a hillside stand of Coulter pines and black and scrub oaks. The trail finds a sandy traverse east and eventually comes upon the south banks of a small sag pond (510.7–3,800'), which lies on the San Andreas Fault. It is commonly dry by fall. The PCT continues east from the pond, ascending gently past a sign notifying you that you have exited Angeles National Forest onto private property. A moment later, you step across seasonally trickling Cow Spring Canyon Creek, which runs into late May in all but the driest years. Next the path swings close to and then crosses paved Pine Canyon Road (510.9–3,839').

A brown signpost marks the road crossing, which leads to a gentle ascent alongside the switchbacking road, soon to reach a large sign diagramming the PCT's course through Tejon Ranch's property. The sign asks that hikers not leave the path for any reason for the next 7 miles and expresses a prohibition against camping and fires.

Now commences a tiring stretch of trail skirting the boundary of Tejon Ranch lands. Up and down you march, north across hillsides of hot, dry, low chamise and manzanita scrub on loose trail tread, marked by frequent tiny, reverse-banked switchbacks. Eventually, you drop steeply down a ridge nose to the verge of a dry grassland in Cow Spring Canyon. Here the ranch boundary, marked by a four-strand barbed wire fence, turns abruptly east, as do you.

The next leg continues on an eastward bearing, ascending up and across a number of small, sunny ridges. In due time, you descend 100 feet from one of the ridges to cross a jeep road in a sandy, buckwheat-dotted wash. Beyond, you climb steeply east out of the wash, pass through a gap, and then traverse a hillside with an overlook of Pine Canyon. Steep, then gentle, descent soon ensues, now turning north to bisect a broad wash. Now heading north again, you amble over a broad saddle, then descend via switchbacks to merge with a good jeep road in a small, narrow valley. Turn right (northeast) along the gently descending road, which passes above a small ranch at the canyon's mouth. Beyond, the road descends north, arrow-straight out onto the alluvial verge of Antelope Valley. Pass some branching fence-line jeep roads, but continue straight ahead, soon reaching busy, paved CA 138 (517.6–3,052'), just west of its intersection with signed 269th Street West. Green metal gates now allow horse and foot traffic access to the pavement. Hurry across—the highway is very busy.

WATER ACCESS

Hikertown, whose fate as a trail-angel property was uncertain at press time, has a faucet just outside its gate that has remained a reliable water source in recent years.

Back on the PCT, you pass through a green gate to regain your fence-side dirt road-trail, still descending easily due north. In less than 0.5 mile you find another sign announcing the special restrictions for using the PCT in the Tejon Ranch. Beyond it, you pass through two stile gates to reach Lancaster–Barnes Ranch Road at its junction with 269th Street (518.1–2,997').

Walk north along this paved road, near the shuttered and fenced-off elementary school. Just north of the school, pavement ends (518.5–2,979'), and the PCT heads right (east) through a gate and onto a sandy dirt road. This road parallels the behemoth California Aqueduct, a veritable concrete-lined river flowing in a channel hidden behind a massive earthen berm to the north. Follow the current path or either of two firmer, more-used roads, just south of the aqueduct, levelly east to a pair of roads. The first of this pair, Three Points Road, is paved and bridges the aqueduct at a siphon (519.5–2,980'). Cross north over the aqueduct, then walk a short distance right (east) through a gate along its northern bank to the historic Los Angeles Aqueduct (519.7–2,979').

Here, the Los Angeles Aqueduct is a huge, buried pipe, and engineers were faced with the rather bizarre problem of routing the larger California Aqueduct under the smaller waterway.

Now the northbound PCT turns left (due north) on a sandy tack just east of the buried Los Angeles Aqueduct. The once-indestructible brown-painted iron posts emblazoned with a large white PCT emblem have disappeared, but your long, shadeless route is laid out before

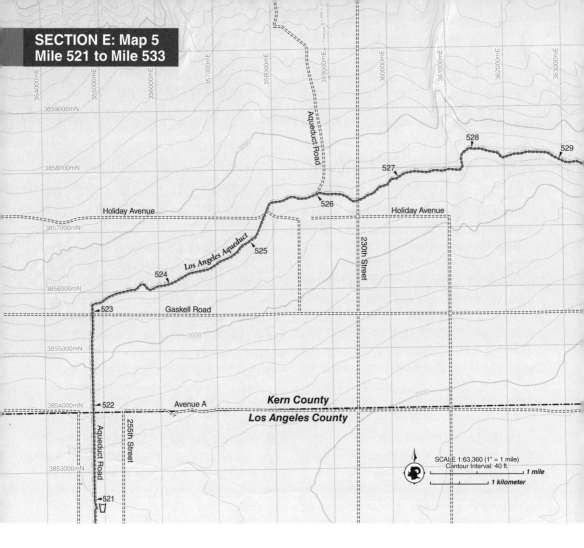

you like a dust-ridden red carpet (many hikers, not unreasonably, refer to this stretch as the death march).

WATER ACCESS

You pass a few habitations, all built in the peculiarly eccentric style of California desert residents, and then, just before the trail crosses a jeep road, a faucet topped by a tall rusty pipe just east of the aqueduct (520.9–2,889'). It's not a mirage, but its flow is controlled by the aqueduct maintenance department; don't count on it, and check the PCT Water Report (pctwater.com) for updates.

For the northbound, the next certain water lies in Cottonwood Canyon, 14 miles ahead. If you're heading south on the PCT, the next water is most likely at Hikertown, whose fate as a trail-angel property was uncertain at press time but which has a faucet just outside its gate that has been a reliable water source in recent years.

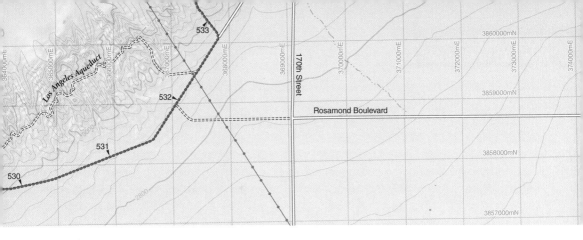

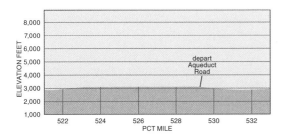

Now the route north leads into a low, scraggly "woodland" of Joshua trees, the hallmarks of the Mojave Desert.

You amble into Kern County, your unimproved way occasionally signed as AQUEDUCT ROAD. Just over a mile later, your straight-north course turns east as the Los Angeles Aqueduct itself bends east, transforming from a black-tarred pipe to an underground channel with a broad, flat concrete roof. (The aqueduct actually lies just north of the main dirt access road that the PCT route follows.) Your way leads east, climbing imperceptibly alongside the aqueduct as it traces a scalloped, contouring route across a succession of broad alluvial fans footing the Tehachapi Mountains. Unfortunately, barbed wire fences make it difficult to stray from the aqueduct. Even more unfortunate is the fact that, although you are walking alongside a buried

About 0.5 mile later you descend to your lowest Antelope Valley point, 2,865 feet, to cross the sandy wash of a seasonal creekbed. Here the shade of a lone tree and wooden trestle supporting the massive, black-tarred, 8-foot-diameter aqueduct pipe offers an unorthodox rest spot amid another quintessentially California desert feature: an ad-hoc garbage dump of cans, household appliances, and an auto carcass or two.

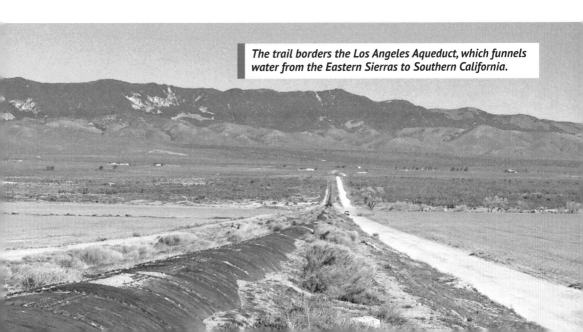

The trail borders the Los Angeles Aqueduct, which funnels water from the Eastern Sierras to Southern California.

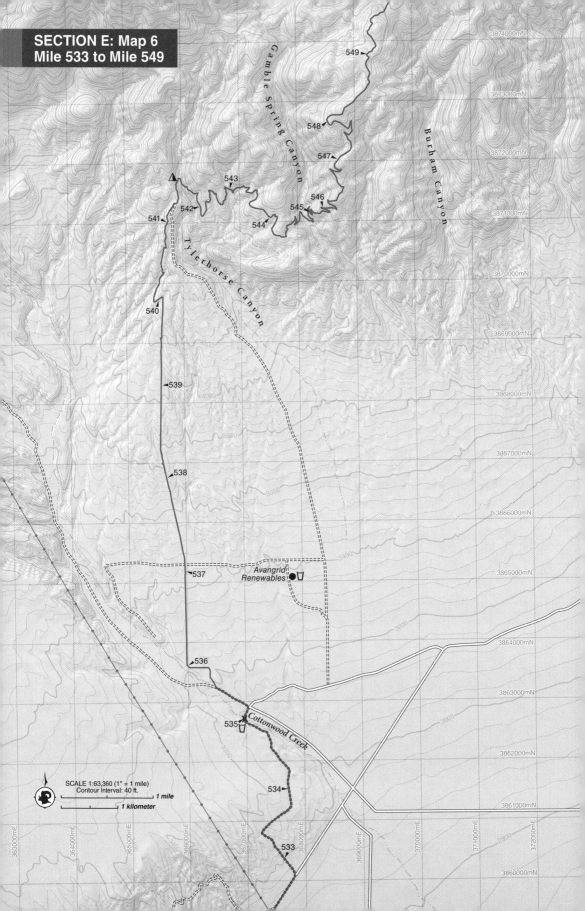

Gamble Spring Canyon

Burham Canyon

549

548

547

546

545

544

543

542

541

540

Tylerhorse Canyon

539

538

537

Avangrid
Renewables

536

535 Cottonwood Creek

534

533

SCALE 1:63,360 (1" = 1 mile)
Contour Interval: 40 ft.
1 mile
1 kilometer

3874000mN
3873000mN
3872000mN
3871000mN
3870000mN
3869000mN
3868000mN
3867000mN
3866000mN
3865000mN
3864000mN
3863000mN
3862000mN
3861000mN
3860000mN

363000mE
364000mE
365000mE
366000mE
367000mE
368000mE
369000mE
370000mE
371000mE
372000mE

river of cool, pristine High Sierra water, there is no way to get to it. The next possible (though not reliable) water for northbound hikers is in Cottonwood Canyon, at mile 534.9.

Forging ahead, you soon find a long stretch of aqueduct that winds across the broad fan of Sacatara Creek, passing innumerable branching dirt roads bound for everywhere and nowhere.

The route now turns across Little Oak Canyon Creek's wide, dry wash, then winds monotonously across a gentle alluvial hillside to an intersection (529.3–3,109') with a good dirt road that crosses the aqueduct via a concrete bridge. Here the PCT is signed to branch right (southeast) via brown metal posts with emblems.

This junction is just a short distance before the Los Angeles Aqueduct disappears altogether at the western foot of a rugged hillside. Now you amble gently down, soon curving east–northeast, then northeast at the pediment of a fascinating badland of steep-sided ravines and ridges. Flash floods have carved the firm red and yellow sediments into a complex of narrow gullies, which has a sparse flora of low juniper trees and rabbitbrush that give color contrast. Eventually, you come to a trio of high-tension power lines marching uphill from the southeast. Ignore the dirt road (532.3–2,895') that runs along their route, and instead continue straight (northeast) on the better road. Very soon you strike a poorer dirt road, your first left turn, at a triangular junction. It takes you gently but directly upslope, soon coming along the southwest side of a small, shallow canyon. Quickly you once again rejoin the Los Angeles Aqueduct, here underground, and turn right (northeast) along its road.

You climb over a low rise, then descend momentarily to resume a nearly level amble, curving north and then northwest into the massive, broad valley of Cottonwood Creek. There are no cottonwoods in evidence along the usually dry creekbed, but there is a nice stand of Joshua trees.

WATER ACCESS

Here you will find a reinforced-concrete horse trough, which is fed by a pipe from the aqueduct. It sits below the southwest end of concrete Cottonwood Creek bridge (534.9–3,086'), just north of a small concrete maintenance lean-to with a walkway that overlooks the wash and below the level of the aqueduct road. (Be aware, however, that water may not be available here year-round—Los Angeles Department of Water and Power may have drained the aqueduct for maintenance at any time between October 1 and May 1.)

Hikers might reach another source of water by exiting the trail at the green equestrian gate near mile 537 and following access roads approximately 1.3 miles to the offices of Avangrid Renewables. The staff welcomes hikers to stop

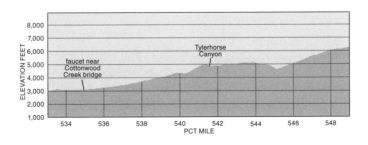

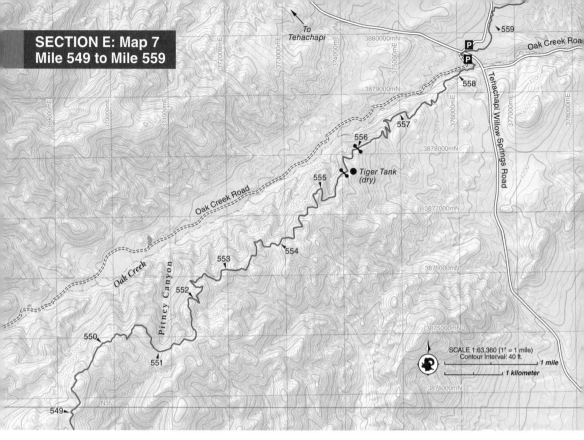

To
Tehachapi

Oak Creek Roa

Tehachapi Willow Springs Road

Oak Creek Road

Tiger Tank
(dry)

Oak Creek

Piney Canyon

SCALE 1:63,360 (1" = 1 mile)
Contour Interval: 40 ft.
1 mile
1 kilometer

in for water and other needs during weekdays; they will also accept resupply packages (see "Supplies" on page 196). After hours, water is accessible at the company's southern fence line (closer to the PCT) via a water tank that is available 24-7. Note that the next reliable water is Tylerhorse Canyon, 6.7 miles away, followed by Oak Creek Canyon, another 23.6 miles away.

Beyond the trough, the bridge carries you across the main wash. This has become a noisy staging area for dirt bikers and ATV enthusiasts.

Walk briefly along the aqueduct to the next dirt road branching left (northwest) up Cottonwood Creek. It is sometimes signed by 4-foot-high brown plastic posts topped with PCT emblems, but they are just as frequently

blown to smithereens by thoughtless target shooters. Follow it gently up through a sunny Joshua tree grove to a resumption of PCT trail tread branching right (north) up the first ravine that cuts the 50-foot-high alluvial embankment above your road. This junction and all others in the next few miles were also originally marked by brown PCT posts, but some dirt bikers have made a project of uprooting them.

Ascend to the top of the slope, emerging on the bajada—a formation consisting of alluvial fans; up through them your route will wind into the Tehachapis. Be aware that dirt bikers have also illegally used the trail to access the Tehachapis, creating many diverging

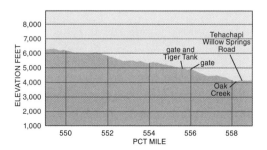

and sometimes confusing paths. At first, you walk north to the lip of another ravine, where posts indicate your turn across two prominent dirt-bike paths to head due west, soon finding another bike path right on a lip overlooking Cottonwood Creek by a pipe. Now turn right (due north), following wooden stakes through the open desert. Soon you parallel and then leapfrog a jeep track on a hot, gentle ascent. Cross an east–west jeep road, then turn a bit west of north to continue up, now with increasing numbers of low junipers and decreasing Joshua trees beside your shadeless path.

Strike more poor dirt roads at a T-junction, after which the trail continues on the same bearing up to a scenic and breezy knoll, where you note your progress and survey the southern flanks of the Tehachapis. Next descend briefly across a pair of ravines to cross a poor jeep road that traces the south boundary of a barbed wire fence. The PCT parallels the four-strand fence, with its steel and wooden posts, as you march due north in sandy, open grassland. Approaching the west side of a large ravine, you join a good jeep road, walk along it 0.1 mile, and then resume your fence-line position to soon find a perpendicular jeep road and the end of the fence.

From here, the path takes a more logical line, and a slightly steeper one, north to the head of the ravine, then over two low ridge noses and across a dry streambed, now in much denser cover of sagebrush, rabbitbrush, and low junipers. A brisk ascent follows, eventually reaching a wide, rough jeep/dirt-bike path that climbs the ridge west of Tylerhorse Canyon.

CAMPING Climb momentarily north along that path to find a post marking PCT tread, which drops steeply down into often cool and shady Tylerhorse Canyon (541.6–4,843'). Often, within a week or two of spring rains, Tylerhorse Creek will be flowing nicely, and tall junipers and Coulter pines will afford a nice quiet camp. **Beware of flash floods during and after storms.**

The PCT continues up into the Tehachapis, turning generally east and making a hot but well-graded ascent across three major ravines, then descends a bit to a saddle overlooking Gamble Spring Canyon (545.1–4,643'). Here you ignore the now-familiar plethora of dirt-bike trails and instead descend almost 400 feet, via sandy switchbacks, to the dry floor of Gamble Spring Canyon. There is often water here in springtime (about 0.3 mile off the trail), but it cannot be relied on, especially in drier-than-average years. Above, the final 1,600-foot leg of your 3,000-foot climb into the Tehachapis awaits: First, eight hot switchbacks, long abused by motocross riders, lead up to a brief respite where you traverse around a 5,716-foot knob. Two more switchbacks attack the next slope, but not nearly as viciously as the dirt bikers have—a huge, rutted swath cuts directly up the ridge, obliterating the PCT in places. Near the top, you round clockwise across a breezy nose that is cut by a jeep road and pocked with prospect pits in a small outcrop of Paleozoic marine metasediments. Here the trail swings northeast, keeping just below the ridgetop and its jeep track, soon finding the welcome shade of stands of junipers and pinyon pines, which frame vistas south over Antelope Valley.

VIEWS On a clear morning, Mount San Antonio, San Gorgonio Peak, and San Jacinto Peak can all be seen, as can the massive buildings of the NASA flight research center in Palmdale.

Soon the PCT begins to undulate between groves of fragrant pinyon and Coulter pines and large junipers, which cover slopes between dry flats of sagebrush scrub and mountain mahogany brush. You stay close to, but rarely see, a good dirt road that serves a scattering of vacation cabins. Without fanfare, you reach the PCT's 6,280-foot high point in the Tehachapi Mountains, then descend easily, winding along the pinyon-forested ridge that forms the south side of Oak Creek Canyon. Beyond a gap at the heads of Burham and Pitney Canyons, you climb for a few minutes and then resume your easy descent.

WILDLIFE Vistas are frequent over Oak Creek Canyon, which is carved along the active Garlock Fault, from which the southern Sierra Nevada rises. Oak Creek Canyon is home to one of the last herds of wild dark-brown horses that once roamed the Antelope Valley area, having descended from horses lost by Spanish explorers.

TRAIL INFO The canyon, like these slopes above, is private property, so no camping is allowed, and hikers must stay on the trail. Anyone who drops into the canyon bottom for any reason will be prosecuted.

Continue winding easily down the ridge, in open groves of juniper, occasionally crossing vague, branching jeep trails.

TRAIL INFO Presently the hum of electric generators and the whoosh of blades are heard, and the way descends to the edge of a vast array of wind turbines. These harvest electrical energy from the nearly incessant breezes that blow across the Tehachapis, spawned by temperature gradients between cool coastal air and the hot Mojave Desert. You will grow used to these mammoth windmills, as you will walk among them all the way to CA 58, but initially their incongruous presence reminds you of an enormous flock of squeaking, flapping seagulls.

At mile 555.6, you'll pass what appears to be a rusty old bathtub with a 5-foot-tall closed pipe next to it, perched incongruously under several large wind turbines. Known as Tiger Tank, it was once a source of water for hikers but has little to offer these days besides a photo op and shadeless rest stop before your final descent to Tehachapi Willow Springs Road.

The wind farms force our route to trace the lip of the canyon wall, then to switchback sandily down it, eventually reaching Oak Creek, in a delightful open stand of white oaks. In a minute you step through a pipe gate, then cross usually dry Oak Creek (558.2–4,070') on a small bridge. This is private land, and camping is not permitted.

Now parallel the stream on its north bank for a moment, then turn left (northwest) up across a gentle ridgetop. Soon pass under a double-pole power line, step across a poor dirt road, and drop a few feet to two-lane, paved Tehachapi Willow Springs Road (558.5–4,145') at its junction with paved Cameron Canyon Road. A parking pullout and a large and welcoming PACIFIC CREST NATIONAL SCENIC TRAIL sign mark the junction and make this an easy place to meet up with family or friends or just regain your bearings.

RESUPPLY ACCESS

Here, most hikers will veer from the PCT to head about 9 miles into Tehachapi (west) or Mojave (east) for resupply. Access to Tehachapi is much easier from here than from CA 58, at the end of this section.

Back on the PCT in Oak Creek Canyon, cross Tehachapi Willow Springs Road and pick up slightly indistinct tread heading right (east), just behind several interpretive signs on the history of the area's wind farms and information and maps related to this particular section of the PCT. Turn north across three dirt roads in quick succession, the first two subserving pole lines. Then gently ascend across a broad, dry, sandy ravine, in open grassland dotted with sagebrush and a few low junipers, to the melodious calls of flocks of meadowlarks. Reaching a hillside, you might lose trail tread momentarily where bulldozers have cut a wide swath, but plastic marker posts show the way across one good dirt road to a second, just below another large windmill plantation. Now you turn north, attacking the hillside at a moderate angle, soon crossing numerous dirt roads of varying quality that serve the wind farm and

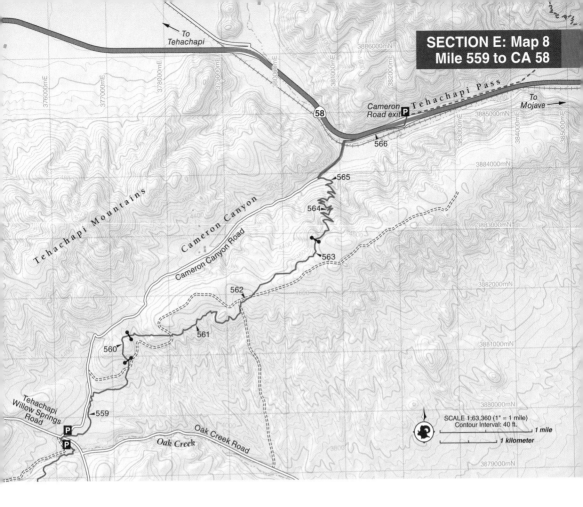

To
Tehachapi

To
Mojave

Tehachapi Pass

Cameron
Road exit

58

566

565

564

Cameron Canyon

Cameron Canyon Road

563

562

561

560

559

Tehachapi
Willow Springs
Road

Oak Creek

Oak Creek Road

Tehachapi Mountains

SCALE 1:63,360 (1" = 1 mile)
Contour Interval: 40 ft.

1 mile

1 kilometer

the double-pole power line that runs along its western boundary.

The climb eventually abates at a small saddle. Here you drop north a few yards, step across a dirt road, and bend east. Open two pipe gates in a barbed wire fence, drop into a gully, then climb steeply east to another gate and again reach a scenic ridgetop. Wide vistas extend south over wind farms, Joshua trees, and desert to the San Gabriel and San Bernardino Mountains.

For the next leg, you undulate east under the propeller-bedecked crest of the Tehachapis on sunny, sandy trail, which crosses dirt access roads three times. At a fourth, good dirt road, you note a guardhouse complex for one of the wind-farming corporations at a road junction just to the north. You pass south of that road, then cross it and ascend gently over

the ridgecrest and down to a saddle with a poor dirt road. The path from here makes its way onto the steeper northern slopes of the ridge, with sweeping panoramas over Cameron Canyon to the Tehachapi Valley and beyond to the southern Sierra. An easy ascent eventually finds a narrow ridge, where you step across a dirt road (563.1–4,769') just below a heavy steel gate, then pass through a barbed wire

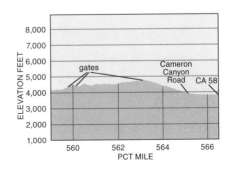

gate in a cluster of junipers. A single switch-back leads to a steep hillside that has been eroded by wild horses.

Below, a dozen well-graded switchbacks lower you to the floor of Cameron Canyon. Reaching the bottom, you turn left (west) momentarily to strike two-lane paved Cameron Road (565.2–3,900') at a pipe gate. Now follow brown plastic PCT markers along that road's south shoulder easily down to cross railroad tracks. From here, the PCT, unmarked, follows Cameron Road east to its overpass of busy four-lane CA 58 at Tehachapi Pass (566.4–3,825'). Welcome to the Sierra Nevada!

Tehachapi, with its extensive facilities, lies 9.2 miles west on CA 58 but is difficult to hitch-hike to from this spot, due to the lack of cars exiting or entering via the Cameron Road off-ramp. It is more easily reached by Tehachapi Willow Springs Road, at mile 558.5, as is Mojave, also 9 miles from the PCT in the other direction.

RESUPPLY ACCESS

The Tehachapi post office is north of CA 58 on Voyager Drive, down the street from a chain hotel.

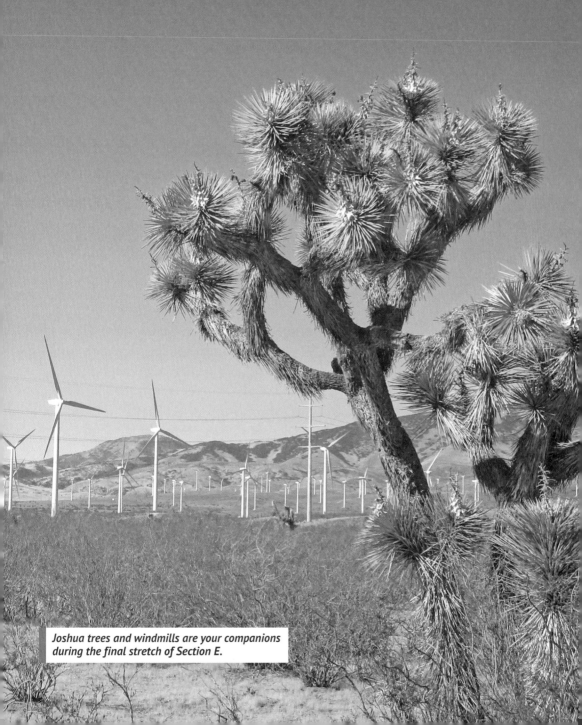

Joshua trees and windmills are your companions during the final stretch of Section E.

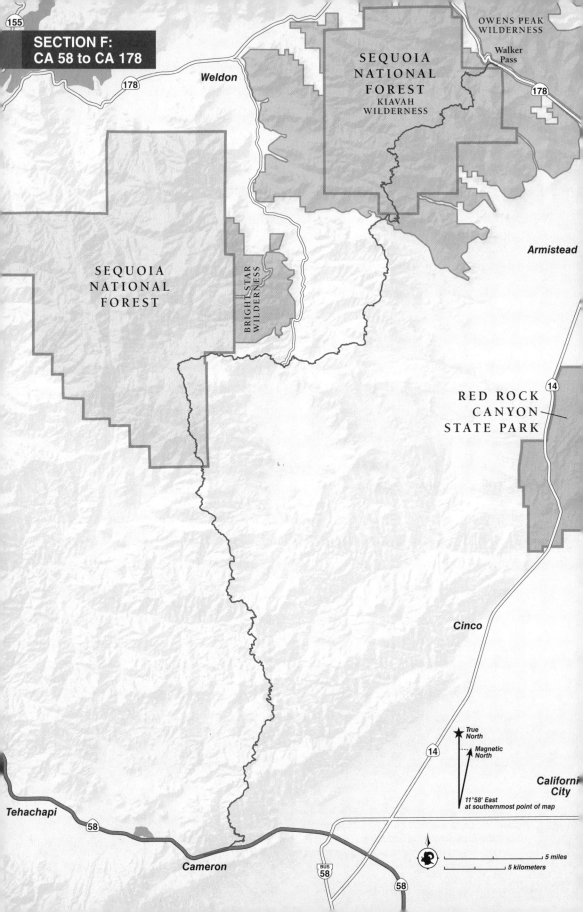

155

178   *Weldon*

OWENS PEAK
WILDERNESS

Walker
Pass

SEQUOIA
NATIONAL
FOREST
KIAVAH
WILDERNESS

178

Armistead

SEQUOIA
NATIONAL
FOREST

BRIGHT-STAR
WILDERNESS

14

RED ROCK
CANYON
STATE PARK

Cinco

14

★ *True
North*

14

⋯ *Magnetic
North*

*California
City*

*11°58' East
at southernmost point of map*

Tehachapi   58

Cameron

BUS
58

58

5 miles

5 kilometers

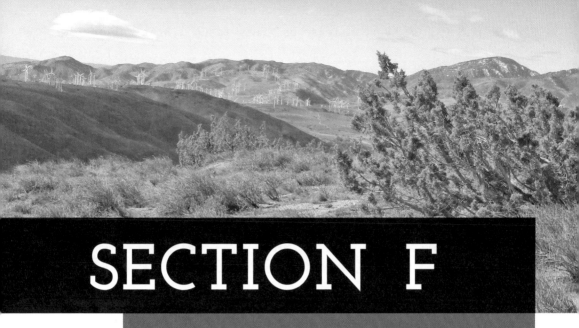

SECTION F

CA 58 near Tehachapi Pass to CA 178 at Walker Pass

SURPRISINGLY TO MANY PEOPLE, most geographers include the Tehachapi Mountains as part of the mighty Sierra Nevada, calling the range the Sierran Tail or the Sierran Hook. The Sierra's southernmost tip, then, is the southwest point of the Tehachapi Mountains below the junction of the San Andreas and Garlock Faults.

In the Sierra north of the Tehachapi range, the Pacific Crest Trail (PCT) immediately climbs onto the Sierra Crest, where it remains for most of this section, traversing the granitic Sierra Nevada batholith, which is exposed so widely. It quickly climbs from a Joshua tree–juniper woodland to a pinyon pine–oak woodland, with five species of oak along the route. A cool Jeffrey pine forest in the Piute Mountains offers a refreshing midsection change before you drop to a desert community of plants, then progress again to a pinyon pine woodland.

Above: The beginning of Section F offers unobstructed views of sharp ridges, deep valleys, and the silhouettes of distant peaks.

The charm of this section lies not only in its diversity of flora but also in its unobstructed views of rows of sharp ridges and deep valleys; of sprawling desert lands and distant peak silhouettes; of faraway pockets of populated, sometimes historical enclaves; of evidence of the human quest for riches and energy to power our lifestyles.

DECLINATION 11°58'E

USGS MAPS

Monolith	Emerald Mountain	Cane Canyon
Tehachapi NE	Claraville	Horse Canyon
Cache Peak	Pinyon Mountain	Walker Pass
Cross Mountain		

POINTS ON THE TRAIL, SOUTH TO NORTH

	Mile	Elevation in feet	Latitude/Longitude
Cameron Overpass at CA 58	566.4	3,825	N35° 05' 54.690" W118° 17' 35.670"
Waterfall Canyon	573.4	6,161	N35° 08' 27.660" W118° 15' 38.040"
Golden Oaks Spring	583.3	5,474	N35° 13' 33.694" W118° 14' 00.586"
Jawbone Canyon Road	602.5	6,609	N35° 23' 25.740" W118° 17' 56.700"
Kelso Valley Road	616.0	4,954	N35° 27' 02.520" W118° 13' 23.580"
Butterbredt Canyon Road	617.8	4,551	N35° 27' 10.440" W118° 12' 15.900"
Dove Spring Canyon Road (to Willow Spring)	621.9	5,285	N35° 27' 51.060" W118° 09' 00.360"
Trail spur to Yellow Jacket Spring	637.0	6,257	N35° 34' 57.960" W118° 07' 25.440"
CA 178 at Walker Pass	652.0	5,264	N35° 39' 47.100" W118° 01' 38.460"

CAMPSITES AND BIVY SITES

Mile	Elevation in feet	Latitude/ Longitude	Number of tents	Feature	Notes
569.4	4,326	N35° 06' 50.700" W118° 15' 27.960"	2	Joshua trees	Wind-prone
570.9	5,156	N35° 07' 07.920" W118° 15' 52.020"	>5	Shade, log benches	
572.9	6,055	N35° 08' 16.260" W118° 15' 59.220"	>5	Waterfall Canyon	Large shaded campsite on saddle with views
592.9	5,018	N35° 18' 02.880" W118° 16' 02.100"	>5		Near private road; heed signs
602.0	6,334	N35° 23' 14.790" W118° 18' 06.490"	>10	Robin Bird Spring	Just west of trail, shade
603.9	6,520	N35° 24' 12.540" W118° 18' 24.600"	>5	Cottonwood Creek	Seasonal water, some shade

CAMPSITES AND BIVY SITES *(continued)*

Mile	Elevation in feet	Latitude/ Longitude	Number of tents	Feature	Notes
608.9	6,249	N35° 27' 18.900" W118° 18' 46.500"	>10	Landers Camp	Seasonal spring, shade, flat areas
634.2	6,885	N35° 33' 50.100" W118° 07' 18.780"	2		
635.3	6,713	N35° 34' 35.280" W118° 07' 48.060"	2		
651.3	5,068	N35° 39' 49.980" W118° 02' 15.060"	11	Walker Pass Campground	Walk-in sites for hikers, picnic tables, fire rings

WEATHER TO GO

Because much of this section is exposed, it can be hot; the beginning can be very windy. The terrain you cover receives snow in winter, with the higher elevations blanketed. Early to mid-spring and mid- to late fall are optimal times to enjoy your trek here. Most thru-hikers arrive at the best time.

SUPPLIES

See pages 196–197 for information on Tehachapi and Mojave. At the end of this section, Onyx has limited groceries and supplies and a post office 16.5 miles west of Walker Pass Campground off CA 178. Also, regional transit for towns around Lake Isabella and Bakersfield reach as far east as the Onyx post office. A KOA Campground is 7 miles west of Walker Pass on CA 178. Haven RV Park in Lake Isabella lets hikers pitch tents on its grassy tree-shaded lawn for discounted rates; it also has a grill/picnic area, a common room with TV and Wi-Fi, and laundry facilities (760-478-4310, haven-rv.com). The small town also has a few motels, a grocery store, and eateries.

Kernville is 36 miles northwest of Walker Pass Campground: take CA 178 and Sierra Way. It has a post office, supplies, motels, and, for your rest and relaxation days, kayak rentals and 1-hour to multiday raft trips on the tumultuous Kern River during adequate water flow.

Ridgecrest lies 26 miles east of Walker Pass and boasts a full lineup of hiker amenities, including motels, restaurants, a Walmart, and a post office near the town center. Buses run Monday, Wednesday, and Friday between Kernville, Lake Isabella, and Ridgecrest. They will stop at Walker Pass with advance notice. Call Kern County Transit at 800-323-2396.

WATER

Year-round water sources are sparse in this section. During periods of extended drought, even usually reliable springs dry up. You will need to boil, filter, or add iodine tablets to render the water available from a series of springs suitable to drink. Both the Bureau of Land Management (BLM) and the U.S. Forest Service (USFS), as well as volunteers from the Pacific Crest Trail Association (PCTA), continue to upgrade the springs. Although there is usually a breeze on this mostly shadeless trail section, days can be hot, and humidity can be low. It is advisable to hydrate yourself well at every water source and to carry a minimum of 3–4 quarts per waterless 10 miles.

PERMITS

The required fire permit can be obtained from the BLM or Sequoia National Forest or online at readyforwildfire.org/permits/campfire-permit. No wilderness permit is needed for this section.

SPECIAL CONCERNS

Refer to page 32 for information about rattlesnakes. For information about ticks, see page 34.

>OFF-HIGHWAY VEHICLES (OHVs)

Be forewarned that the seemingly unlimited open space along some stretches in this section attracts weekend OHVs but very few during the week. They are prohibited on the PCT, except where the PCT joins jeep roads for short stretches.

CA 58 NEAR TEHACHAPI PASS TO CA 178 AT WALKER PASS

>>>THE ROUTE

The closest source of water north on the trail is Golden Oaks Spring, 16.9 miles ahead. Before starting this often windy, exposed section north of Tehachapi Pass, you should hydrate yourself well and carry at the very minimum 3 quarts of water. The trail passes through a crazy quilt of private and BLM lands. Because of private lands, you are asked not to stray from the trail, even for peak-bagging.

You begin your trek at the south end of Cameron Overpass (566.4–3,825'), then cross busy CA 58 on the overpass to the trail on the north side. Hurry past the litter and unpleasant stench. Descend past a metal sign offering local transportation information for PCT hikers; then ignore a wider jeep road pointed north, and head east uphill to a dilapidated gate. Sign the trail register attached to the fence post, and tip your hat to *Wild* author Cheryl Strayed, who began her PCT

hike here in 1995. There may be a thoughtful memo on the amenities hikers will find in both Mojave and Tehachapi. From here, the trail parallels the highway east–northeast along a fenced corridor and through another gate (567.7–3,781'), this one opposite the CAMERON RD EXIT 1 MILE sign. Next you dip through the large wash of Waterfall Canyon and turn northeast to ascend to the right of the flood-control berm next to the wash. Leaving the berm, you progress east while passing groves of juniper trees interspersed with Joshua trees and a few yuccas. Along the foothills, you will find that a dirt road briefly usurps the PCT trail; hike on it.

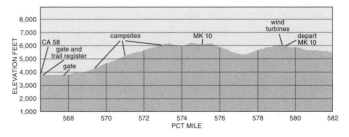

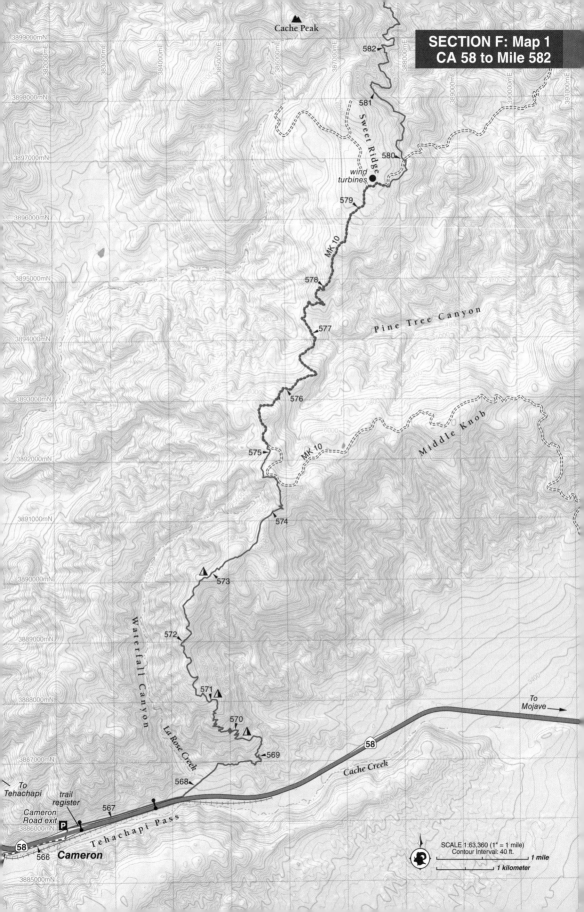

Cache Peak

582

581

Sweet Ridge

580

wind
turbines

579

MK 10

Pine Tree Canyon

578

577

576

Middle Knob

575

MK 10

574

573

572

Waterfall Canyon

571

La Rose Creek

570

569

568

To
Tehachapi

trail
register

567

Cameron
Road exit

P

Tehachapi Pass

58

566

Cameron

To
Mojave

58

Cache Creek

SCALE 1:63,360 (1" = 1 mile)
Contour Interval: 40 ft.

1 mile

1 kilometer

GEOLOGY In the Tehachapi Pass area, you cross over the northeast–southwest Garlock Fault, the second-largest fault in California. Movement along the fault here is approximately 7 millimeters per year. To the north there is no movement; the fault is locked. Seismologists expect a major earthquake in the locked area. (Two major quakes, of magnitudes 6.4 and 7.1, struck nearby Ridgecrest and the surrounding area in July 2019, with reverberations felt as far as Las Vegas and San Diego.) These hills show the fault-zone mishmash of granitics and metamorphics. Geologists identify the rocks as mafic and ultramafic plutonic rocks and associated amphibolite, gneiss, and granulite.

CAMPING Climbing north via switchbacks and some curves, you arrive on a broad slope among scrubby junipers 3 miles into your trip—a level place for a camp if needed.

TRAIL INFO From below you hear the distant chug of locomotives pulling a long chain of freight cars to and from the 17 tunnels and the famous loop at Walong, 12 miles west of the town of Tehachapi. Built in 1875–76, the loop is one of the most photographed railroad sections in the world. It is composed of a tunnel and an ascending circle where an elevation gain of 77 feet puts the locomotives over the caboose if the train is more than 4,000 feet long.

TRAIL INFO Usually you feel the prevailing winds that race through Tehachapi Pass. These winds, the result of cool air rushing in from the coastal west to replace hot air rising from the desert east, activate the forests of windmills strung on ridges seen from this point. The flow of air increases as it compresses against the ridges, resulting in wind speeds recorded here of up to 80 miles per hour.

The wind farms you see were developed as an alternative to energy generated by air-polluting fossil fuels. However, few hikers revel in this section, noting that the windmills are noisy and aesthetically polluting and that the territory around them is gouged with roads. Moving on, you climb a long, tight series of switchbacks that on the map resemble a recorded earthquake on a seismograph. At length you reach gentler slopes along a broad ridge where camping is possible.

VIEWS Looking clockwise from the ridge, you see the Mojave Desert to the east and the isolated features of Soledad Mountain and Elephant Butte rising south of the town of Mojave. Those low volcanic mountains produced millions of dollars' worth of gold and silver extracted from contacts between rhyolite and granitic rock along 100 miles of tunnel. Farther southeast you view the barren expanse of Edwards Air Force Base with Rogers Dry Lake airstrips, whose 7.5-mile-long runway has served as home base for experimental aircraft and as the backup landing site for several space shuttles. To the south loom the Tehachapi Mountains, and to the west their namesake town. The large scar on the north side of Tehachapi Pass resulted from excavations by Monolith Cement Company, still operating more than a century later as Lehigh Southwest. The product was once used in the construction of the Los Angeles Aqueduct, which runs along the east side of the Sierra.

The PCT descends slightly to straddle a narrow ridge between steep canyons, resumes its ascent, and shortly crosses from east-facing to west-facing slopes. In time it encounters pinyon pines.

HISTORY From these trees, in days of yore, the Kawaiisu Indians gathered pinyon nuts. They gathered and hunted from the Tehachapi Mountains north through this area to the South Fork Kern River Valley. To preserve their culture, in 1994 the State of California purchased land surrounding a former village in Sand Canyon, 2.5 air miles west, for a historical park (called Tomo-Kahni, it is open to the public by tour only).

CAMPING Now your trail seeks the crest on ascending slopes. Atop the crest before a descent, a river of sand hidden

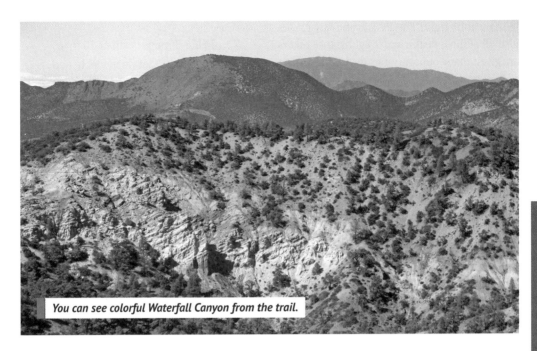

You can see colorful Waterfall Canyon from the trail.

amid pinyon pines offers wind-protected camp-sites (572.9–6,055'). To the west colorful Water-fall Canyon dominates views.

The trail next crosses a jeep road, marked by a wooden fence, then climbs a ridge via three switchbacks and passes a chalky-white hill of tuff protruding at the head of an east-facing canyon. Soon the PCT parallels the jeep road, crosses it again, and curves around the head of Waterfall Canyon (574.7–6,115'). Abruptly the trail ends, and the route joins that jeep road.

You turn left on the seldom-used jeep road (575.1–6,126'), which heads generally north, descends east, and then heads north again. At the bottom of the descent, 2 miles along the road, you curve around a huge gray pine tree on a flat. Again you climb a ridge, perhaps serenaded by a mountain chickadee's clear three-note "how are you"—the "how" a whole note, the "are you" two eighth notes at a lower pitch.

Ahead, as the route eventually descends into a sagebrush swale, you see the first of the 90- and 140-foot wind-turbine towers perched over 5 miles of ridgeline.

TRAIL INFO The Vestas V-27 three-blade turbines, used here for the Sky River Wind project that began in the early 1990s, are far more efficient than the earlier versions you saw previously on ridges. Total output of Sky River exceeds 700 million kilowatt hours per year—enough to supply electricity for more than 23,000 homes. Now the twirling giant pinwheels produce a mechanical hum to accompany the chickadee's serenades.

In this hollow the course crosses a dirt road and forks right where a sign on the locked, gated road sits to the left. In 0.2 mile from the gated road, the PCT branches right (579.5–6,005'), leaving the jeep road where it becomes closed and abruptly descends.

Your route ahead crosses several roads to wind turbines. The company asks that you not venture near the machines.

The PCT, a trail again, zigzags, turns sharply left, and crosses both a wide road to turbines and the ragged jeep road you just left.

VIEWS Here you see your first view of Olancha Peak far to the north over waves of ridges. Beyond, Mount Whitney, the highest mountain in the Lower 48, barely reaches above the waves. Pointy Owens Peak rises southeast of Olancha Peak, with Mount

Jenkins at its right. The PCT eventually passes near all of these peaks, and long-distance hikers are given many opportunities to view this scene as they progress.

Your path, cut on very steep slopes, begins a long, descending traverse around the east side of turbine-bristled Sweet Ridge. It then rounds the flanks of 6,698-foot Cache Peak, the highest peak in the southernmost Sierra north of Tehachapi Pass.

> Miller Springs is about 10 miles ahead, but it's not dependable and requires a steep detour. The next reliable water is at Robin Bird Spring, 18.8 miles farther for northbound hikers. Southbound hikers will have a 16.9-mile trek before the next opportunity for water.

WATER ACCESS

In time the trail, passing slender snowmelt streamlets, descends to cross a jeep road at an offset junction and then arrives at a resurfaced stone-and-cement trough catching a piped-in, year-round flow from Golden Oaks Spring (583.3–5,474'). It's a popular rest stop, with plenty of shade. The PCTA Southern California Trail Gorillas volunteer crew refurbished and upgraded it in recent years by clearing brush, draining the trough, patching cracks, adding fencing, and installing a siphon tube inside the box to improve access. This important water source also serves the cattle and wildlife in the area. Be sure to purify it, and also be aware that the flow can be slow and even dry up by late summer and fall in drought years.

WILDLIFE Springs are important to wildlife, of course, as well as hikers. The area's mule deer, bobcats, mountain lions, and black bears will shy away from this water source while people are near, so it's important not to camp near these shared water sources. Bighorn sheep frequented this spring, as well as other springs in these mountains, as recently as the early 1900s. At that time domestic sheep infected with scabies were released in the area. The scabies spread to the native bighorns, resulting in their demise. In 1978 tule elk were transplanted here from Owens Valley, but most of them migrated to lower elevations and found their way to the alfalfa fields in Fremont Valley.

You head generally northwest, crossing a closed road, then paralleling a wide road to turbines before crossing it. You resume the trail a few paces up the road and on it traverse steep slopes to eventually round prominent Point 5,683. Next, on a pair of switchbacks, you descend below an old jeep road now used to access turbines. You then cross a ravine and climb its west side. Beyond a switchback, a turbine road, and a saddle, you arc west around the extensive drainage of Indian Creek, providing

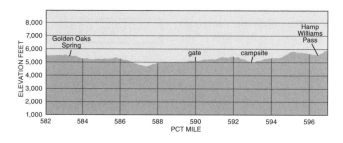

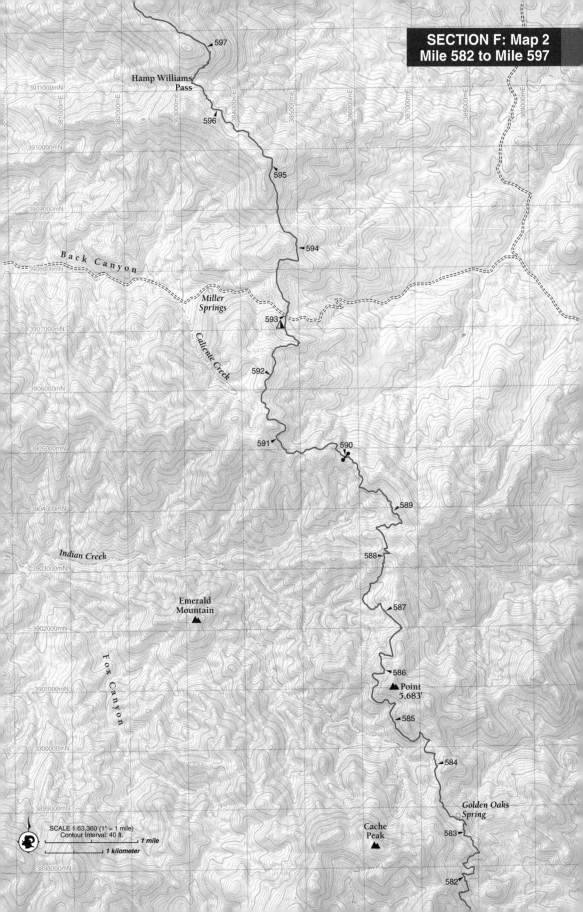

597

Hamp Williams
Pass

596

595

594

Back Canyon

Miller
Springs

Caliente Creek

593

592

591

590

589

588

Indian Creek

587

Emerald
Mountain

Fox Canyon

586

Point
5,683'

585

584

Golden Oaks
Spring

583

Cache
Peak

582

SCALE 1:63,360 (1" = 1 mile)
Contour Interval: 40 ft.
1 mile
1 kilometer

3911000mN
3910000mN
3909000mN
3908000mN
3907000mN
3906000mN
3905000mN
3904000mN
3903000mN
3902000mN
3901000mN
3900000mN
3899000mN
3898000mN

381000mE
382000mE
383000mE
384000mE
385000mE
386000mE
387000mE
388000mE
389000mE

good views of Cache Peak to the south. In time, you reach an east–west ridge, which you cross via a green gate (590.0–5,103') in a cattle fence.

Beyond the gate, the route heads generally west in shade, then swings north to follow a sunny crest, the watershed divide between Caliente Creek to the west and Jawbone Canyon to the east.

VIEWS This crest affords comprehensive views of multicolored Jawbone Canyon and, to the north–northeast, of Kelso Valley and Mayan Peak. (The PCT eventually curves alongside distant Mayan Peak.)

CAMPING The trail undulates near or on the crest, then descends a north-facing ridge to a blue oak savanna with a large grassy area to the left, nicely suited for camping (592.9–5,018'). Be sensitive to fragile plant species, and do not expand existing campsites. Several gleaming quartz rocks form fire rings here. Below the campsite, an east–west road (593.0–5,009') crosses your route.

TRAIL INFO This road connects with other roads to offer passage from CA 14 on the east to CA 58 on the south, but it is a gated and locked private road and extremely rough to the west.

View of desert lands and distant peaks on the trail north of Tehachapi

In a pinch, Miller Springs may offer potable water, but it should not be relied upon, and it requires a 0.75-mile detour down a gorge that is steep in places. To find it, take the jeep road that intersects the PCT at mile 593.0; follow it west down a small gorge to a flat area with a low-lying wooden box to the left. The lid is heavy but can be removed with some muscle. Hikers report that water has been flowing well here in recent years, though some have had difficulty opening the lid to access it.

Back on the PCT, going north, you ascend easily across a grassy ridge with a springtime wildflower sparkle of baby blue eyes, curve around a minor eastward extension, and then hike along a narrow saddle. The path north of the saddle looks ominous, and it is a steep climb by PCT standards. The curious upslope swath cut through scrub oak followed the original trail design. Grateful you are not panting up that route, you ascend north through a scrub oak aisle.

WILDLIFE Scrub oak resembles live oak in miniature: its growth is dense, its branches are ridged, and its forest is impenetrable without the help of cutting tools.

Upon turning northwest, you leave the chaparral oak for the domain of lofty Jeffrey pines and spreading black oaks, the first appearance of these pines and oaks on this section of the PCT. Just beyond the forest you descend to traverse below Hamp Williams Pass (596.5–5,521').

Once again you are faced with a steep climb, lined with scrub oak and relieved slightly by four switchbacks. Breaks in the oak cover offer vignettes of Jawbone Canyon Road below. You will cross that road where it winds in the mountains ahead. Here you make a traverse, a zig and a zag, and climb over a saddle to west-facing slopes, again among welcome Jeffrey pines and black oaks. Just where the Piute Mountains begin in the south is uncertain, but you are surely in the Piutes now. You descend past two peaks and partway around Weldon Peak before the descent increases down a

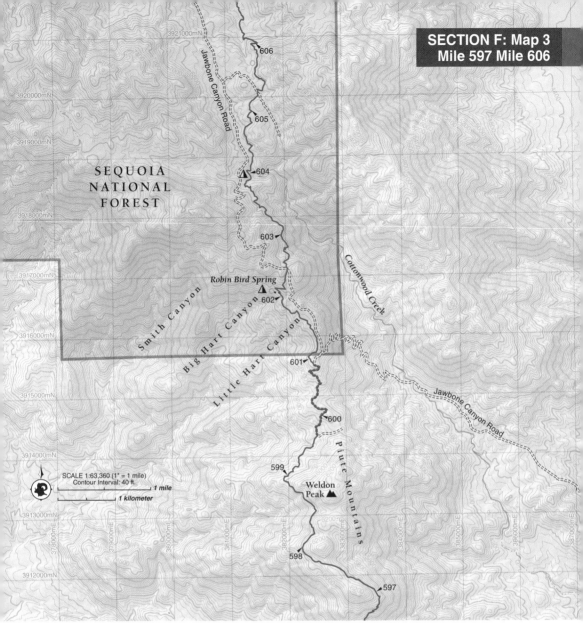

SEQUOIA
NATIONAL
FOREST

606

605

604

603

Robin Bird Spring

602

601

600

599

Weldon
Peak ▲

598

597

Smith Canyon

Big Hart Canyon

Little Hart Canyon

Cottonwood Creek

Jawbone Canyon Road

Piute Mountains

SCALE 1:63,360 (1" = 1 mile)
Contour Interval: 40 ft.

1 mile

1 kilometer

west-facing ridge, then decreases as you turn northeast to enter a cluster of privately owned small parcels. No camping is allowed. Your PCT path ends on a curve of a private dirt road.

Turning right, you proceed up the main private road, permitted for PCT use; be sure to heed the sign and stay on the road. You turn left at the first fork at 0.1 mile, pass several spur roads, ease around a locked cable crossing the road, and then meet a T-junction with a prominent west-descending unpaved road. Here you keep right, then ascend along a tight right

curve and find the PCT path resuming to the left (602.0–6,329'). (The road continues to Jawbone Canyon Road 0.5 mile beyond.)

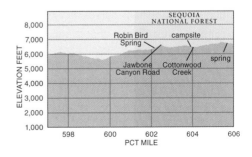

WATER ACCESS

CAMPING A prominent sign directs you to Robin Bird Spring. In 1994 the USFS developed this flowing spring, freed it from cattle contaminants, and piped the water. It also cleared the enormous amount of rubble of a dilapidated two-story house, leaving a flat area for camping. A stile allows easy access through the fence. Follow the galvanized pipe uphill about 20 yards. Hikers should climb over the fence toward the tank and look for a black PVC pipe that feeds the spring. The water in the trough can be silty, and the pipe may be reduced to a trickle by late spring.

Beyond the spring-access road, the PCT switchbacks up to unpaved Jawbone Canyon Road (602.5–6,609').

PCT ACCESS ROUTE This lightly traveled PCT access route, Jawbone Canyon Road, leaves east down the Piute Mountains; crosses Kelso Valley; winds among low, exposed hills; and reaches CA 14, 26.4 miles later. The BLM OHV visitor center is located at the junction. West of the PCT, Jawbone Canyon Road curves north to connect with roads that continue north to CA 178, 33 miles later.

North of Jawbone Canyon Road the PCT descends among scattered Jeffrey pines, white firs, and mistletoe-trimmed black and live oaks. It drops down a few switchbacks and winds along east-facing slopes, where cascades of white-flowered spreading phlox perk up the early-season wayside scenery. The path gently undulates now, passes a magnificent golden oak to your left, and then adds gravel to the dirt tread as boulders surrounded by manzanitas appear.

CAMPING In a short time the trail crosses a willow-lined branch of Cottonwood Creek (604.0–6,467') with possible camping nearby. The stream is often dry by late spring and may be enjoyed by cows as well. The path briefly parallels another willow-hemmed branch of the slender creek, crosses it on a log footbridge, and then proceeds above it.

The well-defined path continues to wind and dip, generally heading north. Strips of Jawbone Canyon Road appear to the west before the PCT turns up a canyon, crosses a logging road, and climbs over a saddle, the watershed divide of Cottonwood and Landers Creeks. Within 0.5 mile, watch for a spring above the trail whose water is caught by a crude cement structure (605.7–6,750').

Back on the trail, you walk above, then switchback down to the headwaters of Landers Creek, a reliable water source after a wet winter (but often a trickle by summer), and through a pocket meadow. Later you switchback down to cross Landers Creek (607.1–6,337') and quickly cross back to the east side again.

Continue heading north. The trail remains in the little canyon until the canyon flares near Landers Meadow, spreading east. After crossing the meadow's outlet stream, the path bridges a trench and crosses Piute Mountain Road (608.1–6,211'). The PCT crosses this road again in about 3 miles.

TRAIL INFO Thanks to a major fundraising effort, the PCTA raised enough money in 2016 to purchase Landers Meadow from a land investment company, thus preserving and protecting the tranquil 245-acre property surrounding the trail from future development. The property had long been a priority acquisition in the PCT Land Inventory,

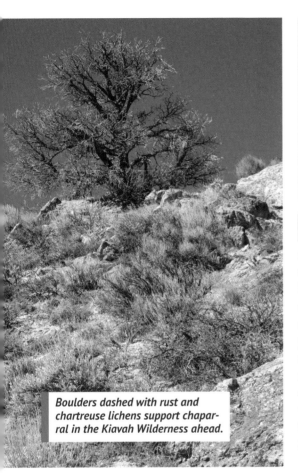

Boulders dashed with rust and chartreuse lichens support chaparral in the Kiavah Wilderness ahead.

Camp) in an area that is safe from fires. A spring above the campground is captured in a tank and piped to splash into a cattle trough, the last source of water for 8.9 miles, and the last reliable on-trail source for 43 miles, when you reach Walker Pass.

PLANTS Returning to the PCT, you head east while aloof wallflowers, standing straight and single, display clusters of bright-orange blossoms in season; blue-purple lupines add a dash of contrasting color. Pinyon pines signal your approach to drier climes, and a logging road crosses your path. In time lichen-splashed boulders appear, along with golden oaks and a few dramatic yuccas. Yuccas grow tough, daggerlike leaves a foot or more long, with sharp tips that puncture the unwary. The stalks, with massive creamy-white blossoms that seem to explode in spring, reach 8–14 feet tall.

Soon you leave the Sequoia National Forest and enter land managed by the BLM. You meet Piute Mountain Road (611.2–6,611') again, this time at the summit of Harris Grade, Piute Mountains' best access. Here you cross both the trail-protecting gate and the road.

In 0.1 mile, as you begin a descent along the north and then east slopes of St. John Ridge, you again see majestic Olancha Peak, far off to the north, reigning over the Kern Plateau.

VIEWS To the northeast, pointed Owens Peak, with curved, serrated Mount Jenkins next to it, divides the desert from the mountains, and all three peaks delineate the Sierra Crest.

While gradually losing elevation, you eventually descend by switchbacks and a long traverse across the slopes of St. John Ridge, passing en route a motorcycle path occupying a gully.

which identifies and ranks potential land acquisitions along the entire PCT.

On the north side of Piute Mountain Road, the USFS has installed more ingenious gates across the PCT, flanked by fences. This discourages motorcyclists, but hikers and horses can easily step over them. The trail beyond gently weaves along a rolling, selectively logged pine flat inland from the creek and then meets graded, unpaved Sequoia National Forest Road 29S05 (608.9–6,313').

WATER ACCESS

CAMPING This road leads left (north) 0.3 mile to a tree-shaded primitive campground (Landers

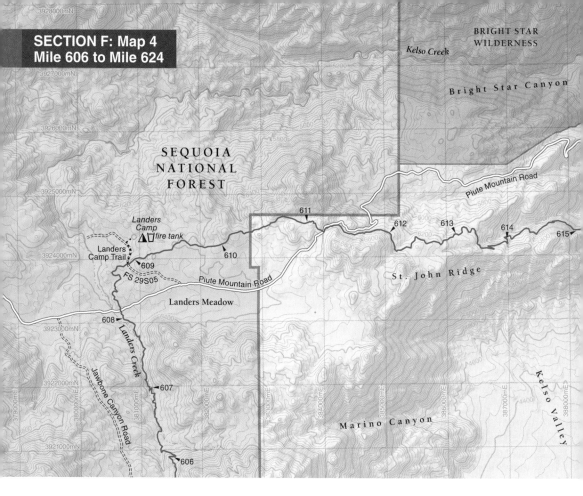

Farther below, a jeep road climbs a steep grade. Soon to the east the serpentine sliver of paved Kelso Valley Road appears. Mayan Peak is to the east, and, to its right, Butterbredt Canyon Road winds up to the Sierra Crest. Your exposed trail descends through bitterbrush and its companion plants to meet Kelso Valley Road at a pass (616.0–4,954'). A trail register is nearby.

After crossing the summit of Kelso Valley Road where it loses its pavement, you approach two distinct paths: an OHV path and the PCT. The OHV path climbs the ridge ahead, becoming one in a web of trails that covers the transitional range you are about to hike: an OHV playground on weekends. These OHV paths cut erosively across your trail. Although the BLM posts signs that clearly indicate the path of the PCT and forbid OHV use of it, it nevertheless receives heavy traffic.

Take the left trail, which heads southeast on a crenulated course across slopes mantled with bitterbrush, sagebrush, and Mormon tea—all dominant brush throughout the range. Next curve across a gully where, downslope to the left, pepper-colored debris excavated from several claims collectively known as the St. John Mine becomes visible.

HISTORY Beginning in 1867, miners extracted gold here for more than 70 years. Most of them lived in the now-vanished settlement of Sageland, just a few miles north.

The route turns left (northeast) to descend on a prominent ridge, curves across a ravine with lines of OHV tracks, traverses north-facing slopes while crossing a band of Joshua trees, and eventually meets Butterbredt Canyon Road near the mouth of its canyon (617.8–4,551').

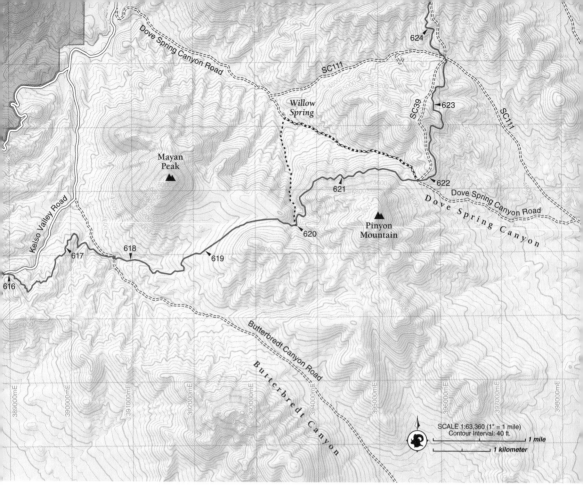

WATER ACCESS

Before continuing, check your water supply. At this intersection, water is usually available at a spring-fed stream 0.7 mile northwest down Butterbredt Canyon Road, then 0.5 mile down paved Kelso Valley Road—a 500-foot elevation loss. A group of cottonwood and willow trees just west of the paved road marks the spring, but the water flows freer just beyond. The next possible water is at Willow Spring (620.0–4,533'), 2.2 miles from the Butterbredt Canyon Road junction, then 1.6 miles downcanyon with 760 feet of elevation drop. Check the PCT water report before attempting this detour, however; access has been inconsistent in recent years.

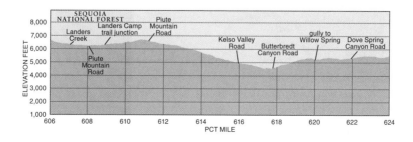

The shadeless, often hot and windy PCT ahead continues from this offset junction at the unpaved road by climbing switchbacks along the ridge between Butterbredt Canyon to the right and an east-trending gulch to the left, then ascending on an easy-to-moderate grade just south of the gulch. The slopes of the gulch eventually flatten as the path traces the valley's elongated curve to the east.

VIEWS The temple of 6,108-foot Mayan Peak to your left rules out northwestward views of the Piute Mountains, but it cannot block out the ribbon of Kelso Valley Road draped on a shoulder of the Sierra Crest.

The trail crosses a bike path on a south saddle of barely discernible Point 5,402; the path west could confuse southbound hikers. The PCT descends to wind around two canyons, then ascends gently to contour past lesser ravines cut in the north slope of Pinyon Mountain. A moderately dense stand of pinyon pines cloaks the north slopes.

WILDLIFE Long-eared owls have been seen on the eastern edge of this forest. Look under the trees by the trail for their pellets, composed of bone and fur regurgitated by the birds.

As you proceed east, the ranks of the forest dwindle, and trees are replaced by xerophytic brush. Still on the slopes of Pinyon Mountain, you reach the junction of multiple roads and paths on a Sierra Crest saddle (621.9–5,285'). Pinyon Mountain, a steep 0.8-mile climb of 900 feet southeast, is protected by boulders and pinyon trees and offers a full view that is especially enticing when the sun hangs low in the southern sky and the shadows stretch long on the desert floor.

WATER ACCESS

If you need water, Willow Spring is 1.6 miles left (downcanyon) on unpaved Dove Spring Canyon Road to the northwest. To find the pond, where there are no willows but plenty of cows, look for a fence above the road to the right

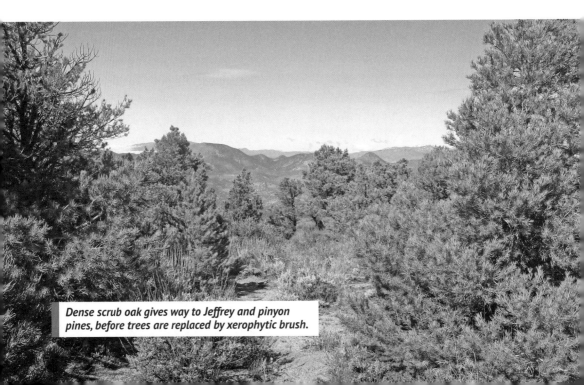

Dense scrub oak gives way to Jeffrey and pinyon pines, before trees are replaced by xerophytic brush.

and the outlet stream that flows on the road from the spring. Dove Spring Canyon Road continues to Kelso Valley Road. Check the PCT water report before attempting this detour, however; access has been inconsistent in recent years. The next potential water source is lower Yellow Jacket Spring, 15 miles from the Willow Spring road junction and 0.7 mile downcanyon with 400 feet of elevation loss.

You leave the saddle to wind north around gullied, east-facing slopes, climbing a little at first and then contouring. Along the way Indian Wells Valley, the El Paso Mountains, and Fremont Valley intercept your gaze as it sweeps the eastern horizon from north to south. Presently you arrive at another multi-road-and-trail junction (623.6–5,385') on a saddle. SC 111 leads west past the Sunset Mine road to connect with Dove Spring Canyon Road just below Willow Spring and the pond, and east to connect with Dove Spring Canyon Road just above Dove Spring.

You walk on a diagonal northwest across the junction saddle, then wind gently upward, staying west of the crest.

HISTORY Glancing downslope you can see the rubble of Sunset Mine: two shafts covered with plywood held in place by iron belt-driven flywheels; a hulk of a rusted bus; and rails from the mine to the chute.

Again, you climb the steep slopes beside and then across a road before reaching a ridge-crest saddle.

HISTORY To the west, prospect digs, a prominent ore chute, and parallel concrete slabs that slash the slope indicate the past activity here at Danny Boy Gold Mine.

Wyleys Knob, the 6,465-foot radio tower–crowned summit to the north, now stands as

a gauge of your progress. From the saddle, the wide PCT path to the right makes a moderate descent northeast via two rounded switchbacks to intersect SC 328 on a crest-line saddle (625.4–5,296'). Ahead the austere journey takes you generally north over a low hill to another crest-line saddle (625.5–5,286'), where SC 47 crosses.

The path gains a low east–west ridge 0.2 mile beyond the saddle. Next the PCT dips to a Joshua tree–covered gap, climbs north on a moderate grade while paralleling a gully, and then curves along a ridge. The gradient eases, and the trail first winds around spur ridges emanating from the Sierra Crest, then crosses a gap in the crest itself. The Scodie Mountains and the granitic outcrop of Wyleys Knob loom to the north. The trail traverses just east of the crest and passes three rounded, weathered crest-line boulders. Below Hill 5,940 a switchback leads you to skirt a hill on the crest, then to cut diagonally across an intersection with unpaved road SC 37 (628.4–5,731').

Now your moderately ascending route curves west, passes granite bluffs, and, below Wyleys Knob, begins a gentle-to-moderate descent. It first drops among pinyon pines but later crosses exposed northeast-facing slopes.

The path travels just downslope from the Wyleys Knob road and quickly reaches a junction with Bird Spring Canyon Road (SC 120) at Bird Spring Pass (630.9–5,355').

WATER ACCESS

Hikers consistently report plenty of water at a cow pond 3.8 miles west of Bird Spring Pass; follow the road until you see the metal silo and water south of it (a few hundred feet off-road). Hikers say this source tends to be reliable even when the springs at Yellow Jacket and McIvers are dry.

SECTION F

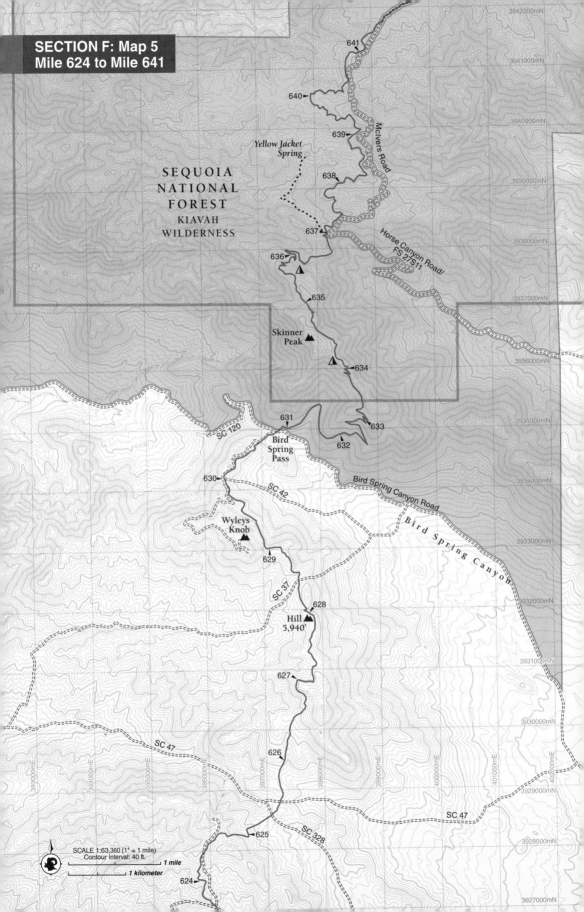

Yellow Jacket
Spring

S E Q U O I A
N A T I O N A L
F O R E S T
K I A V A H
W I L D E R N E S S

McIvers Road

Horse Canyon Road/
FS 27S11

641
640
639
638
637
636
635
Skinner
Peak
634
633
631
632
Bird
Spring
Pass
SC 120
630
SC 42
Bird Spring Canyon Road
Wyleys
Knob
629
B i r d   S p r i n g   C a n y o n
SC 37
628
Hill
5,940'
627
626
SC 47
SC 47
625
SC 328
624

SCALE 1:63,360 (1" = 1 mile)
Contour Interval: 40 ft.
1 mile
1 kilometer

HISTORY This pass was first crossed by Caucasians when in March 1854 John Charles Frémont, on his fifth expedition west, led his party through this passage.

PCT ACCESS ROUTE Unpaved but maintained Bird Spring Canyon Road (SC 120) is the most used access road to the PCT in the transitional mountain range. From the saddle it drops west to paved Kelso Valley Road and east to the aqueduct road, north to SC 65 and east to CA 14.

TRAIL INFO Thanks to the sweeping California Desert Protection Act, signed into law by President Bill Clinton in 1994, you now enter a mostly unbroken network of congressionally mandated wildernesses that takes you through the Sierra. Ahead lies the Kiavah Wilderness. Unlike the "rock and ice" areas of remarkable beauty first encompassed in the National Wilderness Preservation System established in 1964, this designated 88,290-acre area preserves the biota of a semiarid land.

Leaving Bird Spring Pass, you ascend on the PCT northeast into a side canyon along a sandy path ornamented with nosegays of blue penstemons—showy tubular flowers—and reenter Sequoia National Forest and the forest's Kiavah Wilderness.

CAMPING Southwest across the pass, the radio tower, its road, and the PCT slowly recede as you climb moderately up long-legged then short-legged switchbacks and cross over a ridge with a westward orientation.

You can find small flats to sleep on here. After a long, ascending traverse and several short, steep switchbacks, you hike over a ridge, also with room for possible waterless camping, above the Horse Canyon watershed.

VIEWS To the north, the High Sierra rises above the crests of east–west Scodie Mountain ridges, while around you manzanitas and golden oaks join the scattered pinyon pines and numerous spring wildflowers.

The PCT soon reaches its highest point in this section at 7,001 feet near Skinner Peak, then drops along a switchback and descends northwest close to the ridgecrest above a drainage of Cane Canyon.

Across the canyon the northern extension of the Piute Mountains borders the valley of Kelso Creek.

Following two quick switchbacks, your trail turns east across north-facing slopes, allowing glimpses of the eastern reaches of Isabella Lake. Lower on the path you see a mining scar gouged in creamy quartz across the ravine, and a telephone microwave relay tower perched on a point to the northeast. The route's descent eases at a saddle, then traverses 1.3 miles across the grassy slopes of minor Peak 6,455, above sprawling Horse Canyon. Heading north, the PCT cuts across a road that reaches the mine you just saw, then, seconds later, crosses another road (637.0–6,257'), both branching from Horse Canyon Road/Forest Service Road 27S11.

SIDE TRIP Maintained Horse Canyon Road, also a PCT access road, serves the relay station and descends east to CA 14. It is not part of the wilderness.

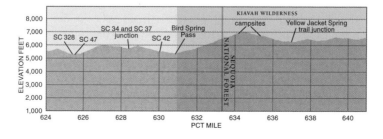

WATER ACCESS

There is usually water seeping at Lower Yellow Jacket Spring. Dig a hole below a seep, let the soil settle, and then filter the water directly from the hole. To get there, hike 0.7 mile down the second branching road at mile 637 to the first broad intersecting canyon. The seeps are on the slope to the left. Upper Yellow Jacket Spring, 0.7 mile upcanyon, is unreliable. The next reliable water source near the PCT is Walker Pass, 15 miles away. McIvers Spring is closer, about 7 miles from the second branching road junction, but it stopped flowing periodically in recent years.

PLANTS Back on the PCT, abundant pinyon pines supply ample shade. The distinguishing characteristics of the pinyon, which grows in high desert ranges, are the single gray-green needle, the blackish-barked trunk, the much-branched crown, and the 2-by-3-inch cones.

HISTORY The fall gathering season of protein-rich pinyon nuts was one of reverence and fellowship for American Indian families. After a solemn ritual, the men shook the trees or loosened the cones with hooks fashioned on willow poles. Children gathered the cones in woven willow baskets for the women to roast. Some nuts were eaten whole, but most were ground into flour. The grinding action created the many holes (mortars) in boulders you find scattered about the mountains.

The PCT gradually gains elevation as it undulates and weaves in and around scalloped slopes, and then travels below the road to McIvers Spring. At length it reaches and joins McIvers Road (641.5–6,681'), arcing east.

PLANTS The "Ichabod Crane" forest of pinyon pines continues to surround you as you walk northeast along the road. The naturally denuded lower branches, gnarled and twisted, make contorted figurations that awaken your imagination. But the forest from here to north of (not including) McIvers Cabin was severely burned in a 1997 fire caused by lightning.

Abruptly the trees give way to a sagebrush–buckbrush expanse, and then forest reappears. In less than a mile after the PCT joined the unpaved road, a short road forks sharply left off your route, and then within the next mile, two spur roads fork right. Some rills cross your road that have early-spring water and late-spring puddles of lavender-flowered, inch-high "belly" plants, and 0.3 mile before the PCT route returns to path, a seasonal brook flows across it.

At a fork (643.8–6,692'), the PCT route leaves the road and resumes as trail heading left (north).

WATER ACCESS

To reach McIvers Spring, head east at the fork and go 0.2 mile. The spring has been mostly reliable in recent years.

McIvers Cabin, a dilapidated batten-board hut, lies among picturesque slabs at the spring. It features a porch and outhouse and was once owned by Murdo McIver, who equipped it with the bare necessities of a 1938 rustic retreat. Though severely run-down, it remains today. Beware of OHV traffic.

At the junction where the trail resumes, you hike on an ascending, undulating path. Manzanita appears, along with a few stands of Jeffrey pine and black oak.

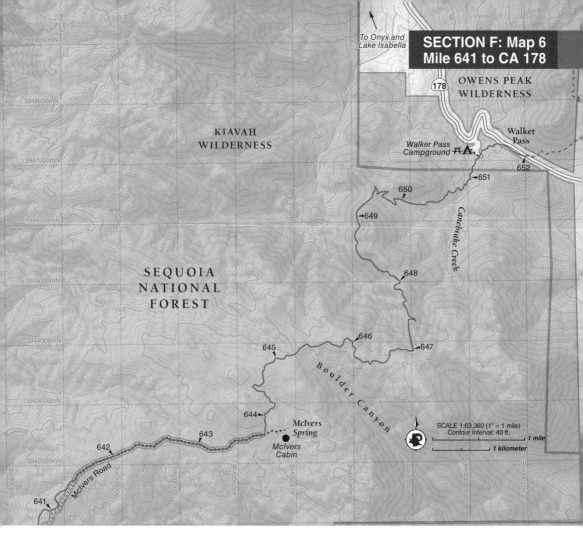

OWENS PEAK
WILDERNESS

(178)

KIAVAH
WILDERNESS

Walker Pass
Campground

Walker
Pass

652

651

650

649

SEQUOIA
NATIONAL
FOREST

648

Canebrake Creek

646

645

647

Boulder Canyon

644

McIvers
Spring

643

McIvers
Cabin

642

SCALE 1:63,360 (1" = 1 mile)
Contour Interval: 40 ft.

1 mile

1 kilometer

McIvers Road

641

The declivitous slopes of Boulder Canyon fall away to the southeast, and vistas of the Mojave Desert and the ethereal San Gabriel and San Bernardino Mountains appear through the haze.

Soon you round some three-story boulders, dashed with rust and chartreuse lichens, supporting a pinyon pine tenaciously growing from a slight crack. Leaving the gentle tableland, you descend on north-facing slopes, with views of the Mount Whitney group in the distant north and, in the northeast, the top of Olancha Peak.

Next the trail curves around a sharp canyon crease. Beyond, the PCT briefly reaches over the ridgetop at a switchback where you catch a fleeting glimpse of the Owens Peak group and the hairpin curve of CA 178, with Walker Pass Campground at the south end of that curve. Far to the north, the slash of Canebrake Road cuts across slopes, and to the northeast the PCT rises above Walker Pass. The trail continues on a long descent across steep west-facing slopes high above Jacks Creek Canyon. In time it passes a use trail angling down the slope to Jacks Creek, crosses a slight ridgeline saddle, and descends on the mountain's northeast-facing slopes.

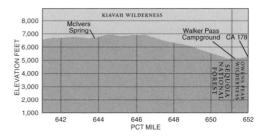

After the second switchback down the mountainside, you round just below a ridgetop, then skirt along the lower slopes of Peak 6,018.

PLANTS Among other plants along this section of the PCT, you may see an occasional large, tissue-thin, white flower of the prickly poppy, resembling a sunny-side up fried egg.

CAMPING Quite soon the trail crosses the often-dry bed of Canebrake Creek, leaves Kiavah Wilderness, and crosses a path (651.3–5,068') leading in 0.1 mile to the comfortable Walker Pass Campground. There are 11 tent sites for hikers and a couple of car-camping sites, plus picnic tables, fire rings, and pit toilets. Hikers report no faucet access in recent years, but it's a popular meeting place for PCT families and trail angels during thru-hiking season. A trail register sits near a PCT sign at the campground entrance. If the camp faucets are turned off, spring water flows from a pipe into a cow trough, left of CA 178, 0.1 mile down, next to the 30 MILES PER HOUR sign. The PCT continues to Walker Pass, winding northeast and exiting at a historical marker (652.0–5,264').

RESUPPLY ACCESS

See page 225 for more information about the several options near Walker Pass.

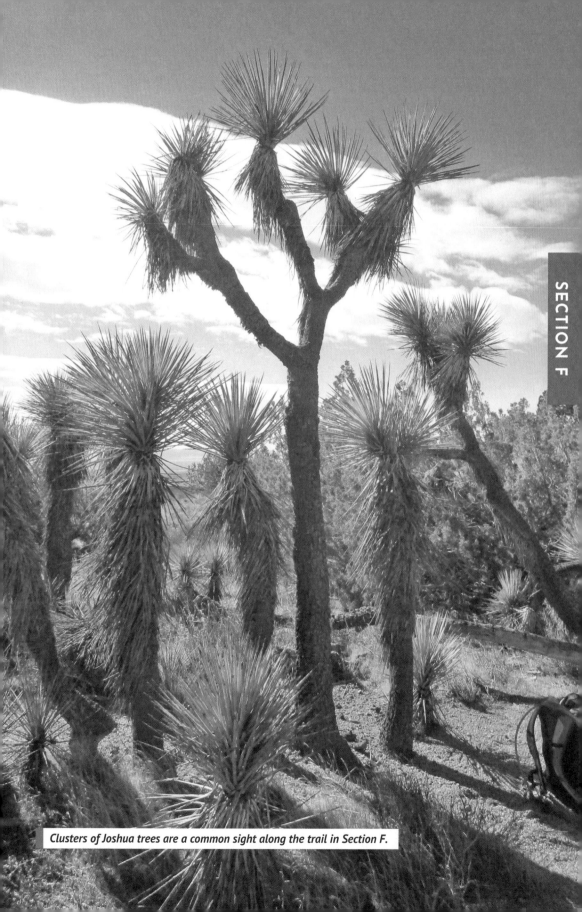

Clusters of Joshua trees are a common sight along the trail in Section F.

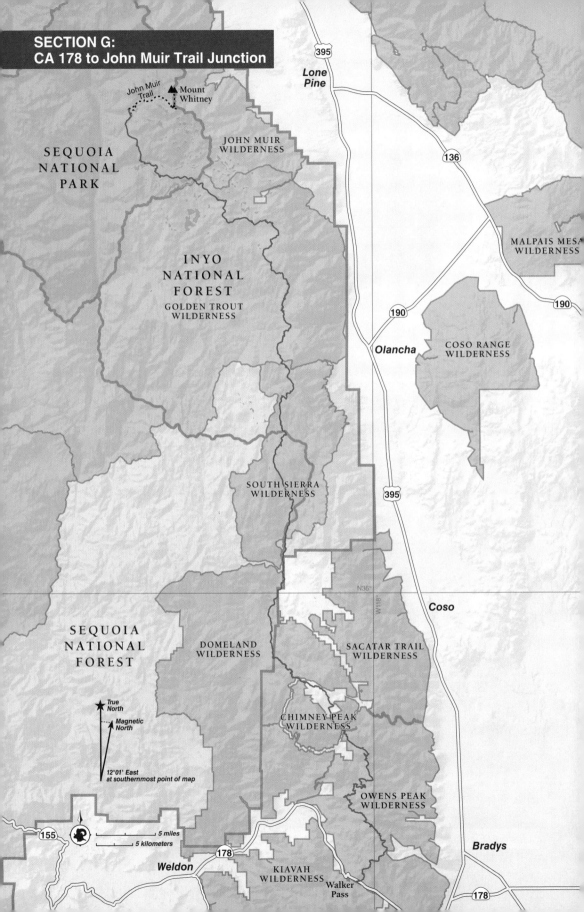

395

Lone
Pine

John Muir
Trail

▲ Mount
Whitney

136

JOHN MUIR
WILDERNESS

MALPAIS MESA
WILDERNESS

SEQUOIA
NATIONAL
PARK

190

190

INYO
NATIONAL
FOREST

GOLDEN TROUT
WILDERNESS

Olancha

COSO RANGE
WILDERNESS

SOUTH SIERRA
WILDERNESS

395

N36°

Coso

SEQUOIA
NATIONAL
FOREST

DOMELAND
WILDERNESS

SACATAR TRAIL
WILDERNESS

True
North

Magnetic
North

CHIMNEY PEAK
WILDERNESS

12°01' East
at southernmost point of map

OWENS PEAK
WILDERNESS

155

5 miles

5 kilometers

178

Bradys

Weldon

KIAVAH
WILDERNESS

Walker
Pass

178

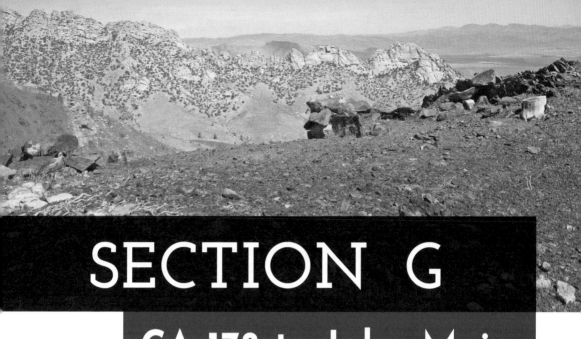

SECTION G

CA 178 to John Muir Trail Junction

NEAR THE END OF THIS SECTION you reach the celebrated High Sierra, with its 14,505-foot Mount Whitney, the highest point in the contiguous United States. Your journey there passes almost entirely within federally designated wildernesses on the Southern Sierra's Kern Plateau, a land of meadows and mountains. Hikers in this nearly pristine country can enjoy the sinuous South Fork Kern River, included in the prestigious National Wild and Scenic Rivers System; sprawling Monache Meadows, the largest meadow in the Sierra; groves of high-elevation, twisted, foxtail pines; and vast lands of solitude where the only sounds are the serenades of nature.

As always, the Pacific Crest Trail (PCT) seeks the high crest whenever possible; hence it traces the semiarid eastern heights of the Southern Sierra. This often-exposed country offers a series of panoramic views.

Above: Ridge near Mount Jenkins

DECLINATION 12°01'E

USGS MAPS

Walker Pass	Crag Peak	Olancha
Owens Peak	Long Canyon	Cirque Peak
Lamont Peak	Monache Mountain	Johnson Peak
Sacatar Canyon	Haiwee Pass	Mount Whitney
Rockhouse Basin	Templeton Mountain	

POINTS ON THE TRAIL, SOUTH TO NORTH

	Mile	Elevation in feet	Latitude/Longitude
CA 178 at Walker Pass	652.0	5,264	N35° 39' 47.100" W118° 01' 38.460"
Morris/Jenkins saddle	656.9	6,509	N35° 41' 41.340" W117° 59' 10.020"
Spanish Needle Creek (first crossing)	668.7	5,105	N35° 46' 08.640" W118° 01' 40.500"
Canebrake Road to Chimney Creek Campground (water)	680.9	5,560	N35° 50' 05.820" W118° 02' 37.620"
Fox Mill Spring	683.1	6,517	N35° 51' 17.460" W118° 03' 49.800"
Rockhouse Basin (seasonal Manter Creek)	693.5	5,846	N35° 55' 28.800" W118° 08' 57.480"
South Fork Kern River	697.9	5,750	N35° 58' 36.720" W118° 09' 18.360"
Road to Kennedy Meadows General Store	702.2	6,009	N36° 01' 25.140" W118° 08' 02.940"
Olancha Pass Trail junction (access to US 395)	720.6	9,106	N36° 13' 27.120" W118° 07' 43.980"
Trail Pass to Horseshoe Meadow/Lone Pine	745.3	10,492	N36° 25' 47.160" W118° 09' 56.340"
Cottonwood Pass Trail to Horseshoe Meadow/Lone Pine	750.2	11,132	N36° 27' 11.460" W118° 12' 56.700"
Crabtree Meadow/Ranger Station/Mount Whitney trail spur	766.3	10,321	N36° 33' 07.170" W118° 21' 29.820"
John Muir Trail junction/access to Lone Pine	767.0	10,779	N36° 33' 31.980" W118° 21' 42.360"

CAMPSITES AND BIVY SITES

Mile	Elevation in feet	Latitude/Longitude	Number of tents	Feature	Notes
656.0	6,579	N35° 41' 13.860" W117° 59' 38.580"	2	Small	
656.9	6,509	N35° 41' 41.340" W117° 59' 10.020"	>5	Morris/Jenkins saddle	Wind-prone, unprotected
672.8	6,761	N35° 46' 55.500" W118° 01' 20.400"	5	Spanish Needle Creek	Seasonal water, shade
676.1	6,899	N35° 48' 12.840" W118° 00' 41.940"	>5	Lamont Peak	Ridge above Spanish Needle Creek, views
680.9	5,560	N35° 50' 05.820" W118° 02' 37.620"	>10	Chimney Creek Campground	Downhill from trail; creek valley with pit toilets, large rocks, and picnic tables
704.7	6,146	N36° 03' 16.200" W118° 07' 49.680"	Dozens	Kennedy Meadows Campground	Pit toilets and sometimes faucet water, reliable creek nearby
709.5	7,026	N36° 06' 30.720" W118° 07' 26.220"	>5	Near Crag Creek	Small tent sites west of trail

SECTION G

CAMPSITES AND BIVY SITES *(continued)*

Mile	Elevation in feet	Latitude/ Longitude	Number of tents	Feature	Notes
713.4	7,996	N36° 09' 08.760" W118° 08' 43.200"	>5	Beck Meadow	Amid trees on either side of trail
716.5	7,832	N36° 10' 55.320" W118° 07' 43.740"	>10	Steel bridge	Sheltered sites on slope south of bridge, exposed sites along river's north bank
719.2	8,321	N36° 12' 47.580" W118° 08' 14.820"	>10	Cow Creek	Campsites along creek
730.8	8,948	N36° 19' 17.460" W118° 07' 51.660"	>10	Death Canyon	Seasonal creek and many trailside campsites
741.7	9,672	N36° 24' 48.180" W118° 08' 15.060"	8	Diaz Creek	
760.5	9,518	N36° 29' 46.240" W118° 20' 14.670"	>5	Rock Creek	Large campsite, bear-proof box nearby
766.3	10,356	N36° 33' 07.170" W118° 21' 29.820"	>5	Several sites	Bear-proof box, seasonal water nearby

WEATHER TO GO

Though you begin this section a mile high in elevation, your start is on the desert (east) side of the Sierra and, therefore, very warm in summer. Summer temperatures moderate after Kennedy Meadows and can be cool (even snowy) as you climb to higher elevations. Mid-spring (or late fall) is best for the first part of this section, and summer, after snowmelt, is ideal from Kennedy Meadows north. Afternoon thundershowers are common in the Mount Whitney area. Refer to the paragraphs about snow under "Special Concerns," on page 251.

SUPPLIES

After leaving Walker Pass, the next provisions are at Kennedy Meadows, a well-known hiker community just off the PCT at mile 702.2. It has a restaurant, tent sites, and a small general store (559-850-5647; open daily, 9 a.m.–5 p.m.) with a grill, laundry, outdoor showers, and a pay phone, and it allows hikers to camp out back. The store accepts hiker resupply packages for a small fee sent by USPS or UPS. Include ETA on your package and address to: Your Name, c/o Kennedy Meadows General Store, 96740 Beach Meadow Road, Inyokern, CA 93527.

Olancha is a tiny town with a post office, a motel, and Gus's Fresh Jerky, which sells specialty jerky and other packaged foods and drinks. Exit the PCT at mile 720.6, and follow the Olancha Pass Trail 6.9 miles to paved Sage Flat Road, which leads to I-395 in 5 miles.

For major resupplying at the north end of the Kern Plateau at Trail Pass, mile 744.5, descend 2.1 miles north to the parking lot at the end of Horseshoe Meadow Road, and hitchhike 22.8 miles down it and Whitney Portal Road to Lone Pine, a small town east of the PCT with a grocery store, motels, restaurants, and other amenities, including an outdoors outfitter and a post office. It is accessible from the Mulkey Pass, Trail Pass, and Cottonwood Pass Trails, or Crabtree Meadow trailhead.

WATER

Each source of water and the mileage to the next water are mentioned in the text. Because this is a high, near-crest trail and, in this section, is on the Sierra's drier east side, it is wise to take advantage of each source, especially during drought years. A spring, where you usually obtain water, is, after all, an accumulation of rain and snowmelt that was prevented from penetrating deeper into the ground. It follows, then, that during a drought, even the dependable springs and the creeks that flow from them could be in trouble. For assurance, you may want to carry extra water from source to source, and check the PCT Water Report (pctwater.com) before hitting the trail, if possible.

PERMITS

All trails accessing the John Muir Trail and PCT in this area require a permit and have quotas. Thru-hikers who have obtained a permit from the Pacific Crest Trail Association (PCTA) are exempt, unless they plan to leave the trail here and return later. Any thru-hiker who exits this stretch to do more than resupply or who plans to reenter at a different point must obtain a new permit from the local land management agency. Permits are issued for the trailhead and date at which you begin your hike.

Short-trip hikers will need a wilderness permit and a fire permit for Golden Trout Wilderness and Sequoia National Park. They will need only a fire permit, good for one calendar year, for the other wildernesses and for nonwilderness areas. A special permit, distributed by lottery between February 1 and March 15, is required if you plan to climb Mount Whitney. Contact the Inyo National Forest Wilderness Permit Office at 760-873-2483, or visit fs.usda.gov/inyo for more information on how to apply.

SPECIAL CONCERNS
>ANIMALS

Bears are present but usually not a problem until Sequoia National Park, provided that you keep a clean camp and use bear canisters. Bear canisters are required in Sequoia National Park and highly encouraged throughout the Sierra Nevada. See page 29 for more details.

Also known as mountain lions, cougars are so infrequently seen that you are fortunate if you catch a glimpse of one. See page 31 for more details.

>WASTE

Along with your permits, you are issued a wag bag—a system for packing out waste. The bags can be obtained in Lone Pine at the Eastern Sierra Interagency Visitor Center and the Crabtree Ranger Station. They include a urine-activated powder to encapsulate and deodorize solid waste. The waste is then contained in a zip-top bag to pack it down the mountain. The bags are required throughout the Inyo National Forest and recommended in all high-traffic areas where the natural environment is threatened.

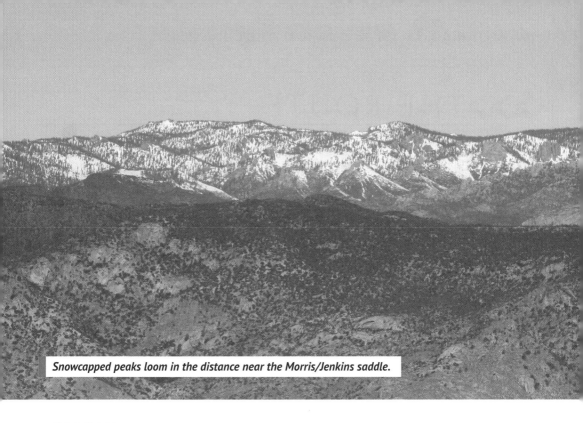

Snowcapped peaks loom in the distance near the Morris/Jenkins saddle.

>SNOW

At any time of year, be prepared for unexpected snowstorms in the Sierra. In some years, hikers will find ice and deep snow when they arrive in the high country. Hiking through the snow-covered Sierra with its wondrous scenery can be an incredible adventure, but it should be attempted only by very competent, strong hikers. In snow conditions an ice ax and crampons are highly recommended. An ice ax has many uses: as a walking stick for balance in snow, as a tool to chop steps in ice or hard snow, and as a brake to stop a slide after a fall. Skill with a compass is also recommended: few markers or signs indicate a snow-obscured trail. Proper clothing is essential, of course, and knowledge of hypothermia symptoms and treatment is a must (see page 21 for more on hypothermia). Snow travel is fatiguing and slow; hiking early in the day, when the snowpack is firm, may be helpful.

Some hikers take the bus through Owens Valley to bypass the Sierra snow, then return to travel the high country last, before the next winter's storms set in (however, challenging snow in the Sierras can often mean that all the northern trail routes are covered). One alternative is to experience the snow until you reach Trail Pass and there decide whether to exit (if the road is open, that is). If exiting, descend to Horseshoe Meadow and hope to hitchhike to Lone Pine to catch a bus. Rides may be scarce before snowmelt, and the road may be closed. However, the 22.8-mile distance down the road offers breathtaking views of Owens Valley and the distant snowcapped mountains. This plan also helps avoid crossing Sierra streams when they are swift and swollen with snowmelt and avoids emerging swarms of mosquitoes. Anticlimactic? Maybe, but think of finishing your PCT odyssey in the High Sierra during its most accommodating season.

Keep in mind, however, that PCT long-distance permits are valid only in the southern Sierra if travel is continuous. If you skip any portion here and wish to return later, you will be required to obtain new permits from local agencies (see Permits, opposite).

CA 178 TO MOUNT WHITNEY

>>> THE ROUTE

You need to hydrate yourself well before starting your hike. The next water is at Joshua Tree Spring, 11.8 miles away. Since the California Clean Water Act passed in 1988, the standard for healthful drinking water has become so stringent that agencies that test their backcountry-piped water seldom find it meets the high level of purity the law requires.

Because of the propensity for winter rockslides on the steep slopes of Mount Jenkins, equestrians are urged to contact the Bureau of Land Management (BLM) in Bakersfield for current conditions.

The PCT resumes north of CA 178 opposite the Walker Pass historical marker (652.0–5,264') and soon enters 74,640-acre Owens Peak Wilderness. There is a trail register nearby and a large sign indicating the trail mileages ahead of you.

TRAIL INFO The Owens and Chimney Peak Wilderness Areas ahead were mandated by Congress in 1994 by the California Desert Protection Act, designed to keep the area in its natural state and to protect its diversity of plant and animal life.

You ascend moderately northeast, where the trail makes a highly visible line across steep, sandy slopes of medium-grained granodiorite, then becomes gentle as it winds above a canyon.

PLANTS A look back showcases pine-clad Scodie Mountain. Below, your gaze follows CA 178 east to the distant El Paso Mountains. In early spring of some years,

the slopes around you are scattered with blue chia, a sage that has two and sometimes three pompons ringing one stem. Chia seeds were roasted by American Indians for food and used by Spaniards for medicinal purposes. Here, too, are lupines and tiny white forget-me-nots that perfume the air.

You veer gradually north on the path and then negotiate six switchbacks in the welcome shade of pinyon pines. Shortly you cross the crest at a saddle and note a few golden oaks added to the pinyon forest.

The trail, now an easy grade near the crest line, crosses a south-facing slope, then regains the crest amid forest. The path proceeds on a long traverse across northwest-facing slopes, over a crest-line gap, and then across west- and north-facing slopes to a saddle with a medium-size campsite southwest of Morris Peak.

CAMPING After rounding Morris Peak you attain the Morris/Jenkins saddle (656.9–6,509'), where a campsite south of the small hill on the crest can accommodate several tents.

Beyond the hill you cross the crest to the east side of Mount Jenkins. Now you ascend slightly to the commemorative plaque (657.1–6,605') cemented to a granite boulder, which has a small seat, formed during trail construction blasting, where you may rest, reflect, and view.

VIEWS Indian Wells Canyon spreads to the desert below, where the towns of Inyokern and, farther away, Ridgecrest

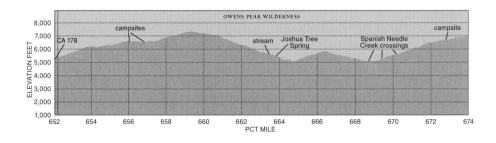

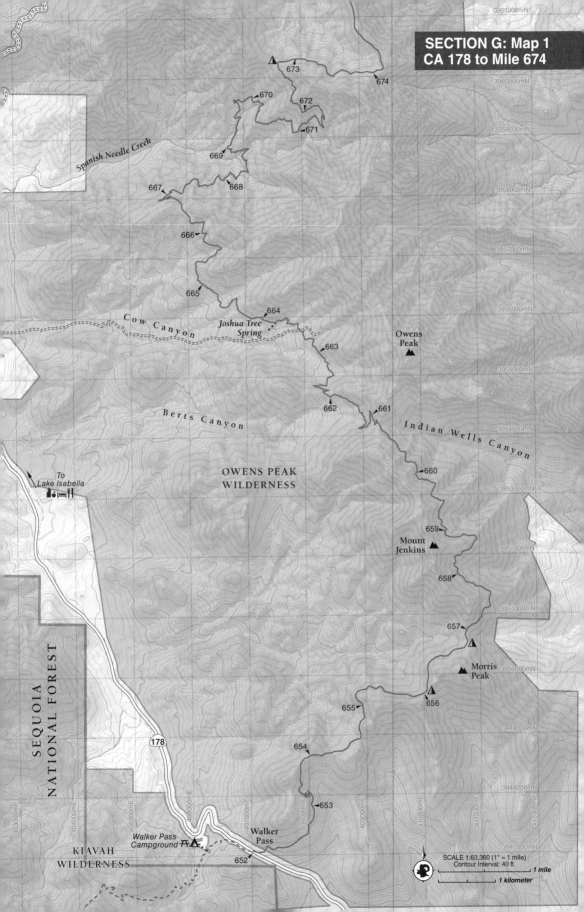

673
674
670
672
671
669

Spanish Needle Creek

667
668
666
665
664

Cow Canyon

Joshua Tree
Spring
663

Owens
Peak

662
661

Berts Canyon

Indian Wells Canyon

660

OWENS PEAK
WILDERNESS

To
Lake Isabella

659

Mount
Jenkins

658

SEQUOIA
NATIONAL FOREST

657

Morris
Peak

656

655

654

178

653

Walker
Pass

Walker Pass
Campground

652

KIAVAH
WILDERNESS

SCALE 1:63,360 (1" = 1 mile)
Contour Interval: 40 ft.

1 mile

1 kilometer

waver in the desert sun. Vast China Lake's Naval Air Weapons Station, where many sophisticated weapons have been conceived and developed, occupies the land north of Ridgecrest.

HISTORY **Mount Jenkins's namesake:** In December 1984 the United States Board on Geographic Names officially named this mountain Mount Jenkins. This sprawling, serrated 7,921-foot mountain on the Sierra Crest commemorates James (Jim) Charles Jenkins, who as a teenager hiked across its steep slopes while helping scout a route for this trail. He had been assigned to write the section of the PCT from the town of Mojave to Mount Whitney for this guidebook.

Jenkins soon expanded his interest. In the following years he hiked over all the trails in the whole Southern Sierra, some several times, no matter how obscure; climbed most of the peaks; covered miles of cross-country; and drove on every bumpy, rutted ribbon of dirt that passed for a road. He gathered information about plants, animals, geology, weather, and the lore of gold miners, cattle ranchers, and the American Indians who preceded them. While doing fieldwork and research, he developed a deep appreciation for these mountains, on which he expanded in his guidebooks, *Exploring the Southern Sierra* (two volumes, with Ruby Johnson Jenkins), now out of print but still available from used-book dealers.

He also became greatly involved in promoting conservation and protection for the Southern Sierra. For his contributions to this area, Mount Jenkins was named in his honor, the culmination of a five-year grassroots effort by his friends. The official record in the archives of the United States Department of Interior reads, "named for James Charles Jenkins (1952–1979), noted authority on the flora, fauna and history of the southern Sierra Nevada who wrote guidebooks on the area."

PLANTS While you hike along the PCT, you may see vivid deep-blue Charlotte's phacelia. This exquisite flower, found beside the plaque when the mountain was dedicated, is uncommon and should be left to propagate. In contrast to the less-than-foot-high velvety phacelia is *Nolina parryi,* reaching 10 or more feet high. This plant is indigenous in the Sierra to only this small corner. Nolina's pliant leaves are sharp-edged but not sharply tipped. Its trunk is broad, and its blossoms when dry resemble creamy parchment paper, lingering until late autumn and sometimes into the following year. Nolinas are often mistaken for yuccas.

The path, weaving around the extensions and recesses of Mount Jenkins, undulates slightly, passes a prominent ridge, curves deeply into the mountain scarred with slides of quartz diorite rocks, and then rounds another ridge. At the rounded point of that ridge, ducks flanking the trail indicate the start of the best route to climb Mount Jenkins.

SIDE TRIP Turn west to scramble up the ridge and follow the ducked use path to and over the skyscraping, nontechnical Class 2+ summit rocks to the highest point, 7,921 feet, where another commemorative plaque rests. The views are spectacular.

Striding along the PCT, you hike over chunks of metamorphic rocks; observe Jeffrey pines, sugar pines, and white firs—uncommon in this high-desert environment—and proceed around another ridge where you see ahead the ragged light granites of Owens Peak. You then gradually descend while crossing more mountain creases.

HISTORY Above the trail, one of these creases marked by a duck, 2.9 miles north of the trail plaque and 0.6 mile south of the Jenkins/Owens saddle, conceals scattered pieces of a Navy twin engine JRB-4 Expeditor. The 1949 crash took the lives of five scientists and two pilots from China Lake's Naval Ordnance Test Station (now known as the Naval Air Weapons Station) who were on their way to Alameda.

Moving on, you reach the Jenkins/Owens saddle (660.8–7,020'). The windy Sierra Crest is the jumping-off point for 8,453-foot Owens Peak, the highest peak fully within Kern County.

The PCT descends west from the saddle, and you see CA 178; distant Isabella Lake; Canebrake Road, which you will cross; and the Domelands. Beyond four switchbacks and several small slides of diorite rock, the path contours northwest, skirts a minor knob, and reaches a lesser saddle east of conical Peak 6,652. After another set of four switchbacks the trail curves around the Cow Canyon watershed. In this canyon it crosses a rough dirt road (663.4–5,500'), which the Civilian Conservation Corps work crews, who built much of this section of PCT, used for access.

SIDE TRIP This rutted road heads west to reach CA 178 in 3.9 miles, at a point 6.7 miles west of Walker Pass.

The unsigned road is closed to vehicles since becoming part of Owens Peak Wilderness.

WATER ACCESS

Beyond the rutted road, you cross a seasonal creek and then reach a 0.25-mile spur trail (663.8–5,481') to year-round Joshua Tree Spring, where a sign warns that the water is unfit for drinking.

At the spring, boughs of golden oak arch over several places to rest near an elongated cattle trough. A pipe brings water from a spring box, affording easy access for hikers. The seasonal creek flows below the spring. Volunteers from the American Hiking Society helped

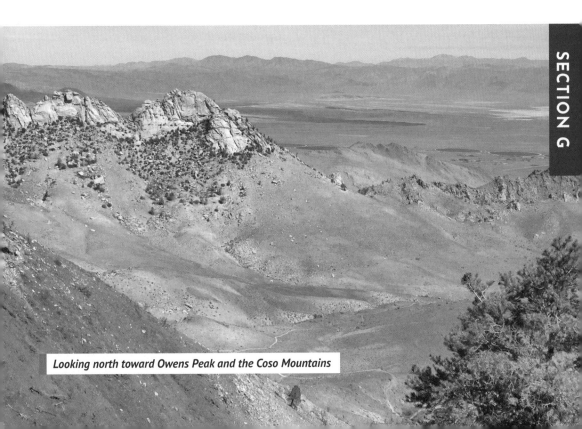

Looking north toward Owens Peak and the Coso Mountains

SECTION G

the BLM develop the spur trail and lay the spring box. The next seasonal water is 4.9 miles ahead at Spanish Needle Creek, and the next nonseasonal water is 17 miles ahead at Chimney Creek.

The PCT loses elevation as it tracks a northwest route around a major ridge from Owens Peak. Then, after ascending to cross this ridge at a saddle, it climbs, sometimes steeply, northeast up a draw before again resuming a northwest direction to still another saddle. Leaving views of CA 178 and the South Fork Valley behind, the path continues in pinyon forest and its associated understory brush. The wide, smooth PCT again loses elevation now by a series of five switchbacks, while below and off to the west the prominent slash of Canebrake Road gains elevation via one lengthy switchback.

VIEWS A summit block of Lamont Peak looms directly north of you, hiding its sheer, jagged north ridge, and Spanish Needle soon appears in the east. At your feet, sometimes in the middle of the path, arrowleaf balsamroot's big yellow flowers bloom— everything about this sometimes 32-inch-tall plant is big.

Beyond the switchbacks, the trail nearly levels before again descending east along the steep slopes. Within your view below, a private, gated road hugs the path of Spanish Needle Creek. After crossing a canyon with early-season runoff, your path bends north, and its gradient eases. Half a mile later it crosses a headwaters branch of Spanish Needle Creek (668.7–5,105').

Usually some water trickles along the Spanish Needle Creek drainage, which is shaded by willows and cottonwoods.

PLANTS While in the drainage you may look for the Spanish Needle onion, *Allium shevockii*, discovered in the 1980s—the tipped-back flower petals are bright maroon above and lime green below.

WATER ACCESS

Leaving the trees momentarily, the trail climbs out of the canyon around exposed slopes and again enters a forest, here with a few alders added, well watered by a spring-fed finger of Spanish Needle Creek (669.4–5,269'), your best source of water in this canyon.

Because water is so scarce along the crest, the PCT was routed to drop into Spanish Needle Creek canyon to take advantage of this series of springs. The trail's circuitous routing adds several extra miles of hiking.

You next climb in a pinyon pine woodland along a minor ridge, where you are likely to startle coveys of mountain quail, seemingly abundant in these mountains. You negotiate a sharp turn in a side canyon, which points you generally east to cross a spring-fed streamlet, this one frocked with wild roses. Then you clamber briefly along a blasted area, cross a seep, and again enter a shady canyon adorned with occasional bracken ferns.

WATER ACCESS

Once more you cross a finger of Spanish Needle Creek (670.2–5,637'); this and the previous streamlet join to form the creek you crossed below. The next reliable water is 10.6 miles away at Chimney Creek.

After a brief stretch south, the trail climbs east across the south-facing slopes of Spanish Needle Creek canyon, then contours around another ridge. Here the first of several white marbleized veins was blasted to carve the path.

VIEWS On this stretch you are treated to open views of jagged peaks bracketing Spanish Needle, which looks like a rounded, protruding thumb on a clenched fist.

The trail again turns southeast, abruptly turns back, climbs a switchback, and ascends out of the canyon. A pair of short switchbacks, 0.3 mile apart, helps you gain elevation to reach the ridge between the Spanish Needle group and Lamont Peak (672.8–6,761').

CAMPING Campsites were developed along the divide, to the left of the trail, to accommodate trail crews, and more are located above the trail.

While looking north and east at the BLM's Chimney Peak Recreation Area below, you see land favored by the Tubatulabal Indians and probably by prehistoric tribes before them.

HISTORY The area is rich in archaeological sites; for instance, some bedrock mortars are within easy access of the trail. Federal law prohibits removing or disturbing any archaeological resource on public lands; even pocketing an obsidian chip is against the law.

The PCT once again curves above a canyon, but this eastward leg takes you through another break from pinyons and live oaks to north-facing slopes of Jeffrey and sugar pines, white firs, and black oaks—a mix of trees found in abundance on the west side of the Kern Plateau. After gaining some elevation, the trail then curves north along the Sierra Crest, where expansive eastern views unfold of Sand Canyon below and the desert beyond.

The trail cuts a nearly straight swath northwest, just below the ridgeline, taking you once again through pinyons, oaks, and brush in sunny, dry country and then swings briefly east into a canyon, where another small stand of Jeffrey pines and firs flourishes.

PLANTS These few patches of pine and fir occur typically on north slopes where moisture lingers longer in this dry climate.

CAMPING Now the trail traverses to a narrow saddle and then climbs a bit to a broader one (676.1–6,899') with camping possibilities.

An extended descent on the PCT to Canebrake Road and Chimney Creek Campground begins. A short switchback leads you northwest to a 0.5-mile leg along Lamont Peak slopes.

PLANTS A couple of rust-brown, fragrant, scaly-needled, shreddy-barked western junipers thrive here and ahead in the most insecure places.

Rounding boulders, the path heads east before turning north onto another Sierra Crest saddle, this one with limited views.

Heading in a general northwest direction again, the PCT leaves the Sierra Crest, not to return until Gomez Meadow, almost 50 trail miles ahead. It slowly loses elevation but occasionally rises briefly as it heads along lower slopes of the north side of the canyon between Lamont Peak and Sawtooth Peak.

Accompanied by its water-loving willows, a seasonal creek crosses the path (678.3–5,950'); its water tumbles down from multicolored, sheer-sided rock canyons high above. Soon Lamont Meadow and a private inholding in this BLM-administered public land, called Chimney Peak Recreation Area, come into view, and then you see Canebrake Road.

WATER ACCESS

Finally, you dip to cross Chimney Creek. Faucets at the campground are sometimes turned off—best to get your water here (680.8–5,539').

Immediately you are ushered by a corridor of late-summer-blooming rabbitbrush to unpaved, maintained Canebrake Road (680.9–5,560'). Canebrake Road heads south 10.7 miles to CA 178 or north 4 miles to Kennedy Meadows/Nine Mile Canyon Road. Take that road east 10.8 miles to US 395 or west 13.4 miles

SECTION G

to Kennedy Meadows, which you reach via the PCT in 21.3 miles.

CAMPING Chimney Creek Campground, 0.2 mile up the road, scorched in parts by wildfires in recent years, has tent sites, pit toilets, and sometimes faucet water. The creek, however, flows much of the year across the center of the linear camping area.

The PCT leaves Owens Peak Wilderness, crosses the unpaved road, and enters 13,700-acre Chimney Peak Wilderness. Your route leaves the rabbitbrush and sagebrush behind for a short while to climb above and parallel to the road and campground amid a flurry of spring blossoms featuring the yellow, daisylike coreopsis. The path, less sandy now, dips to cross a usually dry creek, and then by a small switchback it proceeds up the south-facing slopes of the creek's canyon.

WILDLIFE Often you need to step carefully here lest you harm a horned "toad" blending in with the rocks and sand. It is really a horned lizard, and with its spikes and bumps, it is one of those contradictions: a creature so homely as to appear attractive.

Ahead you top out of this canyon and enter another one above a stream, whose chortle echoes as the precipitous granodiorite walls of the canyon close in.

HISTORY Beyond the canyon, to the left of the route, you find a scattering of debris where the multilevel ruins of a barite mill appear. The mineral barite, used in drilling muds, was mined here until about the early 1950s. Gold and tungsten were also mined in the area.

WATER ACCESS

This clutter overlooks Fox Mill Spring (683.1–6,517') and its usually reliable flowing pipe and trough; just beyond it is a seasonal stream. This is the last water until the sometimes dry creek at Rockhouse Basin, 10.4 miles ahead.

Immediately beyond the spring, the trail crosses a dirt road (683.2–6,581'). The path winds along slopes and gains elevation, while several sagebrush meadows and the dirt roads that snake through them appear to diminish below. Chimney Peak's double points seem just a stone's throw across the canyon to the east–northeast.

Now out of Chimney Peak Wilderness, you cross another dirt road.

PLANTS A few stately old juniper trees grace the path. Junipers can grow from partially digested seeds in bird droppings, far from parent trees.

Next, round a nose about 0.5 mile after the road, and then tramp through a pocket of sagebrush.

FIRE Suddenly, among pinyon pines, you reach the eastern border of the massive Manter Fire. In the summer of 2000 an estimated 816 acres of Chimney Peak Wilderness and an estimated 66,967 acres of Domeland Wilderness ahead—around 75% of that wilderness—were consumed. Two decades later, the damage is still evident. From here to

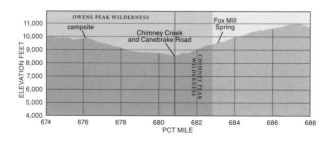

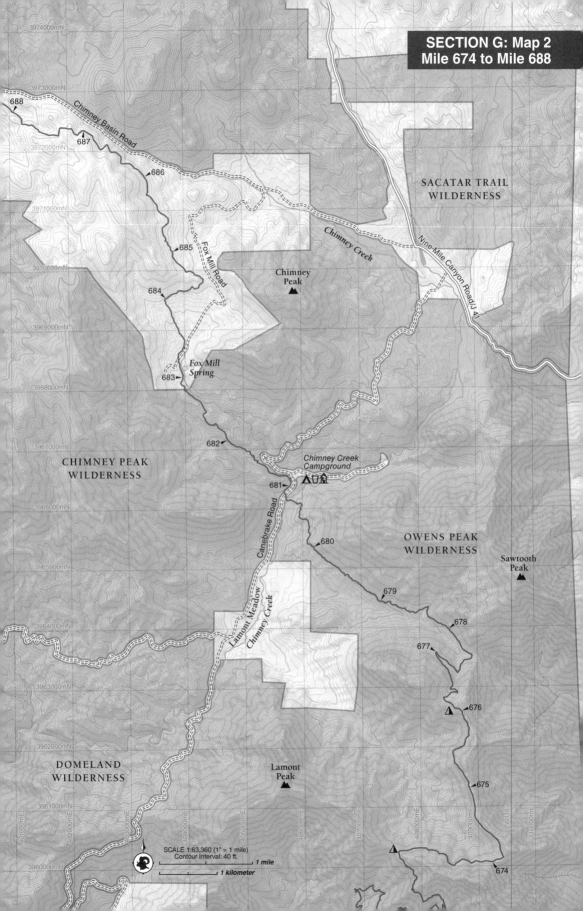

SACATAR TRAIL
WILDERNESS

Chimney Basin Road

688

687

686

685

Fox Mill Road

684

Chimney Creek

Chimney
Peak

Nine-Mile Canyon Road/J 41

683

Fox Mill
Spring

682

CHIMNEY PEAK
WILDERNESS

Chimney Creek
Campground

681

Canebrake Road

680

679

678

OWENS PEAK
WILDERNESS

Sawtooth
Peak

677

676

Lamont Meadow

Chimney Creek

5400

5600

675

DOMELAND
WILDERNESS

Lamont
Peak

SCALE 1:63,360 (1" = 1 mile)
Contour Interval: 40 ft.

1 mile

1 kilometer

674

just beyond Pine Creek, around 14 miles, you will hike in the burned area. This was an especially hot fire that not only burned the vegetation in its path but also scorched the rocks and baked the soil. Nothing seemed to have survived except a few unburned pine cones. But from these pine cones seeds scattered, and some, which settled in crannies along the now barren slopes, have germinated and begun the regeneration of the forest for future hikers to enjoy.

You cross another dirt road and begin a northwestward trek across the steep ridges and dry furrows of 8,228-foot Bear Mountain, slowly ascending over metamorphic soils and chunks of rock among black skeletal trees. To the north, Olancha Peak comes into view. At last reach the top of a minor ridge.

You begin a descent now, bearing west and crossing a road and then immediately crossing another, both leading to large excavations sliced into the red-rock slopes to the left. Several more of these gouges attract attention as you progress down the trail.

VIEWS At one time, the red-brown soil here enhanced the gray-green pinyon forest, and an occasional juniper added to the pleasing weave. This will one day return. Farther ahead the tapestry of Rockhouse Basin appears, with the stark granites of the Domelands weighing the basin's southwest border. The distant blues of Bald Mountain and other Kern Plateau peaks delineate the northwest curve of the basin, where the muted sage greens of Woodpecker Meadow are barely visible. The High Sierra silhouette stretches across the northern horizon, containing the Great Western Divide and the curved summit of Mount Langley.

The trail, curving northwest, crosses a road, then descends along a canyon where a sun-dappled seasonal creek glitters in the recesses. At a bend in this canyon, the path arches over a culvert containing a seasonal stream.

TRAIL INFO You have entered Domeland Wilderness, where a 7,000-acre addition in 1994 and the 32,000 acres added in 1984 considerably enlarged the original "rock" wilderness, which was a charter member of the National Wilderness Preservation System, established by Congress in 1964.

GEOLOGY Domes, spires, and obelisks rise from this semiarid wilderness, now encompassing more than 100,000 acres. Rock climbers practice their skills on the granite. There are meadows and sizable fishing creeks, along with the serpentine South Fork Kern River. The forests will return, but it will take 200 years to replace some of the old Jeffrey pines. A breeze usually moderates the heat of summer in this spacious land.

You cross over unpaved Chimney Basin Road (689.1–7,226') and next climb over a saddle and descend along the southwest side of a deeper canyon. In time you reach a flat on a small northeast-trending spur ridge (691.6–6,600') before entering the broader lands of Rockhouse Basin.

FIRE There are better views now of Woodpecker Meadow, an area burned in the Woodpecker Fire of 1947. The trees there were unable to reestablish themselves and were replaced by sagebrush and buckbrush. Stegosaurus Fin, Domeland's resident dinosaur, which sits prominently in the wilderness interior, displays its fin and curved back. The South Fork Kern River, weaving through the basin below, remains hidden.

You continue to descend, sometimes clinking over loose, rocky slopes, then plodding through sandy soils near the foot of the descent.

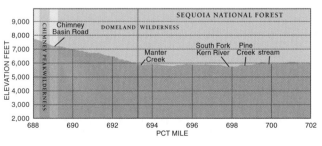

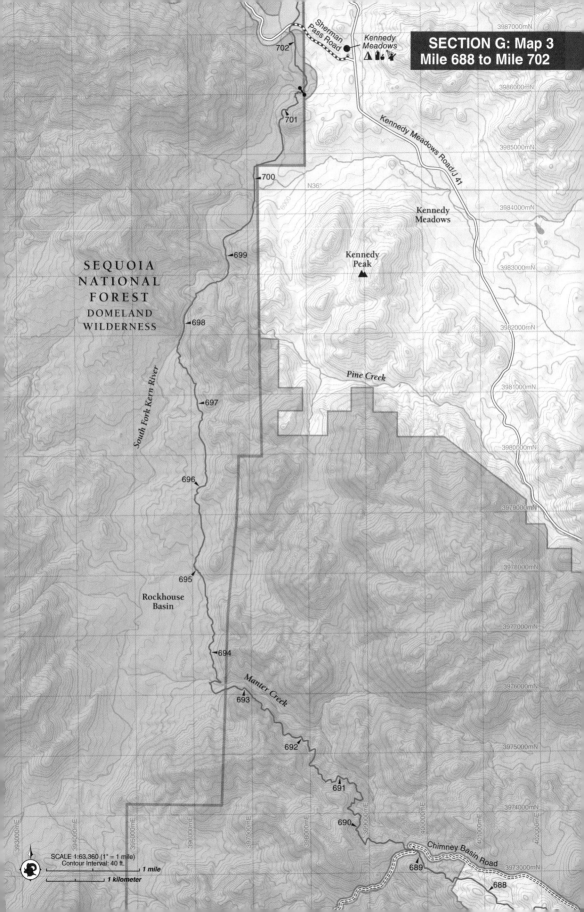

Sherman Pass Road

702

Kennedy Meadows

701

700

N36°

699

Kennedy Meadows Road/J 41

Kennedy Meadows

SEQUOIA
NATIONAL
FOREST
DOMELAND
WILDERNESS

Kennedy Peak

698

Pine Creek

697

South Fork Kern River

696

695

Rockhouse Basin

694

Manter Creek

693

692

691

690

Chimney Basin Road

689

688

3987000mN
3986000mN
3985000mN
3984000mN
3983000mN
3982000mN
3981000mN
3980000mN
3979000mN
3978000mN
3977000mN
3976000mN
3975000mN
3974000mN
3973000mN

393000mE
394000mE
395000mE
396000mE
397000mE
398000mE
399000mE
400000mE
401000mE
402000mE

SCALE 1:63,360 (1" = 1 mile)
Contour Interval: 40 ft.

1 mile

1 kilometer

Now in Rockhouse Basin, you turn right and first cross Manter Creek (693.5–5,846'), then immediately cross a closed road that is returning to nature.

WATER ACCESS

If water is needed and the creek is dry, follow its bed 1.1 miles or continue along the PCT another 4.4 miles to the South Fork Kern River.

Once again in the Sequoia National Forest, now in the Domeland Wilderness, you head upcreek and then switchback to head north, roughly following the South Fork. But, alas, the river is about a mile away for the next few miles. You now scuff along the sandy trail through a forest of pinyon pines. This sandy trail is subject to erosion, but if erosion has made it hard to see, just follow the corridor through the trees scarred by sawed-off branches.

You soon dip through the brushy wash of a waterless basin. After a burn the sagebrush root sprouts and returns rapidly. From here to Pine Creek, you will find sections of unburned forest. Later you cross a northeast-to-southwest-trending closed road, which descends along a gully. Just over a mile from the closed road, you cross a willow-lined, seasonal creek.

PLANTS In late spring you may see dainty, funnellike white evening snow—flowers that fully open when the light wanes—covering these sandy grounds.

Contouring slightly northwest now, you approach a gateway of resistant metamorphic bedrock through which flows the South Fork Kern River (697.9–5,750').

WATER ACCESS

Beginning on the slopes of Trail Peak near Cottonwood Pass, a place you will visit as you travel north on the PCT, the South Fork Kern River flows south, wandering across the Kern Plateau, gathering much of the eastern plateau's drainage, and eventually flowing into Isabella Lake. Most of the year it resembles a placid creek with good fishing holes and refreshing bathing pools, but during snow-melt the river becomes tumultuous, charging wildly through its banks. Then it is dangerous to cross. But during snowmelt this river is in its most unspoiled state and displays its scenic value, illustrating why in 1987 it was included with the North Fork Kern River in the protective custody of the prestigious National Wild and Scenic Rivers System.

Turning north again, the path threads between the willow and wild-rose tangles that edge the river and the boulders composing the cliffs. The trail climbs and dips, generally following the watercourse but not slavishly.

PLANTS Sprinklings of flowers add an artist's touch to the captivating scenery, and the three-needled, vanilla-scented Jeffrey pines, which line the water's edge, though burned, may recover.

Shortly you cross spring-fed Pine Creek; then, about 0.5 mile later, you notice that the trail melds into a closed road and that you are out of the burned area. In time, as you descend with views of a house below, you leave the road at a junction where it curves west toward the river and continue on the path straight ahead (north), following the barbed wire fence on the right. Soon you pass west of the house, then wade through a stream garnished with sedges and watercress and cross a closed OHV road next to the stream (699.9–5,933'). A vast outlying area of sagebrushy Kennedy Meadows stretches ahead, and you begin hiking through it.

Just 0.25 mile later the PCT approaches a fence corner, then leaves the fence and angles off to the northeast, away from the river. In the middle of this meadow, the path crosses another closed OHV road. Not far north of the meadow, the PCT climbs the lower west slope of a hill, where you catch your first sight of paved Sherman Pass Road and a few buildings along it. Pressing near the river again, the trail passes through three cattle gates (please close) and exits Domeland Wilderness. Between the first two gates, it rounds west of outcrops where the path is often washed out by high water or covered with tall grass. Sections of this are privately owned land, and trails or roads may lead away from the river, but you continue ahead. After the second gate, you ascend a couple of low hills, pass through the third gate, and head for the paved road, just east of a bridge (702.2–6,009').

RESUPPLY ACCESS

At this point, if you need supplies, a shower, a washing machine, refreshments, or package pickup; or just wish to sign the PCT register, chat, or catch the Saturday-night movie, continue 0.7 mile right (generally southeast) along the road to tree-shaded Kennedy Meadows General Store. Ride-sharing is often available here.

This road with many names— Sherman Pass, Kennedy Meadows, Nine Mile Canyon, Forest Service Road 22S05, J41, M-152— reaches US 395 in 24.2 miles.

Major supplies are available in Ridgecrest, 25 miles southeast of the junction, off CA 178. The road reaches the Kern River to the west in 44.3 miles and subsequently Kernville 19.5 miles farther, where there are ample supplies and accommodations.

When it is time to move along, you return to the trail where it crosses the road and amble north to Kennedy Meadows Campground. You would walk the same distance if you took the northbound road just beyond the store to reach the campground.

Across the paved U.S. Forest Service (USFS) road, you continue on sandy turf among early-season high-desert flora. Heading north, you dip through washes and cross dirt roads that lead west to riverside campsites, fishing pools, and swimming holes. Occasional junipers offer spots of shade as you pass fences, first on the right and then on the left. Then you go through one gate and soon through another. Enticing murmurs of the river increase as you reach and then hike above the musical South Fork. Slowly you leave the sagebrush meadow that is embraced by the gentle peaks of the semi-arid side of the Kern Plateau and head toward a distant fire-scarred mountain, seen up the river canyon to the north.

Soon the trail crosses the road to the campground and proceeds along higher ground. Here it winds for a short time around boulders among pinyon pines and brush. Then it crosses the road again and bisects Kennedy Meadows Campground (704.7–6,146').

CAMPING No longer run by the USFS, this campground has 39 units and has remained open to hikers and anglers, who fish for golden trout in the river. It is a good place to overnight while you sort through your food packages from home, but it's

SECTION G

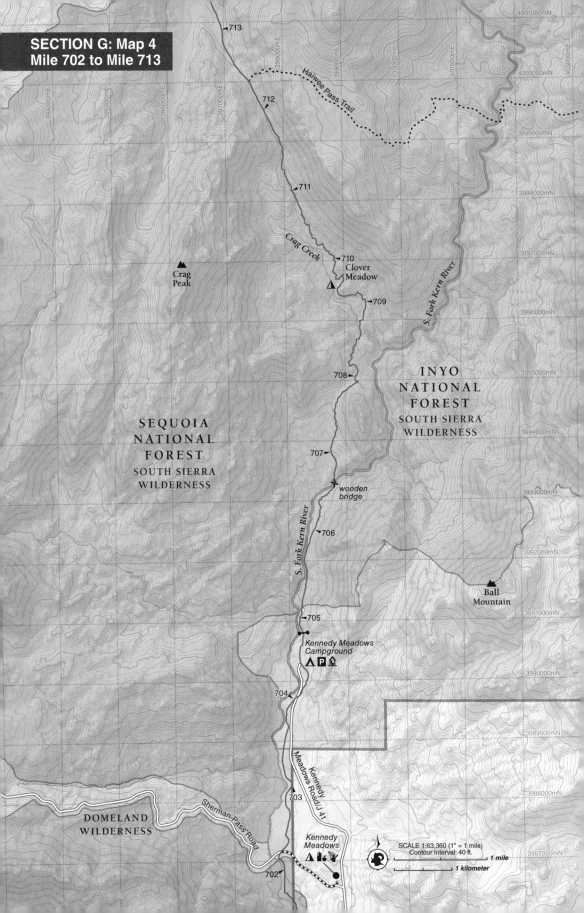

713

712

Haiwee Pass Trail

711

Crag Creek

710
Clover
Meadow

709

Crag
Peak

708

INYO
NATIONAL
FOREST
SOUTH SIERRA
WILDERNESS

SEQUOIA
NATIONAL
FOREST
SOUTH SIERRA
WILDERNESS

707

*wooden
bridge*

S. Fork Kern River

706

S. Fork Kern River

Ball
Mountain

705

Kennedy Meadows
Campground

704

Kennedy
Meadows Road/J 41

703

Sherman Pass Road

DOMELAND
WILDERNESS

Kennedy
Meadows

702

SCALE 1:63,360 (1" = 1 mile)
Contour Interval: 40 ft.

1 mile

1 kilometer

recommended to call the general store before you arrive (559-850-5647) to confirm that the campground is still open.

The PCT leaves the north end of Kennedy Meadows Campground. Pinyon and Jeffrey pines, along with juniper trees, offer shade as the trail immediately dips into a side canyon, then eases through a stock-fence gate, passes several lateral paths to the river, and enters South Sierra Wilderness.

TRAIL INFO This wilderness was one of many established by the comprehensive California Wilderness Act of 1984. Its 63,000 acres closed the gap between Domeland and Golden Trout Wildernesses, giving wildlife a wide, undisturbed area to roam and wildflowers room to spread.

The PCT soon approaches the river and heads right (northeast) to a sturdy yet scenic, steel-girded wooden bridge (706.6–6,288').

Beyond the bridge, the trail climbs north of a knoll and then continues over gravelly terrain. Soon your path gains the slopes of a craggy 7,412-foot mountain whose soils nurture an occasional prickly pear cactus.

PLANTS The prominent yellow-orange blossoms of this spiny plant turn pink to rose as they mature.

Past the ascent, the path switchbacks down once to reach a saddle, and then it makes a weaving traverse above the rumble of the South Fork Kern River, sometimes heard but not seen in its canyon to the east. The PCT then dips to cross Crag Creek (708.6–6,815'). Yellow monkey flowers and cinquefoil luxuriate near the banks of the creek.

After a short ascending hike beyond the ford, you again face the skeletal remains of trees.

FIRE These trees were burned in the 1980 Clover Meadow blaze. Buckbrush ceanothus, rabbitbrush, and associated xerophytic plants have replaced the forest; the pines are slow to regenerate, even four decades later. The stark grays and blacks of the burn contrast sharply with the creek's riparian expanse and the greens of Clover Meadow below.

You pass an unburned pocket of trees and, 1.8 miles into the burn, again reach the welcome shade of forest.

PLANTS Mountain mahogany is abundant here. This woody brush with small, wedge-shaped leaves clustered near branch tips turns silvery in the fall when clad in its corkscrew, feathered plumes.

The path meets the usually dry eastern branch of Crag Creek. A spring appears in the creek's channel just before the path climbs a narrowing, boulder-strewn slot, but a lush growth of willows and wild roses laps up most of the water, leaving a timid flow. The grade abates amid yellow-flowered bitterbrush and ends at a saddle and a T-junction with Haiwee Pass Trail 37E01 (712.3–8,070'), which follows an ancient American Indian path east to the river and through Haiwee Pass to Owens Valley—a route that almost became the eastern leg of a trans-Sierra highway. Damaged by past floods, the trail may be overgrown in parts and difficult to locate.

CAMPING Beyond the saddle, the PCT drops gently to Beck Meadow, a sagebrush finger of Monache Meadows. Campsites can be found at the foot of the grade in the trees on either side of the trail. Please follow Leave No Trace principles and camp at least 200 feet from the trail.

VIEWS A spacious view of Monache Meadows, the largest meadow in the Sierra, includes distant Mount Whitney and its neighbors peering over the plateau peaks. Among the seasonal flowers trailside, the yellow evening primrose, with its heart-shaped petals, makes a dramatic appearance.

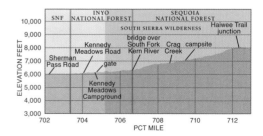

The PCT veers north from northwest-leading Beck Meadow Trail 35E15 (713.4–7,939') and from the all-but-gone grooves of an old jeep road that crossed the path.

HISTORY Jeeps first penetrated into Monache Meadows in 1949, but long before that, horse-drawn buckboards left their parallel treads.

After less than a mile of relatively level hiking north, you veer right (north–northeast) toward hulking Olancha Peak to angle up the lower slopes of nearby Deer Mountain. After crossing a usually dry gulch, you climb through another gully from which you see a cow trough below at the edge of Beck Meadow. A spring sometimes bubbles forth above the trough in the gully. You next pass through another stock-fence gate, and then Mount Langley, framed by Brown and Olancha Mountains, comes into view to the north. Its rounded back side resembles that of Mount Whitney, with which it is often confused. After 0.7 mile from the gate, you top out on Deer Mountain's northern ridge.

From there the path briefly heads southeast to a switchback, then north to drop out of the forest and cross a retired jeep road that bisects a low, broad ridge. The PCT heads northeast along the ridge, turns right, and drops to an arched bridge over the South Fork Kern River (716.5–7,832'). Interestingly, the steel in this bridge was treated to resemble an old, rusted structure, rendering it less conspicuous. The bridge spans shallow water except during snowmelt, when most long-distance PCT hikers pass this way; then it is an important safety factor.

WILDLIFE You will probably cause great commotion among the cliff swallows that return annually to raise their young in the braces under the bridge. Their mud nests are gourdlike, with a narrow, short tunnel entrance into which they dart to feed fat bugs to their families.

CAMPING An ideal campsite is sheltered by trees on the slope south of the bridge, and exposed sites sprawl near

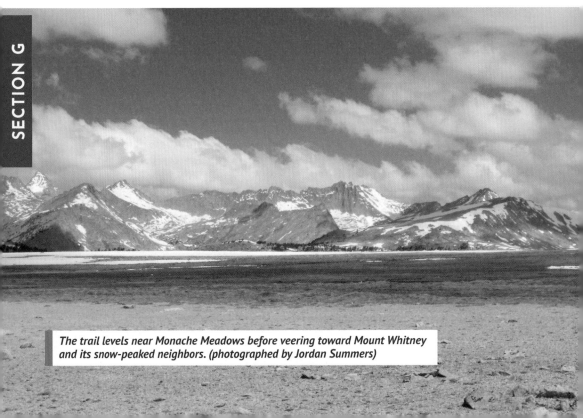

The trail levels near Monache Meadows before veering toward Mount Whitney and its snow-peaked neighbors. (photographed by Jordan Summers)

the river's sandy north bank. Be sure to set up camp at least 200 feet from water and the trail.

Here you leave Sequoia National Forest and enter Inyo National Forest, but you still remain in South Sierra Wilderness.

Resuming its route north of the bridge, here briefly overlapping an OHV road, the PCT passes a southeast-heading trail to Kennedy Meadows, a path that vibrated with motorcycles before the wilderness was established. Immediately your trail passes a dirt road, which leads north into the canyon straight ahead. After paralleling the river a short way, the PCT turns right at a junction, while the road-trail it was on continues to Monache Meadows.

Trail-width now, the PCT climbs northwest above the meadow while jogging laterally around washes and ridgelets to stay within its desired grade of 15% or less.

TRAIL INFO One can usually identify sections of PCT that overlay old trails: on old trails it plunges in and out of washes rather than curving around them.

The trail mounts a low ridge and heads north, leaving open slopes sparsely dotted with chartreuse-lichen-painted boulders.

CAMPING It then enters forested Cow Canyon. Midway up this canyon, the trail resumes on the former PCT path that it left in Beck Meadow and immediately crosses Cow Creek (719.2–8,321'), where you find the first of a spread of campsites along the creek. Expect to share your water here with the many grazing bovines found in the area.

The trail soon crosses the creek again but quickly returns and ascends a canyon where Kern ceanothus debuts.

PLANTS This ceanothus has hollylike leaves and pomponlike blue-to-purple flowers. It is a denizen of the plateau, occurring only in a few other places.

The trail merges briefly with paths of a stock driveway angling in from the left. (North-to-south hikers, take note: an accidental turn

onto a driveway path would take you to the head of Monache Meadows.)

You ford the creek once more and look for a PCT post marking the return ford. Again on the left side of the creek, you find your trail among the multiple twining cow paths paralleling it. Where the creek turns east, almost 1 mile after the last junction, you continue north and quickly reach a trickle from a spring just above. After a short, winding ascent, you turn right to join the Olancha Pass Trail (720.6–9,106'). Vegetation coils about the sometimes slack spring immediately south of this junction.

Your route on the conjoined trail runs east, now on a gentle ascent around the head of Cow Canyon. Along the way it passes disturbed terrain on the canyonside created by stock drives, and then it crosses Cow Creek again just 250 yards before the next trail junction (720.7–9,189'), where the PCT departs left (north).

RESUPPLY ACCESS

The rarely used Olancha Pass Trail continues east over the pass, then descends to Sage Flats Road in 6.9 miles. The paved, lightly traveled road heads east 5.8 miles to US 395. For emergency supplies, the town of Olancha, 5 miles north on the highway, has a post office, BLM fire station, restaurant, and jerky store with limited supplies.

The ascending PCT heads left at the junction, switchbacks, arcs northeast up a rounded ridgelet, and then turns north where a lateral branches off to the trail you just left. Your trail runs across slopes of chinquapin and manzanita, fords Cow Creek, and zigzags many times amid bush currant, a favorite berry of black bears. Now leaving the forest, the PCT

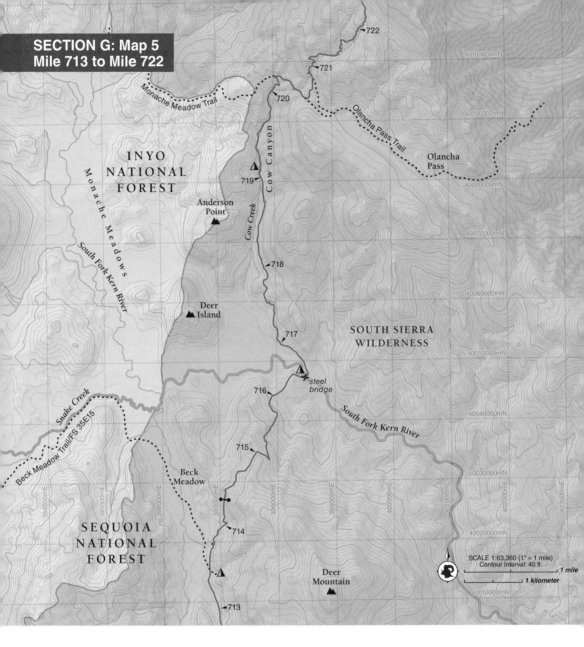

INYO
NATIONAL
FOREST

Monache Meadow Trail

Monache Meadows

South Fork Kern River

Cow Canyon

Cow Creek

Anderson
Point

719

720

721

722

Olancha Pass Trail

Olancha
Pass

718

Deer
Island

717

SOUTH SIERRA
WILDERNESS

steel
bridge

716

South Fork Kern River

Snake Creek

Beck Meadow Trail/FS 35E15

715

Beck
Meadow

SEQUOIA
NATIONAL
FOREST

714

Deer
Mountain

713

SCALE 1:63,360 (1" = 1 mile)
Contour Interval: 40 ft.
1 mile
1 kilometer

continues to parallel the creek, which flows among groups of corn lilies, aptly named plants resembling cornstalks. The open tread is sandy and often very dusty, but it still supports the colorful scarlet gilia, a cluster of red flowers with tubular necks and pointed, starlike lobes. The gradient steepens, and the trail zigzags sporadically as it climbs a side canyon.

It then fords a spring-fed brook and switchbacks among boulders by a foxtail pine, with an extensive view of Monache Meadows and the sandy floodplain of South Fork Kern River.

The PCT's grade diminishes as it leads into the shade of lodgepole and occasional foxtail pines—isolated specimens of the impressive foxtail pine groves ahead.

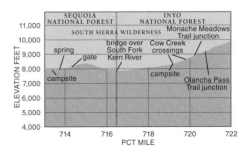

PLANTS The foxtail pine grows in gravelly soils just below treeline, along with very few understory plants. Its short, five-clustered needles surround the branches; a bristly branch end with its tip up resembles a fox's tail. Foxtail pines seem to survive nicely in the extreme weather of the high country where other trees cannot.

Atop a ridge, your trail proceeds past a junction that eventually connects with the Olancha Pass Trail. North of a fallen tree your path ascends gently to moderately, curves northwest, and crosses another open slope with seasonal streamlets and seeps. The farther the trail climbs on this slope, the more remarkable are the Southern Sierra views; Domeland is particularly prominent.

VIEWS In almost 1 mile the trail crosses a flat, forested ridge. Provocative vignettes ahead of (east to west) Olancha Peak, Mount Langley, the Kaweah Peaks Ridge, and Kern Peak may be seen framed by the boughs of the forest.

Continuing to climb, the path curves around a headwaters bowl of Monache Creek and then levels off on a saddle of a ridge that juts out from the west-facing slope of Olancha Peak (724.4–10,580'). This, the highest point along the side of Olancha Peak, is a good departure point for the nontechnical 1,550-foot climb to the top of the most dominant peak on the Kern Plateau.

SIDE TRIP To climb Olancha Peak, ascend northeast on a 0.6-mile cross-country route among foxtail pines to treeline, aiming for the slope north of the summit. There, the rounded and gentler terrain makes for an easy final ascent, but only after you have pulled up and over scores of large boulders. Unexpectedly found among these boulders are vigorous plants of yellow columbine. Then you

---

scale the 12,123-foot summit for the payoff: vistas you won't soon forget.

You might pause to reflect on the fate of the American Indians for whom this summit was named. *Olancha* and *Yaulanchi* were spoonerisms for Yaudanchi, a tribe of Yokuts Indians who probably traded with either the Paiutes north of Owens Lake or the Kosos south of it. The Yaudanchi now reside on the Tule River Indian Reservation.

An alternative to climbing Olancha Peak for plateau views is Point 10,600, west of the saddle and the trail. From there you barely see the rounded back side of Mount Langley fronting the same part of Mount Whitney, but you see the Kern Plateau wonderfully spread before you.

From the saddle, the PCT drops to Gomez Meadow on a gentle-to-moderate grade. Along the way it switchbacks five times and then curves around another headwaters bowl of Monache Creek. The trail leads across a watershed divide, where it leaves South Sierra Wilderness and enters Golden Trout Wilderness.

TRAIL INFO As you saunter along this easy northern descent, you may contemplate some events that involved this area. Before the late 1940s the only way one could reach the gentle Kern Plateau was by foot, animal, or a breathtaking flight in a small aircraft. Then logging began in the southern part and slowly pushed northward. The loggers' roads opened the land to jeeps and their cousins, dirt bikes. All these intrusions resulted in slope erosion, damaged meadows, and silted streams. Environmentalists became alarmed and campaigned to protect the remaining land. They were eventually successful. In 1978 President Jimmy Carter

SECTION G

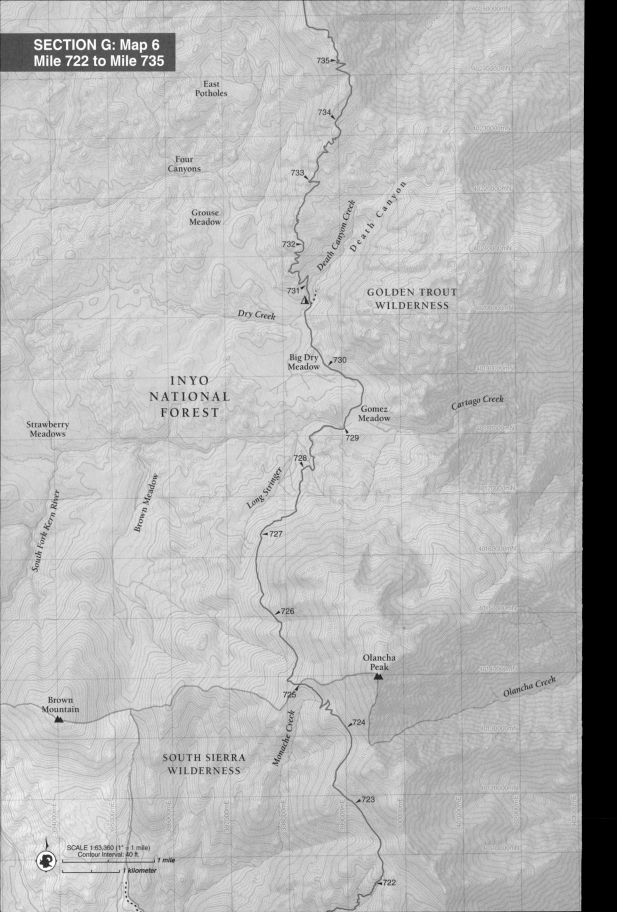

East
Potholes

Four
Canyons

Grouse
Meadow

Death Canyon Creek

D e a t h   C a n y o n

735

734

733

732

731

Dry Creek

**GOLDEN TROUT
WILDERNESS**

730

Big Dry
Meadow

Cartago Creek

Gomez
Meadow

729

**I N Y O
N A T I O N A L
F O R E S T**

728

Long Stringer

Strawberry
Meadows

Brown Meadow

727

South Fork Kern River

726

Olancha
Peak

725

Olancha Creek

Brown
Mountain

724

Monache Creek

**SOUTH SIERRA
WILDERNESS**

723

40250000mN
40240000mN
40230000mN
40220000mN
40210000mN
40200000mN
40190000mN
40180000mN
40170000mN
40160000mN
40150000mN
40140000mN
40130000mN
40120000mN
40110000mN

394000mE
395000mE
396000mE
397000mE
398000mE
399000mE
400000mE
401000mE
402000mE
403000mE

SCALE 1:63,360 (1" = 1 mile)
Contour interval: 40 ft.

1 mile

1 kilometer

722

signed into law the 306,000-acre Golden Trout Wilderness, named for the colorful trout—California's state fish—that evolved in this area. The northern third of the Kern Plateau is part of this wilderness.

You pass above a seasonal spring while hiking across exposed slopes with views of brownish, boulder-topped Kern Peak across the Kern Plateau. This 11,510-foot peak counterbalances Olancha Peak; the two are among the highest points on the plateau.

Now the PCT meanders northwest, dropping in and out of forests and passing seeps and springs that find their way to Brown Meadow and Long Stringer.

The trail gradually curves northeast then bends southeast to cross a creek (728.1–9,045'). This is a better source of water than Long Stringer ahead.

From the creek the PCT leads north and then east on a slightly rolling course. Then it bends sharply north and crosses a meadowside trail at a causeway abutment just west of very level Gomez Meadow (729.0–8,987').

The causeway's 35-yard length elevates the path above the sodden stringer beneath.

PLANTS Shooting stars seem almost airborne across the meadow. The common name of this flower is well chosen because its swept-back crimson or purple petals suggest flight.

The PCT resumes at the north abutment and then immediately crosses another meadowside path. It then curves northeast into a dense forest of lodgepole pines, touching the inconspicuous Sierra Crest, which it last crossed in Owens Peak Wilderness. The trail gradually turns northwest and soon skirts Big Dry Meadow.

CAMPING Beyond this meadow you ford a step-across, all-year creek (730.8–8,951') at the mouth of Death Canyon. To the left are several campsites; to the right (upcanyon),

a path takes PCT equestrians to another in a series of corrals and camping areas built for the PCT trail crews of Inyo National Forest. The corrals are infrequently maintained. The trailside campsites are ideal places to overnight before the nearly 2,000-foot steep climb out of Death Canyon.

Next, in a fine grove of fragrant, gnarled, old mountain juniper trees, you labor up 22 broadly spaced switchbacks and numerous curves on the blocky, spired ridge west of the canyon. You may pause occasionally to view pointed Kern Peak and the broad expanse of Big Dry Meadow. You eventually cross the crest of this ridge for the last time at a slender slot between craggy outcrops. Foxtail pines now shade you, and red mountain-pride penstemons decorate your path as you descend gently to a crest-line saddle from which the eastern slope drops precipitously to Owens Lake bed.

GEOLOGY This alkali flat is usually dry because the Los Angeles Department of Water and Power diverted its inflow to their aqueduct. The pink coloration of the lakebed is due to algae and bacteria.

Next you ascend on seven switchbacks to attain a crest-line prominence, reaching an elevation of 10,700 feet.

VIEWS Here you are rewarded again with grand views of Owens Lake bed and the Coso and Inyo Mountains east of it. Olancha and Kern Peaks dominate the southern half of the horizon.

At length you leave the ridgetop in a descending traverse of west-facing slopes, and

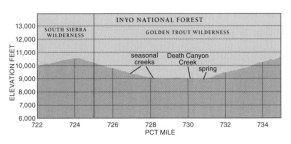

then curve west to a saddle where you meet a junction (736.4–10,364') with a faint, 0.5-mile lateral trail that descends north toward a seasonal spring.

WATER ACCESS

This spring waters a meadow dotted with buttercups in the crease of the canyon about 0.5 mile in on this lateral.

Beyond the faint junction, you ascend mostly northwest, crossing two more crestline saddles. About 0.5 mile later you cross yet another saddle.

TRAIL INFO Here you leave one cattle allotment and enter another. In fact, the whole plateau is a patchwork of these parcels; wilderness designation here does not ban grazing. Most of the cattle people involved have been summering their animals in these allotments for several generations.

The PCT curves north where Sharknose Ridge juts off to the west, then skirts the west edge of wide Ash Meadow on a nearly level stretch of Sierra Crest. The trail leaves the crest to make a brief descent of northwest-facing slopes to a corral in a ravine above Mulkey Meadows.

As the dusty PCT descends, Mount Langley, which is the southernmost 14,000-foot peak in the Sierra Nevada, sinks behind the shoulder of Trail Peak while views of Mulkey Meadows improve. Your path bends east around a spur ridge where you find a rather unusual juxtaposition of foxtail pine, sagebrush, and mountain mahogany. For almost a mile now the path nearly levels and then regains the Sierra Crest at a low saddle.

CAMPING The PCT begins to ascend, but if you need a campsite, leave the trail on a use path (741.7–9,672') to the right (east) to reach Diaz Creek and some open space. A spring issues forth in a side canyon just under 0.5 mile in on this path.

You now climb the crest on a gentle-to-moderate grade gradually heading northwest. After a mile you curve on the crest, then leave it for a short climb north to top a broad ridge south of Dutch Meadow.

You turn sharply left (south) at a corral junction (743.0–9,952'), just below a switchback, but if you need water or a corral, turn right (north) on the 0.2-mile lateral to Dutch Meadow.

The PCT ascends west with two sets of switchbacks to cross the Sierra Crest again. It attains a spur ridge, bends from north to west around a canyon, and then crosses a stock driveway at Mulkey Pass (744.5–10,394'). Beyond the driveway, you travel around the south side of a hill straddling the crest line to reach Trail Pass and a junction with Trail Pass Trail (745.3–10,492').

RESUPPLY ACCESS

If you have a package pickup in Lone Pine or need supplies, descend 2.1 miles north on Trail Pass Trail to Horseshoe Meadow Road and Cottonwood Pass

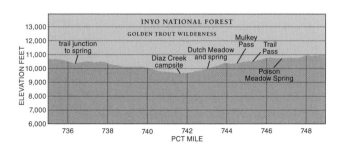

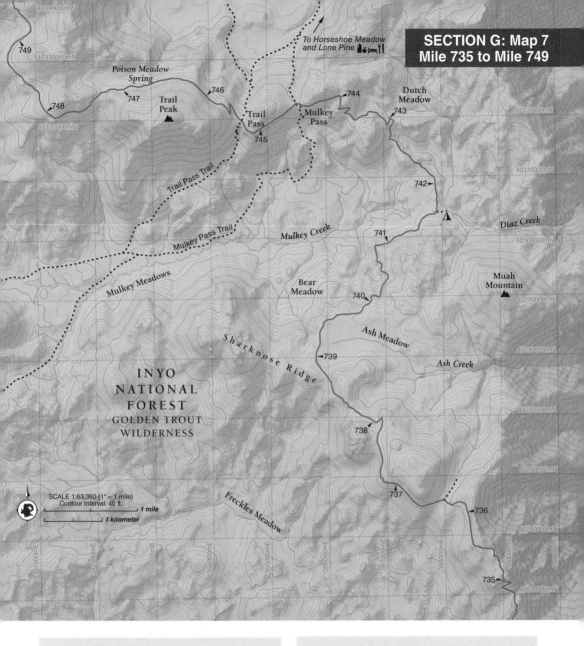

To Horseshoe Meadow
and Lone Pine

749

Poison Meadow
Spring

748

747

Trail
Peak

746

Trail
Pass

745

Mulkey
Pass

744

743

742

Dutch
Meadow

Diaz Creek

Trail Pass Trail

Mulkey Pass Trail

Mulkey Creek

741

Mulkey Meadows

Bear
Meadow

740

Muah
Mountain

Ash Meadow

739

Sharknose Ridge

Ash Creek

INYO
NATIONAL
FOREST
GOLDEN TROUT
WILDERNESS

738

737

736

SCALE 1:63,360 (1" = 1 mile)
Contour Interval: 40 ft.

1 mile

1 kilometer

Freckles Meadow

735

Campground; then hitchhike 22.8 miles to Lone Pine. On most spring weekends after snowmelt and in summer, this place buzzes with activity, but on early-season weekdays, finding a ride at this parking area or the adjacent Cottonwood Lakes parking area may not be easy; in winter, it may be impossible if the road is closed. Nevertheless, this is a far better place to begin a detour to Lone Pine than the detour over Trail Crest to Whitney Portal, where cars are frequent—unless returning to the PCT up Mount Whitney's steep east face toting a heavy pack is of no concern to you.

Continuing beyond Trail Pass, the PCT ascends gently northwest amid foxtail pines and talus, switchbacks two times, and then rounds the north-facing slopes of 11,605-foot Trail Peak.

VIEWS Portals in the forest frame the last exhilarating views of Mount Langley seen from the PCT and the nearer views of Poison Meadow below.

Now the PCT crosses refreshing Corpsman Creek and soon leaves the slopes of Trail Peak to intersect the crest at a saddle. It gently traverses southwest along a route that offers sweeping views of Mulky Meadows below. The path then curves north, passing several small meadows.

GEOLOGY The meadows' seeps and springs combine to become the headwaters of South Fork Kern River, a stream that meanders through three wildernesses on the east side of the gentle plateau until it courses off the south end in a harsh area called The Roughs.

Foxtail pines shade your path, parting occasionally to reveal views of the Great Western Divide. In time you round a watershed divide and pass through a west-facing meadow decked with flowers.

GEOLOGY This meadow's drainage finds its way into Golden Trout Creek, where it travels west to tumble off Kern

Plateau's basaltic rim into the narrow, steep trench of North Fork Kern River—the river's main branch.

After ascending to a spur-ridge saddle, you descend to meet the Cottonwood Pass Trail at Cottonwood Pass (750.2–11,132'). This trail also reaches Horseshoe Meadow Road and Cottonwood Pass Campground to the east.

North of the junction, you climb imperceptibly around the head of an alpine meadow, turn west upon entering forest, and soon reach the outlet stream of Chicken Spring Lake (750.8–11,213'). To catch shoreline views of the lake in its granite cirque, leave the trail before the outlet, and stroll northwest to the shore.

WATER ACCESS

The lake is the last reliable water source before a tarn 2.7 miles onward or a brook that leads into Rock Creek, 9.2 miles ahead. The lake is popular on weekends. On any summer day, though, you will not be alone, since Clark's nutcrackers—black, white, and gray birds—will hop toward you and caw at you.

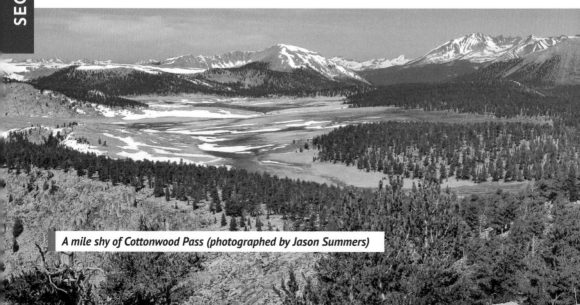

A mile shy of Cottonwood Pass (photographed by Jason Summers)

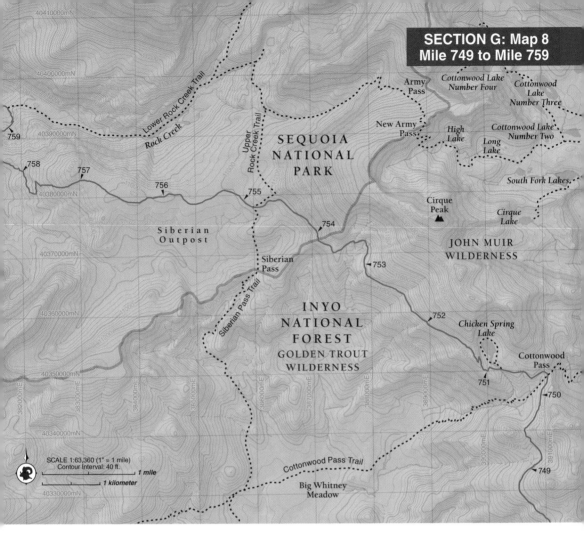

Back on the PCT, you cross the lake's some-times dry outlet stream, climb and switchback above the lake to gain a spur ridge, and then make a seemingly endless treeline traverse of the southwest-facing slopes below 12,900-foot Cirque Peak. Big Whitney Meadow appears intermittently far below you through the forest of foxtail pines. The PCT, at times annoyingly sandy, intersects a seasonal creek (753.3–11,349'), which often flows through summer.

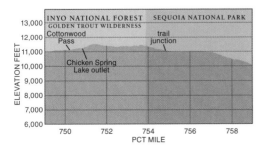

WATER ACCESS

There is no longer a lake in the little basin below the trail here; it is now a meadow. Above the trail, however, a cross-country ascent of 200 feet, alongside the out-let creek, takes you to a fair-size tarn snuggled within a cirque. This sparkling lake and its sandy, sloping beach make an attractive rest stop, but not during a drought, when the lake could be dry.

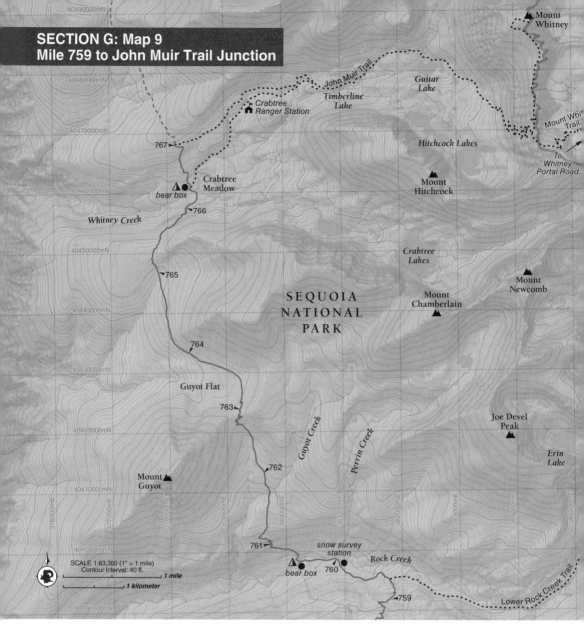

Climbing a little, the trail soon swings around a flat-topped ridge, then begins a descent that, except for some minor ups, does not end until it reaches the Rock Creek ford. The PCT passes an eye-catching fang-toothed rock formation, then enters Sequoia National Park (753.9–11,361'), leaving Golden Trout Wilderness. Pets, firearms, grazing cattle, and logging activities are illegal within the park.

VIEWS On this descent, views of the Great Western Divide appear across Siberian Outpost to the west.

Your downgrade first steepens somewhat, then becomes gentle as the path skirts the northeasternmost prong of Siberian Outpost.

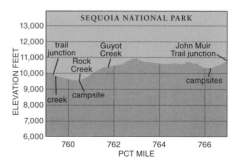

PLANTS The outpost is surrounded by weathered foxtail pine snags with reddish-brown hues.

Now the PCT wanders west, and then crosses the Siberian Pass/Upper Rock Creek Trail (754.8–11,083').

You next head toward the broad, gently rolling ridgetop separating the watershed of Rock Creek to the north from that of stagnant Siberian Pass Creek to the south. The dramatic sky-piercing crags of Rock Creek's headwaters basin are seen to the right (north), and Joe Devel Peak seems but a few steps away. After a 2-mile stroll from the last junction, you start an earnest downgrade. You descend and switchback, then the path levels out to cross a sandy-grassy flat. Lodgepole pines, at first only scattered among foxtail pines, come to dominate the forest as you stroll northwest along a ridgetop, descend moderately via nine switchbacks north, and then hike down to a junction with the Lower Rock Creek Trail (759.3–9,940').

WATER ACCESS

Now your wanderings turn west and zigzag several times more before crossing a brook, the first reliable water since the tarn 5.5 miles back or Chicken Spring Lake, 8.5 miles back.

Pausing, you can easily identify the aromatic wild onions, their pinkish-purple blossoms gracing the banks upstream. Beyond, you follow the south edge of a meadow for a while, cross it diagonally, and then enter forest again.

SIDE TRIP A snow survey station, formerly a ranger station, is nearby. You reach it by first crossing the meadow while paralleling Rock Creek; then, finding the path among the trees, you follow it, hop across a stream, turn right immediately after, and then curve left. It's usually locked tight in summer and fall.

CAMPING On the westbound PCT, you pass some campsites and begin to approach Rock Creek. Use your bear canister here, as well as anywhere in the park. Also, a heavy, metal, rectangular bear-proof box has been placed at the creek crossing. You are asked to share the box, keep it clean, close the door, and always secure the latch.

You ford a rivulet while swerving away from the creek a bit, and finally cross the creek, in low water, on stepping-stones (760.5–9,518'). Just downstream is a log for high-water crossings.

Your path ahead switchbacks, first north and then west–northwest, as it begins to climb a moderate-to-steep grade through stands of lodgepole pine and juniper trees. After passing cold brooks just below their springs, the PCT climbs 10 switchbacks, and then its grade eases.

WATER ACCESS

The trail crosses Guyot Creek (761.8–10,363'), the last source of water until Whitney Creek, 4.5 miles ahead.

After some easy hiking over gravelly terrain, you pass through a wreckage of mature trees on the slopes east of Mount Guyot that were uprooted and broken by a 1986 avalanche. Young, resilient trees survived. Beyond, you labor up and over a pass northeast of 12,300-foot Mount Guyot.

VIEWS As you descend and cross above grit-filled Guyot Flat, you have magnificent views across Kern Canyon of Red Spur and the Kaweah Peaks Ridge, then west–southwest beyond the gap of the Big

SECTION G

Arroyo and the Great Western Divide peaks— notably the pointed summit of Mineral King's monarch mountain, Sawtooth Peak.

Shaded by foxtail pines, you hike along the sandy trail, gradually veering north and passing another gritty flat. Next you ascend a broad, flat-topped ridge, then proceed northeast, dropping abruptly through a series of switchbacks.

Ahead, as you descend the switchbacks, you'll see Mount Young looming. East of it you receive your first near view of 14,505-foot Mount Whitney, the highest mountain in the contiguous United States.

VIEWS PCT thru-hikers have seen Mount Whitney's peak from great distances, as far back as Sweet Ridge north of CA 58. From here its furrowed back side and rounded top are partly hidden by Mount Hitchcock. The grand mountain's most spectacular side, however, is its precipitous east face. Surrounded by other 14,000-foot peaks, the mountain lies on the granitic Sierra Crest.

At the foot of the descent, the PCT travels through a gated fence, levels out, and passes a use path that plummets west next to Whitney Creek and ends at the Kern River.

CAMPING Your path proceeds north, passing to your left a cluster of campsites and a bear-proof box. Then it fords Whitney Creek and arrives at Crabtree Meadow, where it meets a lateral (766.3–10,321') to Mount Whitney.

If you do not plan to climb Mount Whitney, proceed along the winding path north–northwest to a signed junction (767.0–10,779') with the John Muir Trail, the start of Section H.

RESUPPLY ACCESS

To reach Lone Pine, hike east 5.8 miles on the John Muir Trail toward Mount Whitney. At Trail Crest junction, descend 8 miles to Whitney Portal. There, the busy Whitney Portal Road winds down 11.8 miles to Lone Pine, a sizable town. Heavy winter storms have led to rockslides and prolonged closure of this paved road in the past; be sure to check USFS alerts for the Inyo National Forest before depending on it.

Holders of the PCT long-distance permit require an additional permit from the Inyo National Forest to resupply via Whitney Portal (see page 250). Holders of this permit should reenter the wilderness within 48 hours of when they exit to resupply.

SIDE TRIP PCT long-distance permit holders are allowed to day hike from the PCT to the summit of Mount Whitney and back to the PCT. There is no fee, and no additional permits are needed. Few can resist the opportunity to climb such a famous peak, so you turn northeast to ramble along the lateral, favored along the way with views of Mount Whitney's west side. On this path you skirt lush, well-watered Crabtree Meadow, ascend a little canyon beside Whitney Creek, cross the creek, and then recross it to its north side to meet the John Muir Trail.

You do not recross the creek, however, if you are seeking campsites with a bear-proof box or the Crabtree Ranger Station. The campsites are scattered among the trees on the southeast side of Whitney Creek, and the station is 0.8 mile northeast along a replaced section of the John Muir Trail. Long-distance permit holders may not camp east of the Crabtree Ranger Station.

With knowledge that the summit can be bitterly cold, and assessing the time and the weather so as not to be caught on the summit or open slopes in an afternoon lightning storm, you proceed northeast on the John Muir Trail north of the creek. After climbing over granite slabs, you amble near the north shore of placid Timberline Lake.

TRAIL INFO Once heavily used as a base camp for climbing Whitney, these shores have been closed to all camping and stock grazing since before 1970.

Above the lake, your trail passes the last of the forest on a moderate-to-steep grade away from Whitney Creek. Notice the glacial polish on the granite along this ice-carved canyon of spectacular beauty. The path takes on a pattern of climbing slab staircases up granite benches, then traversing around hollows that sometimes hold a tarn or a good-size lake.

CAMPING After topping a ridge, the path approaches Guitar Lake, where many hikers camp among the rocks away from the meadow grasses. Above Guitar Lake, the two tarns at 11,600 feet offer an ideal camp setting, as well, and are the last reliable

sources of water on this summit quest. This area has suffered from huge amounts of human traffic over the decades. Be sure to pack out toilet paper (and consider carrying out your own waste in a wag bag) to minimize the impact.

Here the trail levels briefly, allowing you to pause and catch your breath as you prepare for the high-altitude climb ahead. When the ascent resumes, the Hitchcock Lakes come into view; they were hidden until now in a deep cirque at the foot of 13,184-foot Mount Hitchcock.

The rugged appearance of many glacier-carved peaks contrasted with pockets of delicate deep-pink rock-fringe flowers instills in some a sense of awe and wonder.

A few short switchbacks now signal the onset of nine long-legged switchbacks that wind up the rocky slopes on the highest section of the Sierra Crest to a junction with the eastbound Mount Whitney Trail. Lines of stashed backpacks at this junction make a colorful collage as they lean against the rocky crags.

If you plan on resupplying, from the junction, head east on the Mount Whitney Trail to Whitney Portal and follow the directions under "Resupply Access" on the opposite page.

To reach the summit, turn left, climb north up a pair of switchbacks, pass Mount Muir, and labor breathlessly on a long traverse beside a row of gendarmes.

Your path makes a final few switchbacks up Mount Whitney's back, approaches a stone cabin with its register, and at last attains the summit at 14,505 feet.

HISTORY This mountain was named by members of the Whitney Survey team for Josiah Dwight Whitney (1819–1896), chief of the California State Geological Survey.

TRAIL INFO Strictly enforced quotas on the number of hikers allowed to leave Whitney Portal per day have reduced the population problem here, but it is still possible to find a crowd when you arrive.

HISTORY The stone cabin was built in 1909 by the Smithsonian Institute to be used as an observatory. It was added to the National Register of Historic Places in 1978. In 1990 a fatality occurred when a group of hikers thought the hut a safe refuge during a lightning storm—it was not. It still is not, even though it's fitted with lightning rods.

VIEWS On a clear day you can see almost any of your favorite mountains in the Sierra. Note dim, pointed Owens Peak and rounded Mount Jenkins's tandem silhouette in the southeast, showing the distance you have hiked since Walker Pass. You may be able to see the San Bernardino Mountains as well.

From the summit you backtrack to the junction across the creek from the ranger station. From there you continue on the John Muir Trail, progressing across a sandy flat from lodgepole pines to foxtail pines. A few zigzags and a long westward traverse with lingering views of Whitney lead to a signed junction (767.0–10,779'), where you turn right (north) on the PCT, which joins the John Muir Trail to begin Section H.

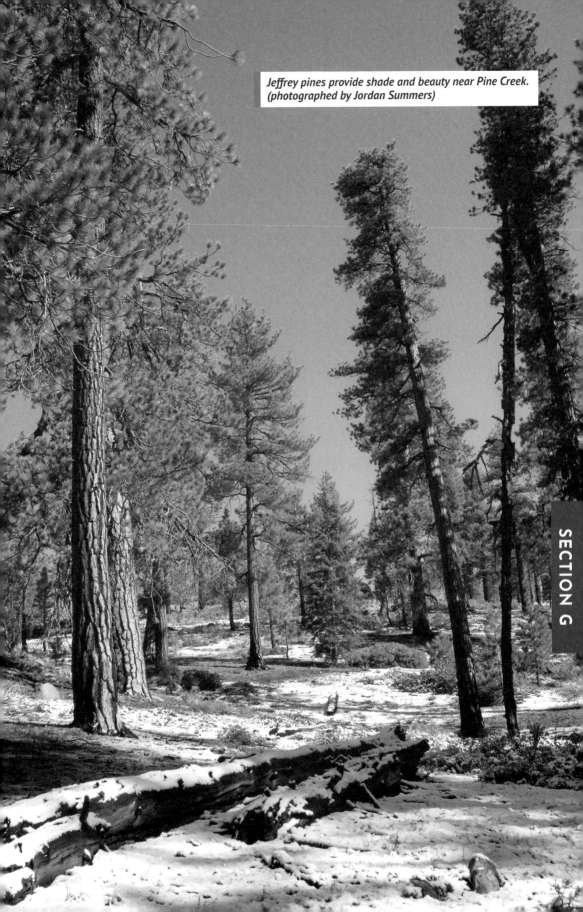

Jeffrey pines provide shade and beauty near Pine Creek.
(photographed by Jordan Summers)

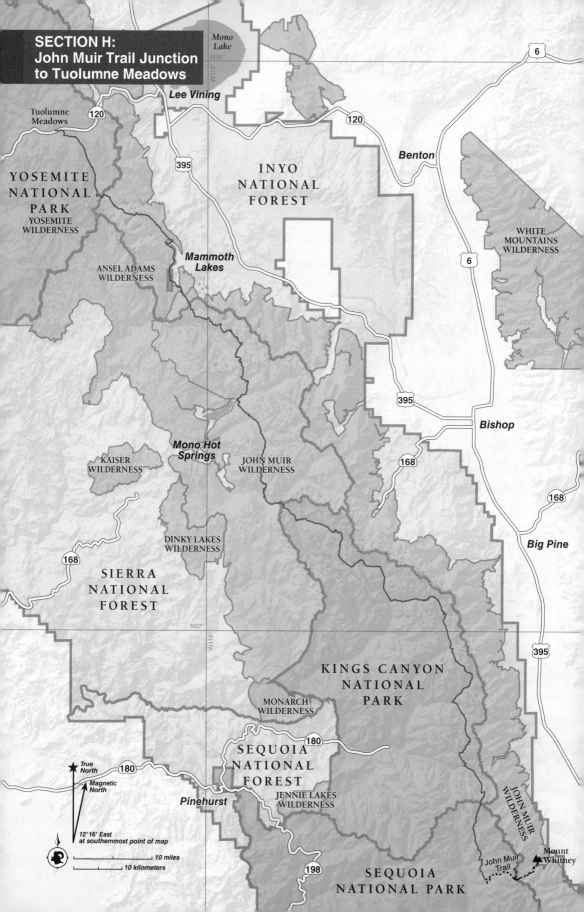

Mono
Lake

6

Lee Vining

Tuolumne
Meadows

120

120

Benton

395

INYO
NATIONAL
FOREST

6

YOSEMITE
NATIONAL
PARK
YOSEMITE
WILDERNESS

WHITE
MOUNTAINS
WILDERNESS

ANSEL ADAMS
WILDERNESS

Mammoth
Lakes

6

395

Bishop

Mono Hot
Springs

KAISER
WILDERNESS

JOHN MUIR
WILDERNESS

168

168

Big Pine

DINKY LAKES
WILDERNESS

168

SIERRA
NATIONAL
FOREST

N37°

W119°

395

KINGS CANYON
NATIONAL
PARK

MONARCH
WILDERNESS

180

SEQUOIA
NATIONAL
FOREST

True
North

180

Magnetic
North

JOHN MUIR
WILDERNESS

Pinehurst

JENNIE LAKES
WILDERNESS

12° 16' East
at southernmost point of map

John Muir
Trail

Mount
Whitney

10 miles

10 kilometers

198

SEQUOIA
NATIONAL
PARK

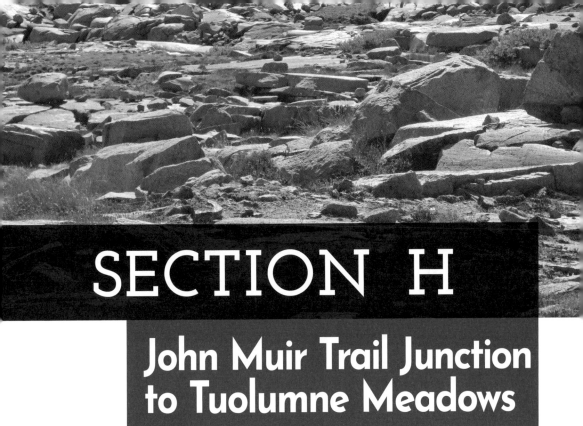

SECTION H

John Muir Trail Junction to Tuolumne Meadows

THE PACIFIC CREST TRAIL (PCT) from the John Muir Trail (JMT) junction to Tuolumne Meadows passes through what many backpackers agree is the finest mountain scenery in the United States. This is a land of 13,000-foot and 14,000-foot peaks, of soaring granite cliffs, of lakes literally by the thousands, of canyons 5,000 feet deep. It is a land where trails touch only a tiny part of the total area, so that by leaving the beaten path you can find utter solitude. It is land rarely crossed by road for 150 airline miles, from just north of Walker Pass to Tuolumne Meadows. And perhaps best of all, it is a land blessed with one of the mildest, sunniest climates of any major mountain range in the world. Though rain and extreme heat are often a part of the summer—and much snow a part of the winter—the rain seldom lasts more than an hour or two, and the sun is out and shining most of the time that it is above the horizon.

Above: Donohue Pass

Given these attractions, you might expect that quite a few people would want to enjoy them. So much so, in fact, that the number of permits available is limited during the season. And it is true that some hikers joke about traffic signs being needed on the JMT, which the PCT parallels for most of this section. But the land is so vast that if you do want to camp by yourself, you can. While following the trail in the summer, you can't avoid passing quite a few people, but you can stop to talk or not, as you choose.

DECLINATION 12°16'E

USGS MAPS

Mount Whitney	North Palisade	Bloody Mountain
Mount Kaweah	Mount Goddard	Crystal Crag
Mount Brewer	Mount Darwin	Mammoth Mountain
Mount Williamson	Mount Henry	Mount Ritter
Mount Clarence King	Mount Hilgard	Koip Peak
Mount Pinchot	Florence Lake	Vogelsang Peak
Split Mountain	Graveyard Peak	Tioga Pass

POINTS ON THE TRAIL, SOUTH TO NORTH

	Mile	Elevation in feet	Latitude/Longitude
John Muir Trail junction (to Mount Whitney)	767.0	10,779	N36° 33' 32.160" W118° 21' 42.420"
Forester Pass	779.5	13,118	N36° 41' 40.260" W118° 22' 24.540"
Vidette Meadow/Bubbs Creek Trail to Cedar Grove	787.3	9,562	N36° 45' 36.830" W118° 24' 44.100"
Kearsarge Pass Trail junction (to Independence)	788.9	10,746	N36° 46' 14.200" W118° 24' 58.670"
Rae Lakes Ranger Station junction	793.9	10,604	N36° 48' 40.860" W118° 24' 02.760"
Pinchot Pass	807.1	12,142	N36° 56' 09.960" W118° 24' 45.120"
Bishop Pass Trail	831.0	8,751	N37° 05' 38.820" W118° 35' 39.540"
Muir Pass/stone hut	838.6	11,974	N37° 06' 43.380" W118° 40' 15.300"
McClure Meadow Ranger Station	848.2	9,652	N37° 11' 16.680" W118° 44' 33.120"
Florence Lake Trail to Muir Trail Ranch	857.7	7,889	N37° 13' 32.880" W118° 51' 40.500"
Bear Ridge Trail junction to Vermilion Valley Resort	874.5	9,874	N37° 22' 57.000" W118° 54' 37.800"
Cascade Valley Trail junction	888.5	9,204	N37° 29' 27.805" W118° 55' 58.382"
Crater Meadow Trail/Horseshoe Lake	903.9	8,660	N37° 35' 28.320" W119° 03' 30.540"
Red's Meadow Resort trail junction (first of two)	906.6	7,718	N37° 36' 35.760" W119° 04' 31.440"
Alternate route through Devils Postpile	907.2	7,480	N37° 36' 50.354" W119° 04' 58.317"
PCT splits with JMT for 13.9 miles	909.0	7,681	N37° 37' 58.440" W119° 05' 20.220"
Agnew Meadows Road	914.8	8,311	N37° 40' 55.090" W119° 05' 10.750"

POINTS ON THE TRAIL, SOUTH TO NORTH (continued)

	Mile	Elevation in feet	Latitude/Longitude
Thousand Island Lake/PCT rejoins JMT	922.9	9,846	N37° 43' 42.660" W119° 10' 16.680"
Rush Creek Trail	925.9	9,645	N37° 44' 37.760" W119° 12' 40.140"
Donohue Pass	929.5	11,073	N37° 45' 39.180" W119° 14' 53.100"
Tuolumne Meadows/CA 120	942.5	8,596	N37° 52' 37.290" W119° 21' 11.060"

CAMPSITES AND BIVY SITES

Mile	Elevation in feet	Latitude/Longitude	Number of tents	Feature	Notes
770.3	10,392	N36° 35' 37.980" W118° 22' 15.540"	>5	Wallace Creek	Water, bear-proof box south of creek
774.1	11,042	N36° 38' 06.580" W118° 23' 07.800"	>10	Tyndall Frog Ponds	Bear-proof box, water
774.7	10,977	N36° 38' 27.272" W118° 23' 18.611"	>10	Tyndall Creek	Bear-proof box, water
778.6	12,502	N36° 41' 26.940" W118° 22' 27.240"	>5	Below Forester Pass	Exposed area, water nearby
784.3	10,480	N36° 44' 02.550" W118° 22' 32.310"	>10	Bubbs Creek	Large campsite, water nearby
787.0	9,554	N36° 45' 32.940" W118° 24' 22.080"	Dozens	Vidette Meadow	Many campsites in upper and lower areas, bear-proof box, water nearby
788.9	10,746	N36° 46' 37.387" W118° 25' 34.410"	>5	Charlotte Lake	Bear-proof box, ranger station nearby
790.0	11,094	N36° 47' 04.800" W118° 25' 15.600"	>5	Below Glen Pass	
793.5	10,570	N36° 48' 24.540" W118° 23' 57.900"	Dozens	Middle Rae Lake	Bear-proof box
795.2	10,315	N36° 49' 39.180" W118° 24' 34.560"	>5	Arrowhead Lake	Seasonal water
799.8	8,532	N36° 52' 25.070" W118° 26' 16.820"	>5	Woods Creek	
808.6	11,158	N36° 56' 42.360" W118° 25' 43.140"	>10	Lake Marjorie	
811.7	10,189	N36° 58' 29.310" W118° 26' 33.380"	>10	South Fork Kings River	
820.5	10,608	N37° 03' 36.660" W118° 29' 17.820"	2	Lower Palisade Lake	
824.0	8,843	N37° 03' 21.900" W118° 31' 33.120"	2	Palisade Creek area	Several camping areas near Palisade Creek
827.5	8,091	N37° 03' 10.680" W118° 34' 49.980"	>5	Middle Fork Kings River	
833.0	9,310	N37° 06' 48.530" W118° 36' 40.730"	>5	Middle Fork Kings River	
840.5	11,443	N37° 07' 40.860" W118° 41' 45.240"	>10	Wanda Lake	
848.4	9,642	N37° 11' 18.050" W118° 44' 46.440"	>5	McClure Meadow	Seasonal ranger cabin, water nearby
853.3	8,375	N37° 12' 11.460" W118° 48' 03.180"	>10	South Fork San Joaquin River	Camping near steel bridge

continued on next page

SECTION H

CAMPSITES AND BIVY SITES *(continued)*

Mile	Elevation in feet	Latitude/ Longitude	Number of tents	Feature	Notes
854.6	8,207	N37° 12' 51.060" W118° 49' 04.160"	>10	Aspen Meadow	
863.7	10,200	N37° 16' 12.240" W118° 52' 35.400"	>10	Sallie Keyes Lake outlet	
866.3	10,582	N37° 17' 54.000" W118° 52' 17.520"	>10	Marie Lake	
870.9	9,236	N37° 21' 03.830" W118° 52' 40.730"	>5	Bear Creek	Adequate camping east of trail
878.7	7,877	N37° 24' 44.590" W118° 55' 25.650"	>10	Mono Creek	Campsites on either side of bridge
885.1	10,937	N37° 28' 12.060" W118° 55' 23.080"	>5	Silver Pass	
888.5	9,211	N37° 29' 34.560" W118° 55' 58.260"	>5	Fish Creek	Campsites near junction with Cascade Valley Trail
901.0	9,115	N37° 33' 49.020" W119° 02' 01.410"	5	Deer Creek	Lodgepole shade
903.9	8,660	N37° 35' 27.730" W119° 03' 30.000"	<5	Crater Creek	
906.6	7,709	N37° 37' 07.920" W119° 04' 24.600"	Dozens	Red's Meadow Campground	Campsites and cabins with hot showers, resupply
911.0	7,688	N37° 39' 06.696" W119° 04' 34.151"	Dozens	Upper Soda Springs Campground	Water, pit toilet
914.8	8,311	N37° 40' 53.926" W119° 04' 52.352"	Dozens	Agnew Meadows Campground	Water, pit toilet; standard, equestrian, and group sites available
920.0	9,677	N37° 43' 20.280" W119° 07' 50.040"	<10	Campsites amid boulders	
926.9	10,069	N37° 44' 58.620" W119° 13' 13.530"	>5	Rush Creek ford	Campsites by stream amid rocks
932.1	9,651	N37° 46' 39.660" W119° 15' 43.620"	10–12	Lyell Creek ford, bridge	Large campsite before bridge amid trees and logs

WEATHER TO GO

High Sierra weather is mostly dry from June to September—especially in September—but afternoon showers are fairly common, and it may even rain at night. A tent and good raingear are mandatory. Snow and high water levels are often serious concerns until the middle of July.

SUPPLIES

This section does not allow easy resupply. To reach any kind of civilization you must—except at Red's Meadow—walk at least 18 miles round-trip. Even then, if you have major needs, you will have to hitchhike many miles farther. At the beginning of this section, you can take the JMT and the Mount Whitney Trail 15.5 miles to Whitney Portal, where there is a very small store (with food and supplies), or hitchhike from the portal 13 miles to Lone Pine, which has almost everything you might want. About 20 miles into Section H, at the Bubbs Creek Trail, you can hike 14 miles west to Cedar Grove, with another very small store, a modest café, and a post office. To hitchhike from there to Fresno would be a major project. About 2 miles farther, at the Kearsarge Pass Trail, you can hike 9 miles east to Onion Valley and hitchhike from there 15 miles out of the mountains to Independence, which has just one store, albeit a rather large one for such a small town. About 42 miles farther, at the Bishop Pass Trail, you can hike northeast 12 miles to South Lake, which has nothing, and hitchhike 19 miles to Bishop, which has everything. Then, 25 miles farther, at the Piute Pass Trail, you can hike northeast 18 miles to North Lake, which has nothing, and hitchhike 18 miles to Bishop. About 2 miles farther, you can hike north 1.5 miles along the Florence Lake Trail to Muir Trail Ranch, which accepts packages and sells emergency supplies. Then 21 miles farther, from where you bridge Mono Creek, you can walk 6 miles west, or take a boat shuttle on Lake Edison, to Vermilion Valley Resort, again with a small store, plus meals, showers, and a package-holding service. Seven miles west by road from there is Mono Hot Springs, also reached by a 1-mile paved spur road off the PCT, with meals, supplies, and a post office.

About 29 miles farther, you are at Red's Meadow, with a somewhat more than minimal store and a café. Just down the paved road is Red's Meadow Campground, which has a nearby, free public bathhouse fed by a hot spring. If you need more than a few supplies, go to Mammoth Lakes, a recreation-oriented town. From a choice of stops along the Red's Meadow–Agnew Meadow stretch of road, you can take a shuttle bus for a fee up over Minaret Summit and down 1 mile to expansive Mammoth Mountain Inn, opposite the ski area. You can also take a taxi from the inn to central Mammoth Lakes, another 4.5 miles farther. The shuttle bus operates from about the weekend before July 4 through the weekend after Labor Day. Note that the charge is for one way only—from the inn over to the Red's Meadow–Agnew Meadow area. Going the opposite way is a free ride. Out of season, the shortest walk to downtown Mammoth Lakes is an 8-mile route starting from Upper Crater Meadow, and this is described in the trail text. On the other hand, you may be able to hitch a ride in the Red's Meadow–Agnew Meadow area if the road is open.

Finally, in the Tuolumne Meadows area, at the end of this section, you can get hot meals and showers at seasonal Tuolumne Meadows Lodge, a mile east of the principal meadow, or you can stop at a good store, with a café and post office, just southwest of the entrance to Tuolumne Meadows Campground.

Be aware that the facilities at Whitney Portal, Florence Lake, Lake Edison, Mono Hot Springs, Red's Meadow, and Tuolumne Meadows may close by early or mid-September.

WATER

The only possible water problem in this section is that you might have to melt some snow if you hike here very early in the season—in spring and well into summer, runoff is everywhere.

PERMITS

If you are northbound, you can get permits for most of this section by contacting Sequoia and Kings Canyon National Park; contact Inyo National Forest for eastside trailheads. If you are southbound, contact Yosemite National Park. (Refer to "Federal Government Agencies" in chapter 2, page 25, for websites and mailing addresses.) Be aware that during the summer season (about late June to mid- to late September), user quotas are in effect for the three national parks and the wildernesses between them. Popular trailheads do reach their quotas, especially on weekends, so plan accordingly. Thru-hikers who plan to leave the trail in this section other than to resupply or those who plan to reenter at a different point must obtain a new permit from the local land management agency. See "Permits" in chapter 2, page 13, for more information.

SPECIAL CONCERNS
>SNOW

For hikers trying to do the whole PCT in one year, the biggest problem in the High Sierra is swift waters. If you leave Campo in late April, you will reach the Sierra before the snow has melted. In most years there will be a lot of snow in the High Sierra in May and June. What you will need for the snowy sections is crampons and an ice ax, and the knowledge of how to use them. And you need a basic understanding of avalanches—where they tend to occur, why they tend to occur, and what to do if caught in one. Bruce Tremper's *Avalanche Essentials: A Step-by-Step System for Safety and Survival* (Mountaineers Books, 2013) is a good primer. Finally, where the trail is hidden by snow, you need some skills with a map and compass to follow the route. You also need physical strength, risk tolerance, and a lot of perseverance.

>COLD

Even in midsummer it may freeze on any given night, so you need appropriate warmth. You will need a tent and plenty of warm clothing, including gloves or mittens.

>FORDS

In late spring and early summer, when runoff is at a maximum, many stream fords can be lethal for hikers. Do not underestimate the risk. It's better to turn around and delay your trip until after peak runoff than risk a dangerous crossing.

If possible, plan your hike to cross the major streams early in the day, when their discharge is less than in the midafternoon or early evening. Cross with a group, if possible; group crossing techniques are considered to be one of the safest and most successful approaches. Practice techniques with your fellow hikers before crossing: Stay close together, and work your way slowly across the stream as a team. A large group that is practiced and works well together can form a wedge that breaks a significant amount of current.

If a stream crossing looks too deep or swift, take the time to find a safe place to cross. This may entail going 100 or more yards up- or downstream. Maybe you'll find a fallen log or some safe boulders to cross, though keep in mind that wet or unsteady logs hold their own risks and dangers. If you must ford, doing so in chest-deep slow water is preferable to waist-deep fast water. Never ford just upstream from dangerous fast water, especially rapids or cascades. Trekking poles or a suitable branch may help you balance.

Because there is always a chance that you might slip—even when the water is only waist-deep—be sure that at least your sleeping bag and electronics are wrapped in waterproof material, such as a plastic trash bag. Some experts recommend that you unlatch the buckle on your backpack's waist

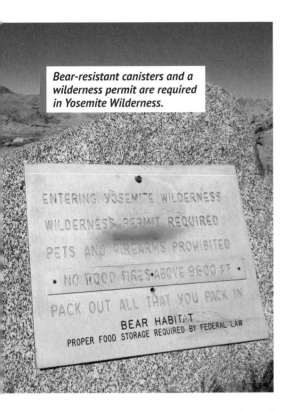

Bear-resistant canisters and a wilderness permit are required in Yosemite Wilderness.

belt, so that if you have to abandon your pack in a hurry (to save your skin), you can do so.

Keep your shoes on: though nobody likes wet shoes, your chances of slipping and falling increase significantly when you're barefoot.

Finally, consider taking a swift-water rescue class ahead of your hike to enhance your backcountry expertise.

>BEARS

Black bears are very intelligent (one might daresay more so than some humans), and evidence for this may be in how adept they are at outwitting us to steal our food. Bears know that where there are backpackers, there is food, and the High Sierra seems to have an endless supply of backpackers from about June through September. So just as we head to the highlands during the summer season, so do the bears. Black bears, as well as strategies to safeguard your food from bears, are discussed in "Animal and Plant Concerns," page 28. What follows here are special issues for those hiking in Section H.

Hikers are required to carry portable bear-resistant canisters, which are available for sale or rent at visitor centers and permit offices throughout the parks (see page 30 for more information). This has proved successful at preventing bears from accessing food. Permanent metal food-storage boxes are also available in campgrounds and other areas of Sequoia and Kings Canyon National Parks, but don't rely on them.

>RANGER STATIONS

A number of summer rangers patrol areas along or near the trail in Sequoia and Kings Canyon National Parks from about July 4 to Labor Day. The route description tells where they are. If you go to a summer ranger station to report a friend in trouble and the ranger is out, please realize that the ranger may be gone for several days, so leave a note and walk out for help yourself.

>CAMPFIRES

Rules for campfires vary throughout this section, depending on your location. Inyo National Forest prohibits all campfires or stove fires; a California Campfire Permit allows you to use portable stoves or lanterns containing gas, jellied fuel, or pressurized liquid fuel. Gas or propane stoves are permitted in Sequoia and Kings Canyon National Parks. In Yosemite National Park, fires must be below 9,600 feet and in an existing fire ring. California campfire permits may be obtained online at readyforwildfire.org/permits/campfire-permit.

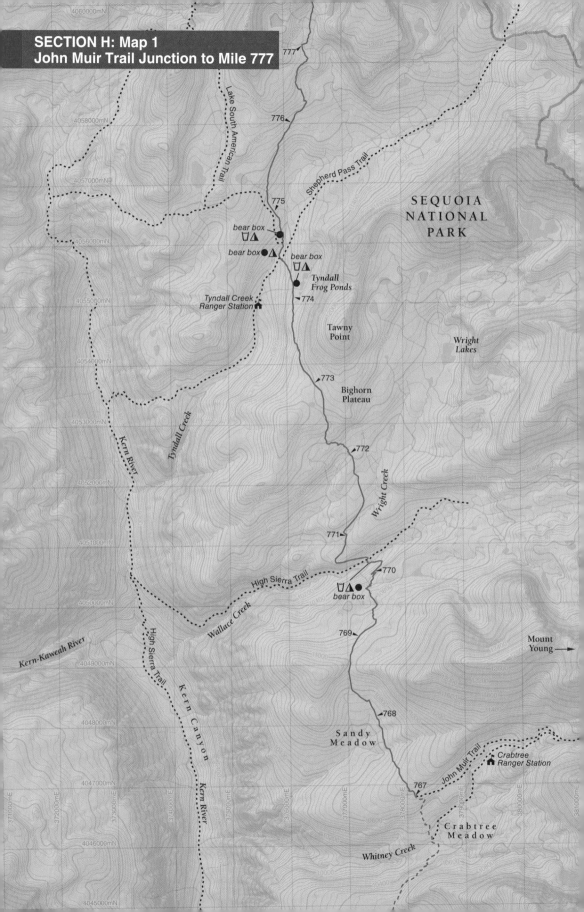

777

776

Lake South American Trail

Shepherd Pass Trail

775

bear box

bear box

bear box

Tyndall
Frog Ponds

774

Tyndall Creek
Ranger Station

SEQUOIA
NATIONAL
PARK

Tawny
Point

Wright
Lakes

773

Bighorn
Plateau

Tyndall Creek

Kern River

772

Wright Creek

771

770

High Sierra Trail

bear box

Wallace Creek

769

Kern-Kaweah River

High Sierra Trail

Mount
Young

768

Sandy
Meadow

Kern Canyon

John Muir Trail

Crabtree
Ranger Station

767

Kern River

Crabtree
Meadow

Whitney Creek

MOUNT WHITNEY TO TUOLUMNE MEADOWS

>>>THE ROUTE

In this trail section, you will be on the JMT almost all the way to Tuolumne Meadows, 175.5 miles ahead. Northbound on the combined PCT/JMT (767.0–10,779'), you skirt Sandy Meadow and ascend to a high saddle (768.7–10,964'). Beyond it the trail winds among the huge boulders of a glacial moraine on the west shoulder of Mount Young and brings you to excellent viewpoints for scanning the main peaks of the Kings–Kern Divide and of the Sierra Crest from Mount Barnard (13,990') north to Junction Peak (13,888'). Soon you descend moderately, making several easy fords, and then switchback down to Wallace Creek and a junction (770.3–10,392') where the High Sierra Trail goes west toward a road-end near Giant Forest and a lateral trail goes east to Wallace Lake.

CAMPING The Wallace Creek ford, just north of the popular campsites, is difficult in early season. There is a bear-proof box south of the creek.

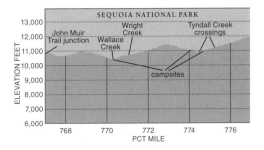

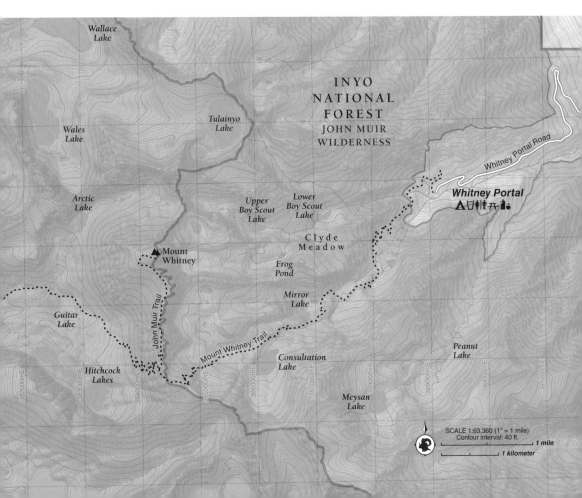

Now your sandy trail climbs to a forested flat, crosses it, and reaches the ford of Wright Creek (771.0–10,700'), which is also difficult in early season.

You then trace a bouldery path across the ground moraines left by the Wright Creek glacier and rise in several stages to Bighorn Plateau. Views from here are panoramic. An unnamed, grass-fringed lake atop the gravelly, lupine-streaked plateau makes for great morning photographs west over it. Now the PCT descends the talus-clad west slope of Tawny Point past many extraordinarily dramatic foxtail pines.

CAMPING At Tyndall Frog Ponds (774.1–11,042'), tiny lakes beside the trail, there are fair campsites, warmish swimming, and a bear-proof box.

At the foot of this rocky slope a trail departs southwest for the Kern River, and 200 yards past the junction you come to the Shepherd Pass Trail (774.6–10,923') going northeast.

CAMPING Not far beyond is a formidable, often-freezing ford of Tyndall Creek, on the other side of which are many highly used campsites and a bear-proof box (774.7–10,977'); campfires are prohibited within 1,200 feet of the crossing.

From these gathering places, your trail makes a short climb to the signed junction with the Lake South America Trail (774.9–11,049') and rises above treeline.

As you tackle the ascent to the highest point on the PCT, you wind among the barren basins of high, rockbound—but fishy—lakes to the foot of a great granite wall, then labor up numerous switchbacks, some of which are literally cut into the rock wall, to Forester Pass (779.5–13,118'), reportedly the highest spot on the entire PCT and on the border between Sequoia & Kings Canyon National Parks. The south side of Forester Pass can be dangerous when snow-covered.

Wearing your wind garment, you will enjoy the well-earned, sweeping views from this pass

before you start the (net) descent of 9,000 feet to Canada. Down the switchbacks you go, unless they are buried under snow, and then stroll high above the west shore of Lake 12,248.

The trail soon doubles back to cross the lake's outlet and then descends. You ford Bubbs Creek just below that lake, then ford it twice more within a mile. Soon you reach tree cover.

CAMPING Now you ford Center Basin Creek (high in early season), pass several overused campsites (with a bear-proof box) below the trail, and then pass the unsigned junction with the Center Basin Trail (784.3–10,480'), marked only by a line of rocks.

You stay on the PCT and ford more tributaries of Bubbs Creek.

Wood is scarce, so take a minimal amount. Wood fires are *not permitted* above 10,000 feet.

CAMPING Continuing down the east side of dashing Bubbs Creek, you pass Upper Vidette Meadow (786.1–9,912'), where there are good, if well-used, campsites and a bear-proof box. At Vidette Meadow (787.0–9,554'), long a favorite camping spot in these headwaters of South Fork Kings River, you find more bear-proof boxes. High use has made the place less attractive, but its intrinsic beauty has not been lost, and the mighty Kearsarge Pinnacles to the northeast have lost only a few inches of height, if that, since Sierra Club founders such as Joseph Le Conte camped here at the turn of the 20th century. Camping is limited to one night in one place from here to Woods Creek. A summer ranger may be in Vidette Meadow east of the trail to assist traffic flow.

Beyond the meadow, the Bubbs Creek Trail goes west to Cedar Grove (787.3–9,562'). The PCT turns north to fiercely attack the wall of

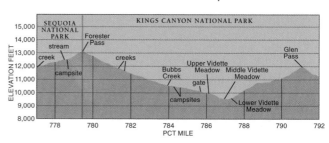

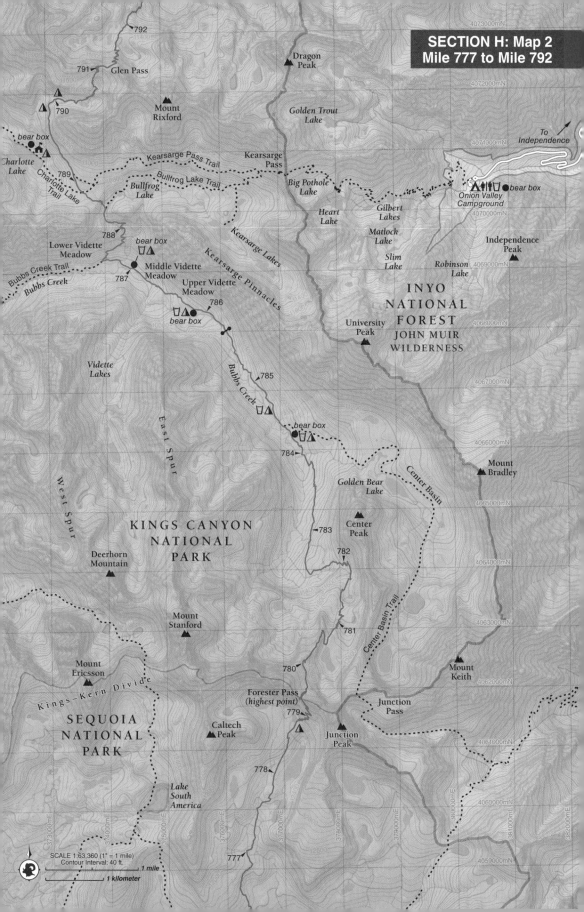

792

791 Glen Pass

Dragon Peak

Golden Trout Lake

To Independence

Mount Rixford

790

bear box

Charlotte Lake

Kearsarge Pass Trail

Kearsarge Pass

789

Charlotte Lake Trail

Bullfrog Lake Trail

Bullfrog Lake

Big Pothole Lake

Onion Valley Campground

bear box

Heart Lake

Gilbert Lakes

Matlock Lake

Independence Peak

Kearsarge Lakes

Slim Lake

Robinson Lake

788

bear box

Lower Vidette Meadow

Bubbs Creek Trail

Middle Vidette Meadow

787

Kearsarge Pinnacles

INYO NATIONAL FOREST

JOHN MUIR WILDERNESS

Bubbs Creek

Upper Vidette Meadow

786

bear box

University Peak

Vidette Lakes

Bubbs Creek

785

East Spur

784

bear box

Golden Bear Lake

Center Basin

Mount Bradley

West Spur

KINGS CANYON NATIONAL PARK

783

Center Peak

782

Deerhorn Mountain

781

Center Basin Trail

Mount Stanford

Mount Ericsson

Kings–Kern Divide

780

Mount Keith

SEQUOIA NATIONAL PARK

Forester Pass (highest point)

779

Junction Pass

Caltech Peak

Junction Peak

778

Lake South America

777

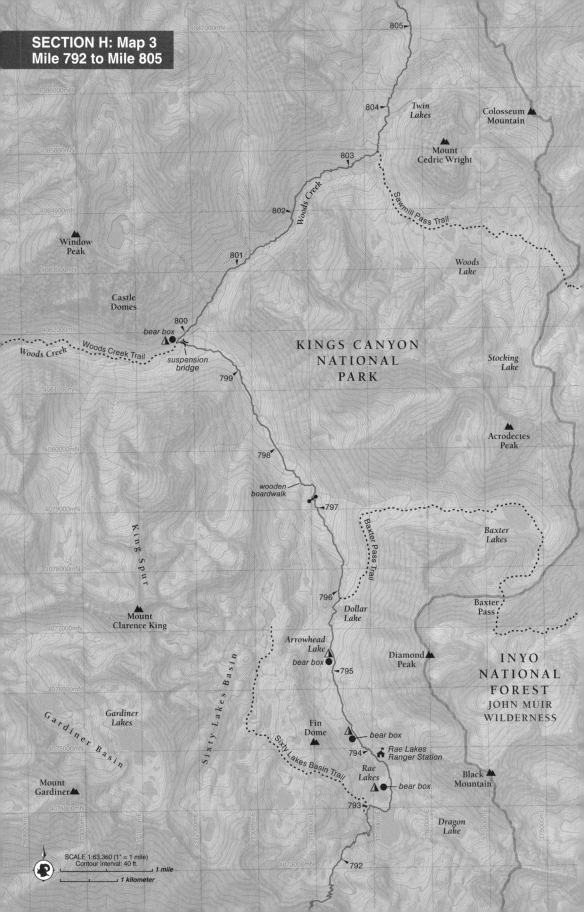

805

804

Twin
Lakes

Colosseum
Mountain ▲

803

Mount
Cedric Wright ▲

802

Woods Creek

Sawmill Pass Trail

Woods
Lake

801

Window
Peak ▲

Castle
Domes

Stocking
Lake

800

bear box
⛺●

KINGS CANYON
NATIONAL
PARK

Woods Creek

Woods Creek Trail

suspension
bridge

799

Acrodectes
Peak ▲

798

wooden
boardwalk

797

Baxter
Lakes

Baxter Pass Trail

King Spur

796

Dollar
Lake

Baxter
Pass

Mount
Clarence King ▲

Diamond
Peak ▲

INYO
NATIONAL
FOREST
JOHN MUIR
WILDERNESS

Arrowhead
Lake
⛺●
bear box

795

Sixty Lakes Basin

Gardiner Basin

Gardiner
Lakes

Fin
Dome

⛺● bear box

794

Rae Lakes
Ranger Station

Sixty Lakes Basin Trail

Rae
Lakes

⛺● bear box

Black
Mountain ▲

Mount
Gardiner ▲

793

Dragon
Lake

792

SCALE 1:63,360 (1" = 1 mile)
Contour Interval: 40 ft.

1 mile

1 kilometer

Bubbs Creek canyon. You come to the junction with the Bullfrog Lake Trail (788.5–10,525'), which travels to Bullfrog and Kearsarge Lakes and is a scenic alternate route to Kearsarge Pass for northbound hikers, then finish off the climb at a broad, sandy saddle that contains the junction of the Charlotte Lake and Kearsarge Pass Trails (788.9–10,746').

RESUPPLY ACCESS

Kearsarge Pass Trail heads east 7.6 miles to its Onion Valley trailhead. From there, you can hitchike 13 miles to Independence, which has just one large store.

CAMPING At Charlotte Lake, you'll find plenty of good camping, bear-proof boxes, and a summer ranger station on its north shore.

You pass a shortcut (for southbound hikers) to the Kearsarge Pass Trail (789.1–10,775') and then traverse high above emerald Charlotte Lake. As the PCT veers east, it ascends gently to the foot of the wall that is notched by Glen Pass.

It is hard to see where a trail could go up that precipitous blank wall, but one does, and after very steep switchbacks, you are suddenly at Glen Pass (791.1–11,946'). The view north presents a barren, rocky, brown world with precious little green of tree or meadow visible. Yet you know by now that not far down the trail ahead there will be plenty of willows, sedges, wildflowers, and, eventually, groves of whitebark, lodgepole, and foxtail pines. To be sure you get there, take

special care on your descent from Glen Pass as you switchback down to a small lake basin, ford the lakes' outlet, and switchback down again.

When you are about 400 vertical feet above Rae Lakes, you will see why Dragon Peak (12,995'), in the southeast, has that name.

At the intersection with Sixty Lakes Basin Trail (792.9–10,563'), the PCT turns right (east), crosses the "isthmus" between the upper and middle Rae Lakes, fording the connecting stream en route (difficult in early season); passes the old Dragon Lake Trail; and winds above the east shore of the middle lake, passing a signed trail (793.9–10,604') to the summer ranger station. The middle and lower Rae Lakes have campsites and bear-proof boxes. Wood fires are not allowed between Glen Pass and 10,000 feet, well below Dollar Lake.

CAMPING Beyond Rae Lakes your gently descending trail passes above an unnamed lake and drops to the northeast corner of aptly named Arrowhead Lake, where there are good campsites. Be sure to scope out developed sites, and don't expand or degrade them.

Then it fords gurgling South Fork Woods Creek and reaches scenic Dollar Lake, where camping is severely restricted to protect its fragile environment. Just north of Dollar Lake, the unsigned Baxter Pass Trail heads northeast across the lake's outlet (795.9–10,217').

GEOLOGY The lower slopes just east of Dollar Lake are composed of Paleozoic sediments that were later metamorphosed to biotite schist. Granitic rock separates these metasediments from a higher north–south band of Triassic-Jurassic lava flows that have been changed into metavolcanic rocks.

The metamorphism of all these rock types probably occurred during the Cretaceous period, when bodies of molten granite rising up into them deformed and altered them. As you progress north to Yosemite, you'll see many more examples of similar metamorphosed rocks.

KINGS CANYON NATIONAL PARK

ELEVATION FEET

15,000
14,000
13,000 — Upper Rae Lakes / Ranger Station
12,000
11,000 — creek / Arrowhead Lake Dollar Lake
10,000 — boardwalk / streams
9,000 — bridge over Woods Creek / stream and gate / creek
8,000

792   794   796   798   800   802   804
PCT MILE

SECTION H

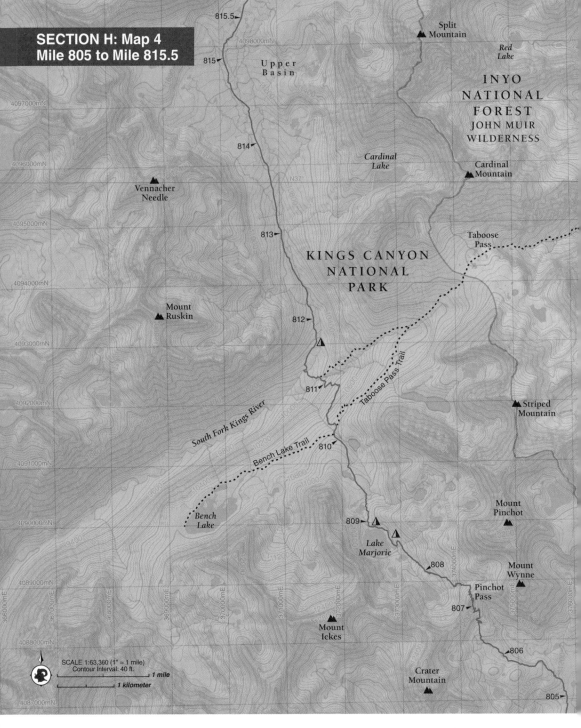

815.5

815

Upper
Basin

814

813

812

811

810

809

808

807

806

805

Split
Mountain

Red
Lake

INYO
NATIONAL
FOREST
JOHN MUIR
WILDERNESS

Cardinal
Lake

Cardinal
Mountain

Taboose
Pass

KINGS CANYON
NATIONAL
PARK

Vennacher
Needle

Mount
Ruskin

South Fork Kings River

Taboose Pass Trail

Striped
Mountain

Bench Lake Trail

Bench
Lake

Lake
Marjorie

Mount
Pinchot

Mount
Wynne

Pinchot
Pass

Mount
Ickes

Crater
Mountain

SCALE 1:63,360 (1" = 1 mile)
Contour Interval: 40 ft.
1 mile
1 kilometer

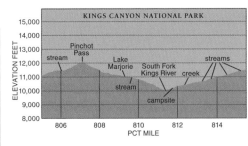

KINGS CANYON NATIONAL PARK

ELEVATION FEET		
15,000		
14,000		
13,000	Pinchot	streams
12,000	Pass	
	stream	Lake
11,000	Marjorie	South Fork
10,000		Kings River creek
	stream	
9,000		campsite
8,000		

806   808   810   812   814
PCT MILE

From the Baxter Pass Trail junction you
descend gently on open, lightly forested slopes,
crossing several good-size though unnamed
streams. The reward for all this descent is a
chance to start climbing again at Woods Creek
(799.8–8,532'), crossed on a narrow suspension bridge.

CAMPING Here you'll find good but much-used campsites with bear-proof boxes.

Just beyond the bridge, the Woods Creek Trail heads south down the creek to Cedar Grove.

WATER ACCESS

As you perspire north from the crossing up the valley of Woods Creek, there is no drinking-water problem, what with the main stream near at hand and many tributaries, some of good size, to ford, jump, or boulder-hop.

After the signed junction of the Sawmill Pass Trail (803.4–10,369'), the grade abates, you soon pass a use trail northeast to Twin Lakes, and you reach the alpine vale where this branch of the Kings River has its headwaters, bounded by glorious peaks on three-and-a-half sides. With one last, long spurt you finally top Pinchot Pass (807.1–12,142'), one of those passes that is regrettably not at the low point of the divide.

CAMPING From this pass the PCT swoops down into the lake-laden valley below, runs along the east shore of Lake Marjorie, where you'll find campsites; touches its outlet (808.9–11,137'); and then passes four lakelets, fording several small streams along the way. A summer ranger station (actually a canvas tent) is sometimes located beyond the fourth lakelet, just south of the signed Bench Lake Trail junction (810.1–10,770').

Just beyond this junction, you ford the outlet of Lake Marjorie and in 200 yards meet the Taboose Pass Trail (810.2–10,778') at the upper edge of a lodgepole forest. Another downhill segment of forested switchbacks brings you to the South Fork Kings River, which is best crossed a few yards downstream from the trail (811.4–10,039'). On the far bank, you turn northeast upstream, then climb steadily and cross several unnamed tributaries, which can slow you down at the height of the melt. Then you ford the infant South Fork (813.7–10,835').

GEOLOGY To the east, on the Sierra Crest, looming Cardinal Mountain (13,397') is named for the color red but is in fact half white and half dark, in a strange mixture of metamorphosed Paleozoic rocks.

West of this peak, you cross grassy flats and hop over numerous branches of the headwaters of South Fork Kings River in the expansive Upper Basin.

This ascent finally steepens and zigzags up to rockbound Mather Pass (816.9–12,097'), named for Stephen Mather, first head of the National Park Service. The view ahead is dominated by the 14,000-foot peaks of the Palisades group, knifing sharply into the sky.

Your trail now makes a knee-shocking descent to a bench above long, blue Palisade Lakes. Midway above the upper lake, you reach a sometimes-difficult ford of Palisade Creek (819.3–10,842'), which drains a high basin to the east–northeast.

CAMPING Spartan yet adequate campsites sit exposed on the bench north and south of this ford and offer good views. The north shore of the lower lake has poor to fair campsites.

Knees rested, you descend again on the "Golden Staircase," built on cliffs of the gorge of Palisade Creek. This section was the last part of the JMT to be constructed, and it is easy to see why. In 0.5 mile, from the bottom of the "staircase," you cross multibranched Glacier Creek and immediately arrive at Deer Meadow (823.4–8,892'), which is more lodgepole forest than meadow but pleasant enough anyway.

Beyond the campsites here, the downhill grade continues, less steeply, across the stream draining Palisade Basin and several smaller streams to reach the confluence of Palisade Creek and Middle Fork Kings River (827.4–8,038'), where a trail takes off downstream for Simpson Meadow.

SECTION H

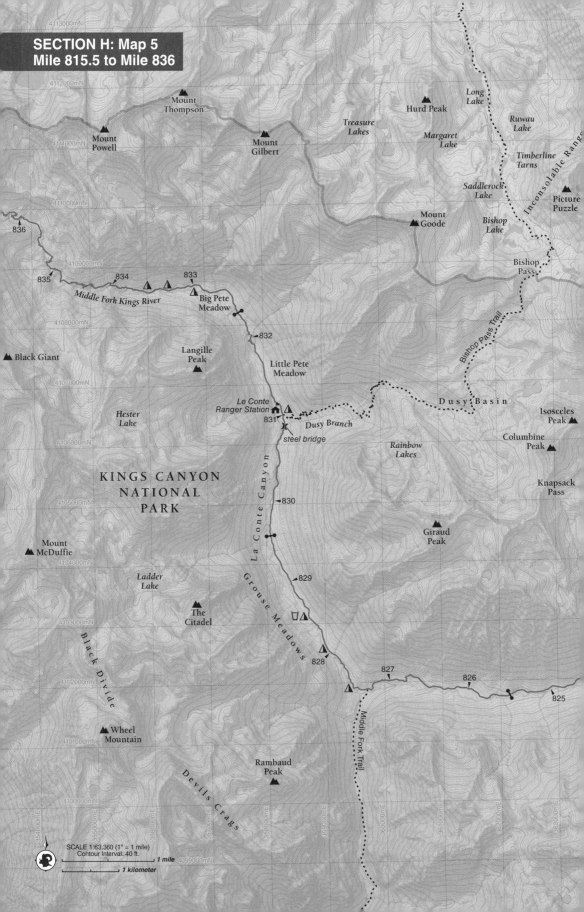

4113000mN

4112000mN

Mount Thompson

Long Lake

Hurd Peak

Ruwau Lake

Treasure Lakes

4111000mN

Mount Powell

Mount Gilbert

Margaret Lake

Timberline Tarns

Inconsolable Range

Saddlerock Lake

Picture Puzzle

4110000mN

Mount Goode

Bishop Lake

836

Bishop Pass

835

834

833

Big Pete Meadow

4109000mN

Middle Fork Kings River

832

Bishop Pass Trail

4108000mN

Langille Peak

Little Pete Meadow

Dusy Basin

Black Giant

4107000mN

Hester Lake

Le Conte Ranger Station

831

Dusy Branch

Isosceles Peak

steel bridge

Rainbow Lakes

Columbine Peak

4106000mN

KINGS CANYON NATIONAL PARK

830

Knapsack Pass

4105000mN

La Conte Canyon

Giraud Peak

Mount McDuffie

829

Ladder Lake

4104000mN

The Citadel

Grouse Meadows

828

4103000mN

827

826

825

Black Divide

Wheel Mountain

4102000mN

Middle Fork Trail

4101000mN

Rambaud Peak

Devils Crags

4100000mN

354000mE

355000mE

356000mE

357000mE

358000mE

359000mE

360000mE

361000mE

362000mE

363000mE

4099000mN

SCALE 1:63,360 (1" = 1 mile)
Contour Interval: 40 ft.

1 mile

1 kilometer

CAMPING The PCT turns north up Le Conte Canyon, staying well above the Middle Fork, and passes more campsites a couple of switchbacks north of the confluence, as well as on a flat uphill from the trail and just north of a dashing double cascade.

The ascent continues past a series of falls and chutes to Grouse Meadows, a serene expanse of grassland.

Up the canyon from these meadows, you can see repeated evidence of great avalanches that crashed down the immense canyon walls

and wiped out stands of trees. The trail climbs gently to turbulent Dusy Branch, crossed on a steel bridge, and immediately encounters the Bishop Pass Trail (831.0–8,751') to South Lake and what is considered the easiest route to the town of Bishop. Near this junction is the Le Conte ranger station, occupied in summer.

Our route upcanyon from this junction ascends between polished granite walls past lavish displays of a great variety of wildflowers.

The trail passes through sagebrushy Little Pete and Big Pete Meadows and swings west to

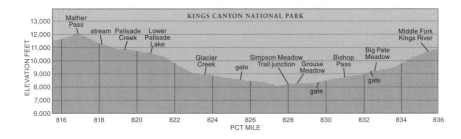

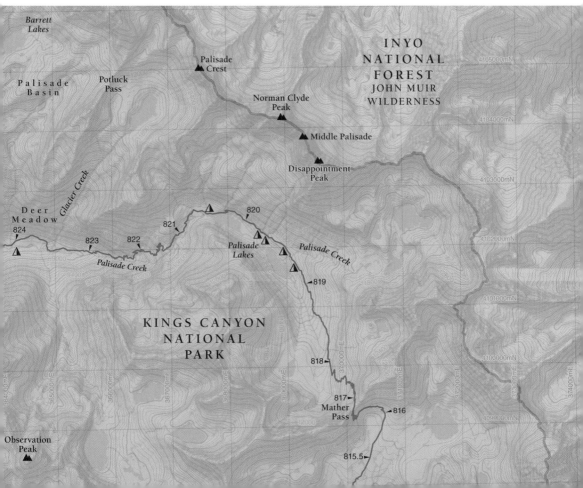

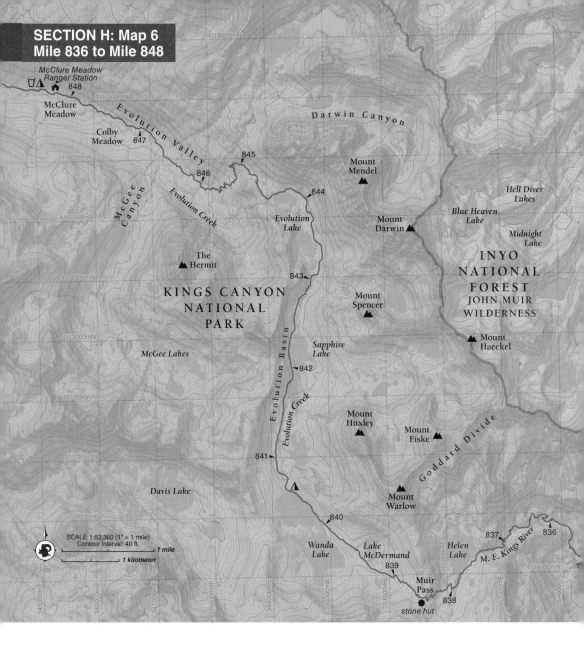

McClure Meadow
Ranger Station
848

McClure
Meadow

Colby
Meadow 847

Evolution Valley

845

846

844

Darwin Canyon

Mount
Mendel

Hell Diver
Lakes

Blue Heaven
Lake

Mount
Darwin

Midnight
Lake

Evolution
Lake

The
▲ Hermit

McGee Canyon

Evolution Creek

843

KINGS CANYON
NATIONAL
PARK

Mount
Spencer
▲▲

INYO
NATIONAL
FOREST
JOHN MUIR
WILDERNESS

Mount
Haeckel

McGee Lakes

Sapphire
Lake

Evolution Basin

842

Evolution Creek

Mount
Huxley

Mount
Fiske ▲

Goddard Divide

841

Davis Lake

840

Mount
Warlow

837

836

SCALE 1:63,360 (1" = 1 mile)
Contour Interval: 40 ft.
1 mile
1 kilometer

Wanda
Lake

Lake
McDermand
839

Helen
Lake

M. F. Kings River

Muir
Pass
838
stone hut

---

assault the Goddard Divide and search out its breach, Muir Pass.

Up and up the rocky trail winds, passing the last tree long before you reach desolate Helen Lake (837.4–11,631')—named, along with Wanda Lake to the west, for John Muir's daughters. This east side of the pass is under snow throughout the summer in some years.

From the outlet, the PCT travels southwest along the shore of Helen Lake, which is near the headwaters of the Middle Fork Kings River, and then shortly begins a switchbacking

ascent to nearby Muir Pass (838.6–11,974'), where a stone hut honoring Muir, built in 1930 and restored in recent years, would shelter you fairly well in a storm. Camping is prohibited in the hut's vicinity.

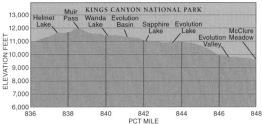

KINGS CANYON NATIONAL PARK

Muir
Pass
Helmet
Lake

Wanda
Lake

Evolution
Basin

Sapphire
Lake

Evolution
Lake

Evolution
Valley

McClure
Meadow

PCT MILE

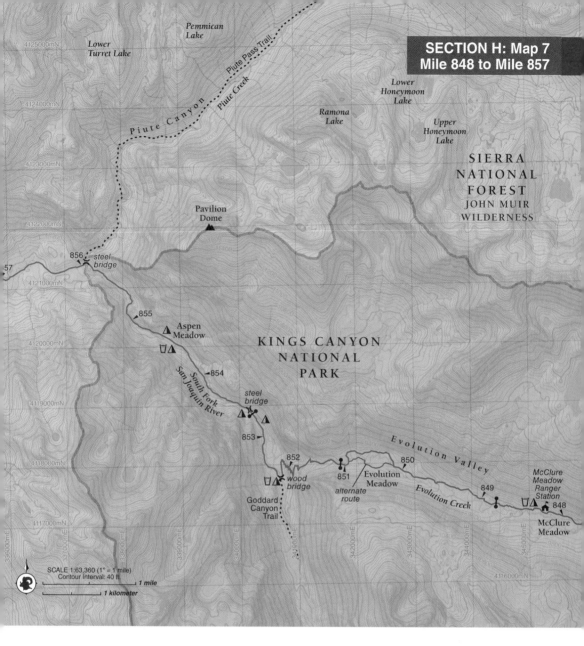

Pemmican
Lake

Lower
Turret Lake

Piute Pass Trail

Piute Creek

Piute Canyon

Lower
Honeymoon
Lake

Ramona
Lake

Upper
Honeymoon
Lake

SIERRA
NATIONAL
FOREST
JOHN MUIR
WILDERNESS

Pavilion
Dome

856   steel
bridge

57

855

Aspen
Meadow

854

South Fork
San Joaquin River

steel
bridge

853

KINGS CANYON
NATIONAL
PARK

852

wood
bridge

Goddard
Canyon
Trail

851

alternate
route

Evolution
Meadow

Evolution Valley

850

Evolution Creek

849

McClure
Meadow
Ranger
Station

848

McClure
Meadow

SCALE 1:63,360 (1" = 1 mile)
Contour Interval: 40 ft.

1 mile

1 kilometer

VIEWS The views from here of the solitary peaks and the lonely lake basins are painted in the many hues of the mostly Jurassic-age metamorphic rocks that make up the Goddard Divide.

From the hut your trail descends gently past Lake McDermand and Wanda Lake. (Wood fires are banned from Muir Pass to beyond Evolution Lake, due to the ban on fires above 9,600 feet.) You then ford Evolution Creek (840.8–11,372') and descend into Evolution Basin, where there are almost no campsites. There is simply not enough ground that is dry, flat, large enough, and stone-free enough to lie down on between Wanda and Evolution Lakes.

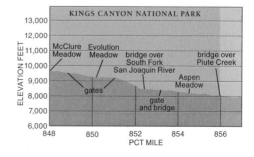

KINGS CANYON NATIONAL PARK

ELEVATION FEET

McClure   Evolution
Meadow   Meadow

bridge over
South Fork
San Joaquin River

bridge over
Piute Creek

gates

Aspen
Meadow

gate
and bridge

PCT MILE

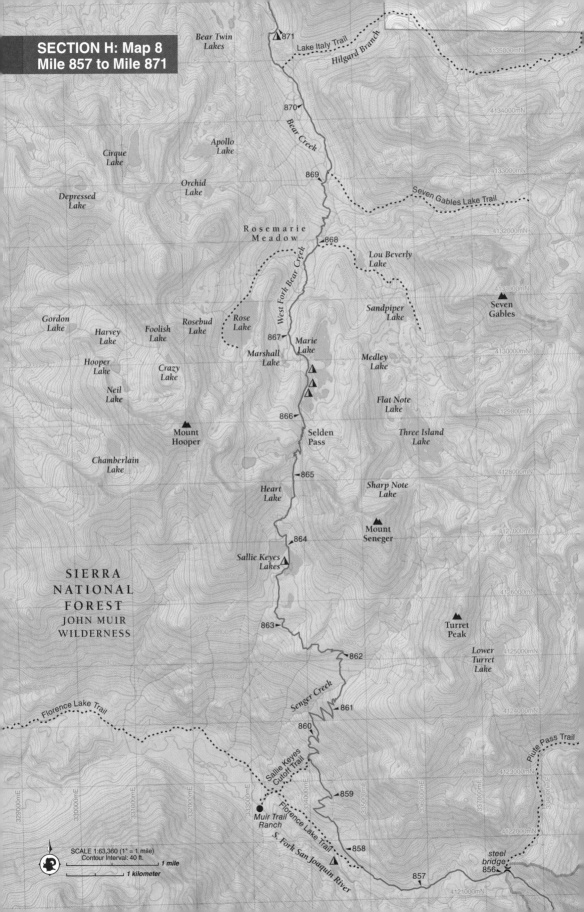

871

Bear Twin Lakes

Lake Italy Trail

Hilgard Branch

4135000mN

870

Bear Creek

4134000mN

869

Apollo Lake

Cirque Lake

4133000mN

Seven Gables Lake Trail

Orchid Lake

868

Depressed Lake

Rosemarie Meadow

4132000mN

Lou Beverly Lake

West Fork Bear Creek

Seven Gables

Sandpiper Lake

4131000mN

Gordon Lake

Rosebud Lake

Rose Lake

867

Marie Lake

Foolish Lake

Harvey Lake

Medley Lake

4130000mN

Marshall Lake

Hooper Lake

Crazy Lake

Flat Note Lake

Neil Lake

866

Selden Pass

Three Island Lake

4129000mN

Mount Hooper

Chamberlain Lake

865

4128000mN

Heart Lake

Sharp Note Lake

864

4127000mN

Mount Seneger

Sallie Keyes Lakes

SIERRA NATIONAL FOREST

JOHN MUIR WILDERNESS

863

4126000mN

Turret Peak

862

Lower Turret Lake

4125000mN

Senger Creek

861

Florence Lake Trail

4124000mN

Piute Pass Trail

860

Sallie Keyes Cutoff Trail

4123000mN

859

Muir Trail Ranch

Florence Lake Trail

858

4122000mN

S. Fork San Joaquin River

steel bridge

856

857

4121000mN

329000mE   330000mE   331000mE   332000mE   333000mE   334000mE   335000mE   336000mE   337000mE   338000mE

SCALE 1:63,360 (1" = 1 mile)
Contour Interval: 40 ft.

1 mile

1 kilometer

GEOLOGY The land here is nearly as scoured as when the ice left it more than 10,000 years ago, and the aspect all around is one of newborn nakedness. To the east is a series of tremendous peaks named for Charles Darwin and other major evolutionary thinkers, and the next lake and the valley below it also bear the name Evolution.

The trail fords the stream at the inlet of Evolution Lake, skirts the lake, and then drops sharply into Evolution Valley.

TRAIL INFO The marvelous meadows here are the reason for rerouting the trail through the forest, so the fragile grassland can recover from overtramping by earlier backpackers and horsepackers.

CAMPING After crossing the multi-branched stream that drains Darwin Canyon, you pass Colby Meadow, with many good campsites. Farther along, at McClure Meadow (848.2–9,652') you will find a summer ranger midway along the meadow and more campsites.

After further descent and several boulder fords of tributaries, you meet the head of Evolution Meadow and begin looking for a good spot to ford the wide, placid waters (which may be difficult in early season) of Evolution Creek (850.9–9,201').

After passing overlooks of some beautiful falls and cascades on the creek, the trail switchbacks steeply down to the South Fork San Joaquin River's canyon floor and detours upstream to cross a log footbridge (852.4–8,482') over the South Fork San Joaquin River to reach the junction with Goddard Canyon/Hell for Sure Pass Trail.

CAMPING Staying on the PCT northwest-bound along the west bank of the river, heading downstream, you pass numerous campsites, recross the river on another bridge, and stroll past Aspen Meadow, where you'll find a few more campsites.

From this hospitable riverside slope, you roll on down and out of Kings Canyon National Park at the steel-bridge crossing of Piute Creek. Here, where you enter John Muir Wilderness, the Piute Pass Trail (855.9–8,072') starts north toward North Lake. Our trail continues west down the South Fork San Joaquin River canyon, away from the river, to a junction with the Florence Lake Trail (857.7–7,889').

RESUPPLY ACCESS

The Florence Lake road-end is 11 miles west down this trail; the private Muir Trail Ranch is 1.5 miles down it. The latter is a possible package drop. It accepts hiker resupply packages and sells stove fuel and a few emergency supplies (but no food unless you are an overnight guest). Packages are delivered to the ranch via pack animals. The company has specific packing requirements and a substantial fee due to the remote location. For details, visit muirtrail ranch.com/resupply.html.

CAMPING Shortly before the ranch, and about 200 yards west of signs that indicate the JMT is 1.5 miles away, both to the east and to the north, an unsigned trail goes south 0.25 mile down to riverside campsites. From the campsites on the south side of the river, a faint trail leads 150 yards southwest to

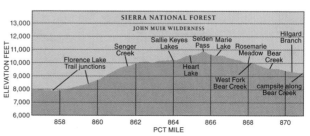

a natural hot spring—great for soaking off the grime, though the river crossing to get to it can be dangerous at high flow.

From the Florence Lake Trail junction, the PCT/JMT veers right to climb the canyon wall. It rises past a lateral trail down to the Sallie Keyes Cutoff Trail (859.5–8,411'), crosses little Senger Creek (861.6–9,748'), and levels off in a large meadow below Sallie Keyes Lakes, in which a trail crosses their outlet creek and then descends south to the canyon floor. Shortly, the trail briefly ascends to the southeastern Sallie Keyes Lake, parallels its west shore, and then crosses the outlet (863.7–10,200') of the northwestern lake.

CAMPING Fair campsites are located at both lakes.

Leaving the forest below, the trail skirts small Heart Lake and presently reaches barren Selden Pass (865.6–10,910'). At this pass, many-islanded Marie Lake is the central feature of the view north, and soon you boulder-hop its clear outlet and then descend moderately to the green expanses of Rosemarie Meadow.

CAMPING From this grassland a trail forks left (867.9–10,037'), soon climbing southwest to Rose Lake, and about 0.25 mile beyond, a trail departs east for Lou Beverly Lake (and eventually Sandpiper Lake). Both Rose and Lou Beverly Lakes provide good, secluded camping; avoid expanding or degrading the sites.

About 200 yards past the last junction, you bridge West Fork Bear Creek (avoid a use trail westward on this ford's north side), and then you make a 1-mile descent in lodgepole forest to a boulder ford of Bear Creek (very difficult in early season), where blueberry bushes line the banks and may provide a welcome snack in late summer.

On the creek's far bank you meet the Seven Gables Lake Trail (869.2–9,578'), which goes up East Fork Bear Creek, but you turn left (downcanyon) and descend gently to the log

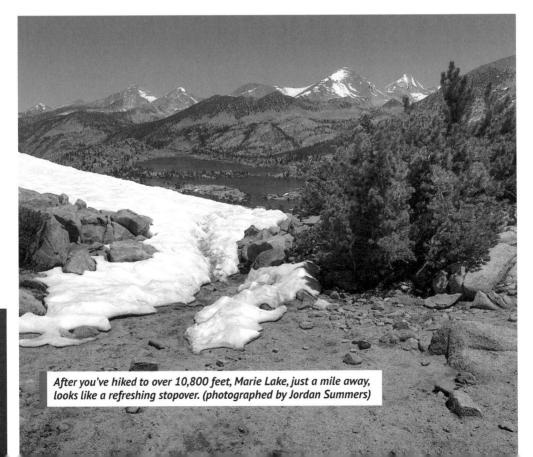

After you've hiked to over 10,800 feet, Marie Lake, just a mile away, looks like a refreshing stopover. (photographed by Jordan Summers)

SECTION H

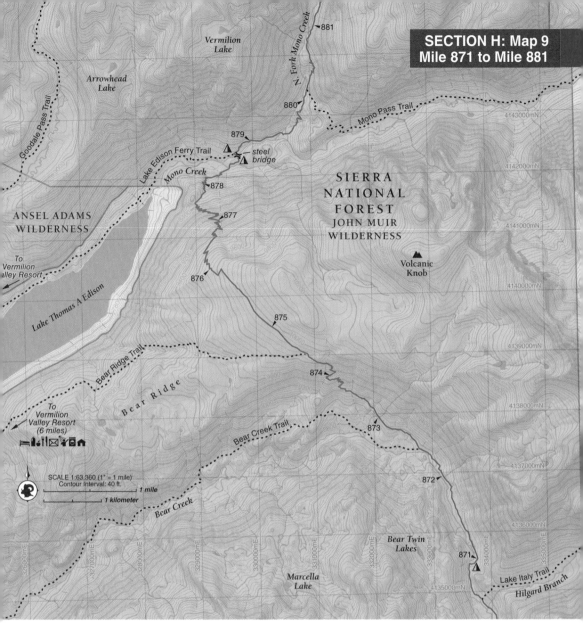

ford of refreshing Hilgard Branch. Immediately beyond, the Lake Italy Trail (870.4–9,328') climbs east, and your trail continues down through the mixed forest cover, always staying near rollicking Bear Creek.

SIDE TRIP Below Hilgard Branch, you reach a junction with the Bear Creek Trail (872.4–8,944') to Bear Diversion Dam. (Those wishing to go to Mono Hot Springs can take this

13-mile trail west to an off-highway vehicle route that leads in 2.5 miles to a paved road; the short spur road

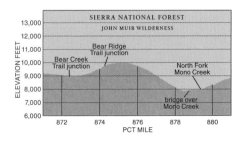

to Mono Hot Springs and its post office lies about 1 mile south on the paved road.)

The PCT gradually veers west as it follows the contour line, fords a difficult tributary, and then turns north at the foot of a tough series of switchbacks. The south-facing hillside gets plenty of sun but is surprisingly wet even in late season. At the crest of Bear Ridge the Bear Ridge Trail (874.5–9,874') begins a dry descent west to the east end of Lake Edison's dam. You can hike 6 miles on the Bear Ridge Trail to Vermilion Valley Resort, or continue a little farther and take the ferry (see "Resupply Access," below). Along the PCT the north side of Bear Ridge is incised with 53 dusty switchbacks.

PLANTS Here you begin in a pure lodgepole forest but successively penetrate the realms of mountain hemlock, western white pine, red fir, Jeffrey pine, aspen, white fir, and, finally, cottonwoods at Mono Creek (878.7–7,877').

RESUPPLY ACCESS

After you cross the footbridge over Mono Creek, you reach a junction with the trail that goes left (west) to Lake Edison and Vermilion Valley Resort, 1 mile and 6 miles away, respectively. Seasonal ferry service (fee) at Lake Edison's head, reached by a signed spur trail, can cut 4.5 miles off your hike to the resort. Campsites lie several hundred yards west down this trail to the resort. Vermilion Valley Resort (559-259-4000; edisonlake.com) accepts hiker resupply packages, UPS only. Address to: Vermilion Valley Resort, c/o Rancheria Garage, 62311 Huntington Lake Road, Lakeshore, CA 93634. Place the hiker's name and ETA on all four sides of the package.

Beyond the bridge, the PCT turns right (east), soon crosses North Fork Mono Creek—a difficult crossing in early season—and climbs to a junction with the Mono Pass Trail (880.1–8,356'). Your steep trail levels briefly at Pocket Meadow, passes a junction with a trail to Mott Lake, and again fords North Fork Mono Creek (881.5–8,993')—very difficult early in the season due to swift, deep, icy water and a rocky streambed (it's one of the JMT's more dangerous fords, where a fall could be fatal). Then you resume climbing steeply on a narrow, rocky, exposed track up the west wall of Mono Creek's canyon.

The first ford of Silver Pass Creek is very difficult in early season. The combination of slippery boulders and icy cascades make this another of the more dangerous fords on the present JMT route; a slip here could be fatal. Above a large meadow, you reford the creek and then rise above treeline. The trail bypasses Silver Pass Lake and then ascends to broad Silver Pass (884.9–10,747'), with a lakelet immediately

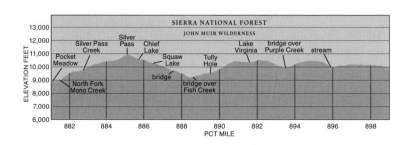

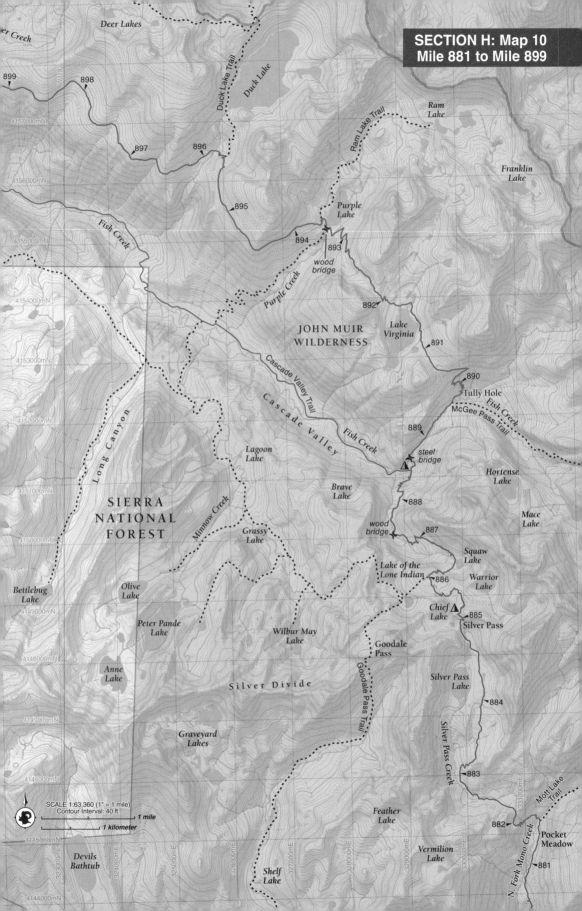

Deer Lakes

Duck Lake Trail

Duck Lake

Ram Lake Trail

Ram Lake

899

898

4157000mN

897

896

Franklin Lake

4156000mN

895

Purple Lake

4155000mN

Fish Creek

894

893

wood bridge

Purple Creek

892

Lake Virginia

891

JOHN MUIR WILDERNESS

4154000mN

4153000mN

Cascade Valley Trail

890

Tully Hole

Fish Creek

McGee Pass Trail

Cascade Valley

889

4152000mN

Long Canyon

Lagoon Lake

Fish Creek

steel bridge

Hortense Lake

Minnow Creek

Brave Lake

888

Mace Lake

4151000mN

SIERRA NATIONAL FOREST

Grassy Lake

wood bridge

887

Squaw Lake

4150000mN

Lake of the Lone Indian

886

Warrior Lake

Bettlebug Lake

Olive Lake

4149000mN

Chief Lake

885

Silver Pass

Peter Pande Lake

Wilbur May Lake

Goodale Pass

Anne Lake

Silver Divide

Goodale Pass Trail

Silver Pass Lake

4148000mN

884

Silver Pass Creek

4147000mN

Graveyard Lakes

883

Mott Lake Trail

SCALE 1:63,360 (1" = 1 mile)
Contour Interval: 40 ft.

1 mile

1 kilometer

Feather Lake

882

Pocket Meadow

4145000mN

N. Fork Mono Creek

881

Devils Bathtub

Shelf Lake

Vermilion Lake

4144000mN

west below it. The descent north passes Chief Lake and then the Goodale Pass Trail (886.0–10,538'), switchbacks northeast down to ford the outlet of Squaw Lake, passes a small meadow whose outlet it crosses on a footbridge, and shortly fords the outlet.

CAMPING It then makes a long, hemlock-lined descent to the beautiful valley of Fish Creek, where there are good campsites near the sometimes hard-to-spot junction with the Cascade Valley Trail (888.5–9,204').

ALTERNATE ROUTE Via the PCT, you are now 18.5 miles from the Rainbow Falls trailhead parking lot near Red's Meadow. Via the Cascade Valley/Fish Creek/Rainbow Falls trail, you are 19.4 miles from it. Some backpackers who aren't committed to following the PCT every step of the way prefer this lower, easier, mostly downhill, less-crowded route. Camping opportunities are greater and, if you're experiencing bad weather, you'll find this lower, well-forested route far more hospitable.

If you stay on the PCT, turn right from the Cascade Valley Trail junction and ascend northeast, soon crossing Fish Creek on a steel bridge. Staying above this good-size creek, the route ascends gently to Tully Hole (889.5–9,524'), a well-flowered grassland where the McGee Pass Trail departs eastward. Now the PCT climbs steeply north up a band of Mesozoic metavolcanics that sweep east and grade into the Paleozoic metasediments of dominating Red Slate Mountain (13,163').

Beyond the crest of this ascent you reach deep-blue Lake Virginia (891.6–10,350').

Early in the season you will have to wade across the head of the lake or detour rather far north. From this boggy crossing, your trail climbs to a saddle below the nearly vertical northeast face of Peak 11,147 and then switchbacks down to heavily used Purple Lake (893.5–9,917'). Just beyond the lake's outlet a trail begins its descent into deep Cascade Valley. Camping is prohibited within 100 yards of the outlet, making camping in this area impossible. In late summer and in dry years, you may not have any trailside water until Deer Creek, 7.5 miles ahead, so plan accordingly.

From Purple Lake the rocky trail climbs west and then bends north as it levels out high on the wall of glaciated Cascade Valley. Soon you reach a trail (895.7–10,174') to Duck Lake and beyond, which could be used to escape bad weather or to resupply at Mammoth Lakes.

Just beyond the Duck Lake Trail, you ford Duck Creek before traversing first southwest and then northwest.

VIEWS If you sharpen your gaze, you will see both red firs and Jeffrey pines above 10,000 feet on this north wall of Cascade Valley, well above their normal range. You also have views of the Silver Divide in the south as you slant northwest and descend gradually through mixed conifers.

CAMPING From the south slopes of Peak 10,519, the trail begins a westward descent, crossing about a mile of lava-flow rubble before turning north for a rambling drop to Deer Creek (901.0–9,115'). Here you'll find fair, lodgepole-shaded campsites.

In the next 0.7 mile the trail starts west, climbs briefly over a granitic ridge, and then descends north to a creek crossing in a long, slender meadow. Heading north through it you have views of The Thumb (10,286'), then

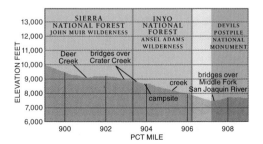

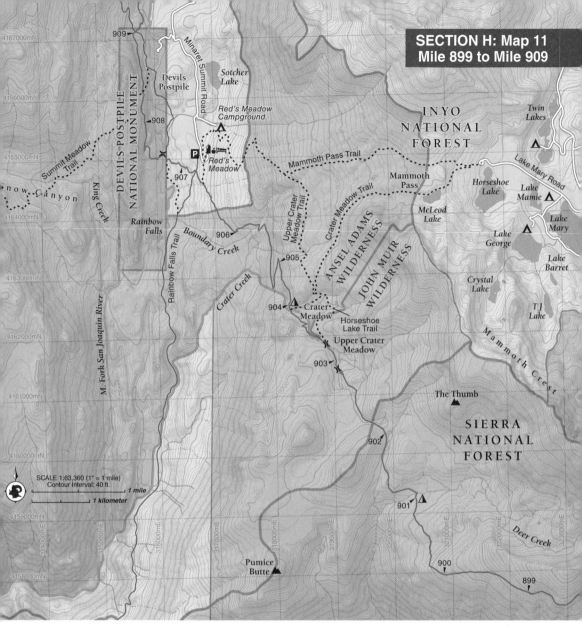

SECTION H: Map 11
Mile 899 to Mile 909

leave this county-line meadow as you cross a seasonal creeklet. You parallel this freshet for about a mile as you descend a bit to Upper Crater Meadow (903.0–8,931').

RESUPPLY ACCESS

In the northwest part of the meadow, two trails (903.9–8,660'), 0.6 mile apart, head northeast to popular Horseshoe Lake. From it,

Lake Mary Road starts a 4.9-mile descent to a junction with Minaret Road in bustling, recreation-oriented Mammoth Lakes. See "Supplies" on page 287 for the seasonal shuttle bus route to the town. If you would rather hike to it and back, then take the following 7.25-mile route, of which the first

5 miles are on trails and lightly used roads.

You can start from either of the two junctions in Upper Crater Meadow. Both trails go about 1.5 miles before a junction, from which you take the Crater Meadow Trail about 1 mile northeast to broad Mammoth Pass. Just east beyond it, you reach the north shore of McCloud Lake, and beyond it continue ahead about 0.5 mile down to a road on the northwest shore of Horseshoe Lake. Walk over to the north end of the lake, from which you could take the aforementioned Lake Mary Road to town.

A shorter, quieter way to town, however, is to go 0.25 mile east on the road, take a spur road 0.25 mile north past houses to its end, and, on a trail, head east, dropping about 300 feet to the west end of Twin Lakes Campground. Continue east through the campground to a road that parallels the east shores of the Twin Lakes. You take this road about 0.5 mile north to Lake Mary Road, on which you walk 2.25 miles to town.

CAMPING Those adhering to the PCT start down along the creek you've been following, cross it in 0.5 mile, and then descend to a recrossing with a good campsite (903.9–8,660'), the last one before Red's Meadow. Here a trail heads northeast to Horseshoe Lake.

Also, this is where you leave John Muir Wilderness for good and enter Ansel Adams Wilderness for a short spell.

GEOLOGY This creekside campsite lies between the two Red Cones, products of very recent volcanic eruptions. The northern one is easy to climb and offers a fine view of the Ritter Range and Middle Fork San Joaquin River's deep canyon. You'll also see Mammoth Mountain (11,053') in the north–northeast, on whose north slopes tens of thousands of skiers, most of them from Southern California, may be found on a busy day. This mountain is a volcano that began to grow just over 100,000 years ago. The area around it, including the upper canyon of Middle Fork San Joaquin River, has been volcanically active for more than 3 million years; the last eruption occurred less than 1,000 years ago. It is the Sierra's "hot spot"—ironic, considering that it is also a mecca for skiers due to its large, late-melting snowpack.

Beyond the creekside campsite between the Red Cones, the PCT makes lazy switchbacks down to Boundary Creek (905.7–8,039'). Roughly midway between it and the next junction, you cross a smaller creek, where you exit from an east lobe of Ansel Adams Wilderness. Through a fir forest your well-graded route descends to an abandoned stagecoach road (906.6–7,718').

RESUPPLY ACCESS

CAMPING Now on a broad path, you can walk about 300 yards north on it to Red's Meadow Pack Station. Another 230 yards north on a paved road takes you to Red's Meadow Resort, with a store and café, at road's end. Beyond that is Red's Meadow Campground. From the resort, and from a number

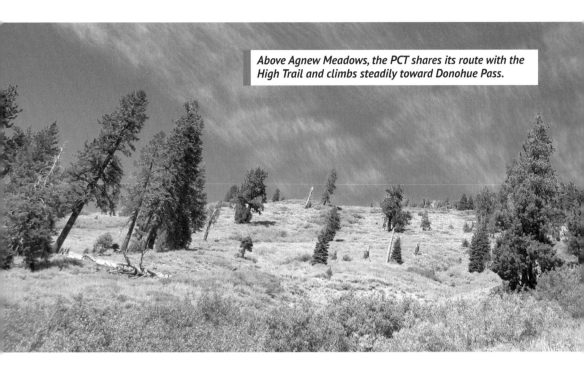

Above Agnew Meadows, the PCT shares its route with the High Trail and climbs steadily toward Donohue Pass.

of roadside stops as far north as Agnew Meadows, you can take a shuttle bus to the Mammoth Lakes area (see "Supplies" on page 287).

Past the abandoned stagecoach road, you immediately cross a horse trail that climbs briefly north to the pack station, reaching it at a switchback in the paved road. Just past this horse trail the PCT descends to a crossing of the Rainbow Falls Trail (906.8–7,629').

SIDE TRIP This popular trail starts from the Rainbow Falls trailhead parking lot, about 250 yards north of the PCT. If you have the time, hike 1 mile south on this trail for a view of Rainbow Falls. Afternoon is the best time to see and photograph this waterfall, as well as the columns of Devils Postpile, just ahead.

Beyond the Rainbow Falls Trail, you curve southwest over to a low, nearby crest from which an old trail, essentially abandoned, heads north, and then you meander northwest down to a trail junction (907.2–7,480') by the east boundary of Devils Postpile National Monument.

ALTERNATE ROUTE Here you can leave the PCT and head 0.5 mile north to a junction, crossing a creek from Sotcher Lake just before you reach it. From this junction, at the base of a Devils Postpile lava flow, you can head 0.25 mile east to the paved road mentioned earlier, then hike a few yards north on it to the entrance to Red's Meadow Campground, which has public restrooms and a freshwater spigot nearby.

From the lava-flow junction the alternate route climbs 0.25 mile northwest to a ridge, from which

SECTION H

you can take a short trail up to the glacially polished top of the Devils Postpile. The main trail skirts along the base of this columnar lava flow, reaching a junction in about 0.25 mile, just beyond a junction with a trail from the top of the lava flow. If you were to continue straight ahead from this second junction, you'd reach the monument's small visitor center and its adjacent campground in about 0.3 mile. Instead, to regain the PCT, you turn left at the second junction, descend to a nearby bridge over the San Joaquin River, and in a minute reach a junction. From here, head 0.4 mile north to the PCT.

Back at the monument's east boundary, PCT purists immediately cross the San Joaquin River on a sturdy bridge, wind west past two seasonal ponds, and then make a struggling climb north through deep pumice to an intersection with the Summit Meadow Trail (908.3–7,710′). Northbound, this trail descends 0.25 mile to meet the alternate route, while the PCT contours along pumice-laden slopes, soon reaching the end of the alternate route (909.0–7,681′). Here the JMT and PCT, which have coincided through most of this hiking section, diverge for about 13 miles, becoming one tread again near Thousand Island Lake. On their divergence, both quickly reenter Ansel Adams Wilderness, though the PCT briefly leaves it in the Agnew Meadows area.

ALTERNATE ROUTE Briefly, the 12.9-mile JMT segment—the more popular of the two—climbs to a trail junction near Minaret Creek, quickly crosses the creek, and winds over to another junction by Johnston Meadow, 1.4 miles from the PCT junction. The JMT climbs past knee-deep Trinity Lakes, then later makes a three-stage descent to Shadow Lake, dropping to shallow Gladys and ideal Rosalie Lakes along the way (6.1 and 6.8 miles, respectively, from the PCT junction). You can camp at either lake but not at Shadow Lake. However, good-to-excellent campsites abound in the 0.7-mile JMT stretch west of the lake, up along Shadow Creek. No campfires are allowed along this stretch, but stoves are permitted. From the creek the JMT climbs 1.9 miles to a high ridge, then drops 0.75 mile to the east end of Garnet Lake, which is off-limits to camping. Ruby Lake, about 1.3 miles farther, offers one campsite, as does Emerald Lake, just beyond it. Emerald, however, is probably the best lake along this 12.9-mile route for swimming. No camping is allowed near the east end of Thousand Island Lake.

Back where the JMT and PCT split, the pumice-lined PCT winds down to the tributaries of Minaret Creek (909.6–7,617′), which must be waded except late in the season, just below dramatic Minaret Falls. Still in pumice, the trail bends northeast and almost touches the Middle Fork San Joaquin River before climbing north away from it over a lava-flow bench that overlooks Pumice Flat. In a shady forest of lodgepole pines and red firs, you make a brief descent to a bridge across the Middle Fork. From the far side of the bridge, a trail heads just around the corner to the west end of Upper Soda Springs Campground. Beyond the bridge you head upriver, having many

To Agnew Pass
and Clark Lakes

922

Summit
Lake

921

Emerald
Lake

Badger
Lakes

920

San Joaquin
Mountain ▲

OWENS RIVER
HEADWATERS
WILDERNESS

Thousand
Island
Lake

Ruby
Lake

John Muir Trail

Altha
Lake

River Trail

919

▲ Two Teats

Garnet
Lake

Clarice
Lake

918

Laura
Lake

Shadow Creek Trail

Olaine
Lake

917

Deadman
Pass

Nydiver Lakes

Shadow
Lake

Shadow Creek

M. Fork San Joaquin River

916

Agnew
Meadows

High Trail
Trailhead

Ediza
Lake

Cabin
Lake

Rosalie
Lake

Gladys
Lake

914

915

To Mammoth
Lakes and
203

INYO
NATIONAL
FOREST
ANSEL ADAMS
WILDERNESS

Lois
Lake

Emily
Lake

Vivian
Lake

913

Iceberg
Lake

Volcanic Ridge

Castle
Lake

912

Starkweather
Lake

Cecile
Lake

Minaret
Lake

Upper
Soda Springs
Campground

911

Deadhorse
Lake

Minaret Creek Trail

Minaret Creek

John Muir Trail

910

Pumice Flat

SCALE 1:63,360 (1" = 1 mile)
Contour Interval: 40 ft.

1 mile

1 kilometer

Johnston
Lake

Minaret
Falls

Superior Lake Trail

909

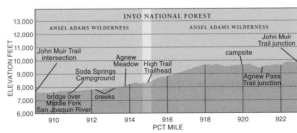

INYO NATIONAL FOREST

ANSEL ADAMS WILDERNESS

ANSEL ADAMS WILDERNESS

John Muir
Trail junction

John Muir Trail
intersection

Agnew
Meadow

High Trail
Trailhead

campsite

Soda Springs
Campground

Agnew Pass
Trail junction

bridge over
Middle Fork
San Joaquin River

creeks

ELEVATION FEET

13,000
12,000
11,000
10,000
9,000
8,000
7,000
6,000

910   912   914   916   918   920   922
PCT MILE

opportunities to drop to nearby eating, drinking, and chilly swimming spots along the dashing Middle Fork. After crossing a stream, the trail bends from north to northwest and crosses a second stream. Then, just past a small knoll, it reaches a junction (913.6–8,078').

Leaving the river route, the PCT first parallels it northwest, then climbs via short switchbacks to a junction with the River Trail (914.1–8,285'). You start east up it and in 80 yards meet a fork. The left fork goes 0.4 mile northeast to Agnew Meadows Campground. From here you can walk another 0.4 mile east on a winding dirt road, along which you'll find the PCT's resumption by a trailhead parking area.

WATER ACCESS

Taking the right (southeast) fork, you hike through a long, narrow trough before curving northeast around a meadow, almost touching the ranger's trailer (with a parking area) before reaching Agnew Meadows Road (914.8–8,311'), which has water and a pit toilet by the High Trail trailhead parking area.

RESUPPLY ACCESS

The main road to Red's Meadow lies 0.25 mile east, and at that junction is the first of several stops made by shuttle buses from Mammoth Mountain Inn (see "Supplies" on page 287).

From the Agnew Meadows road, the PCT shares its route with the signed High Trail,

which switchbacks upward about 400 vertical feet before climbing northwest.

WATER ACCESS

Creeks, creeklets, and springs abound along this section of the PCT. The volcanic-rock formations above us store plenty of water, which they slowly release throughout the summer.

GEOLOGY Views are relatively few until about 2.5 miles beyond the top of the switchbacks, and then the Ritter Range explodes on the scene, with Shadow Lake and the Minarets, both across the canyon, vying for your attention. Views and water abound over the next 2 miles of alternating brushy and forested slopes.

Soon you arrive at a junction with a trail (920.4–9,735') that climbs easily over Agnew Pass to good camps near the largest of the Clark Lakes, about 1.1 miles distant. Summit Lake, just before the pass, is good for swimming but a bit short on level camping spots.

From the junction, the High Trail runs concurrent with the PCT and now descends, crossing Summit Lake's seasonal outlet creek before climbing briefly to an intersection (921.0–9,507'). Westward, your climb abates and in 0.3 mile you reach a de facto trail, which you'll find just past a lakelet on your left.

CAMPING This trail goes 0.2 mile southeast to good camps—the last legal campsites on the PCT this side of Rush Creek—beside the largest of the Badger Lakes, which is the only one that is more than waist-deep. It is one of the best lakes in the entire Ansel Adams Wilderness. Be sure to set up camp at least 200 feet from the shore to help preserve the lake's beauty.

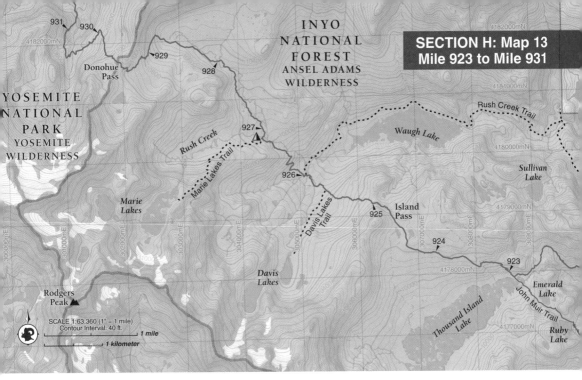

INYO
NATIONAL
FOREST
ANSEL ADAMS
WILDERNESS

YOSEMITE
NATIONAL
PARK
YOSEMITE
WILDERNESS

931 930
929
Donohue
Pass
928
927
926
Rush Creek
Marie Lakes Trail
Marie
Lakes
Waugh Lake
Rush Creek Trail
Sullivan
Lake
Island
925 Pass
924
923
Davis Lakes Trail
Davis
Lakes
Rodgers
Peak
Thousand Island
Lake
Emerald
Lake
John Muir Trail
Ruby
Lake

SCALE 1:63,360 (1" = 1 mile)
Contour Interval: 40 ft.
1 mile
1 kilometer

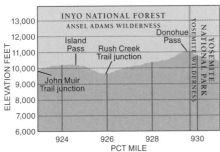

Elevation profile: INYO NATIONAL FOREST / ANSEL ADAMS WILDERNESS / YOSEMITE NATIONAL PARK / YOSEMITE WILDERNESS. Labels: John Muir Trail junction, Island Pass, Rush Creek Trail junction, Donohue Pass. ELEVATION FEET axis 6,000–13,000; PCT MILE axis 924–930.

Leaving the Badger Lakes area, you continue west, passing a third trail to the Clark Lakes in 0.25 mile. Soon you make a brief descent to a junction with the River Trail (921.9–9,610'), then climb moderately northwest before rambling southwest to a reunion with the JMT near the east end of spreading Thousand Island Lake (922.9–9,846').

CAMPING Camping is prohibited within 0.25 mile of this lake's outlet but is legal elsewhere. Keep in mind that it gets so busy here in summer that some like to call it Thousand Hiker Lake.

The PCT climbs moderately through a thinning forest to two lakelets, reached just before Island Pass (924.6–10,227'). The trail then traverses 0.3 mile to a ridge before descending to a sometimes obscure junction (925.6–9,699').

SIDE TRIP From here the Davis Lakes Trail climbs 0.8 mile south to the tip of lower Davis Lake. Campsites by it are small and quite exposed, but the beauty of this lake and its surroundings makes them a worthy goal.

About 250 yards past the Davis Lakes Trail junction, you reach the first of several Rush Creek forks. Along the 0.5-mile trail segment that ensues, early-season hikers may have three wet fords to make. You may want to keep your boots off until the last ford, just before a junction with the Rush Creek Trail (925.9–9,645').

RESUPPLY ACCESS

This trail descends a lengthy 9.5 miles to popular Silver Lake on well-traveled CA 158 (June Lake Loop Road). As such, you will want to take it only for emergency reasons. While you can get supplies in the town of June Lake, the effort is not worth it.

CAMPING Leaving the forks, you quickly make some short, steep switchbacks northwest up to a ridge, then cross the ridge and ease up to a junction with the Marie Lakes Trail (926.9–10,062'). Just beyond the junction, you'll find some campsites by Rush Creek, which is best crossed at an obvious jump-across spot slightly downstream.

After the ford, the trail winds excessively in an oft-futile attempt to avoid the boulders and bogs of the increasingly alpine environment. Whitebark pines diminish in number and stature as you climb toward a conspicuous saddle—easily mistaken in early season for Donohue Pass. After a wet slog across the tundra-and-stone floor of your alpine basin, you veer southwest toward a prominent peak and ascend a sometimes obscure trail past blocks and over slabs to the real, signed, tarn-blessed Donohue Pass (929.5–11,073'), where you leave Ansel Adams Wilderness.

The Yosemite high country unfolds before you as you descend northwest, partly in a long, straight fracture (southbound hikers take note). You then curve west to a sharp bend southwest, a few yards from which you can get a commanding panorama of Mount Lyell, at 13,114 feet Yosemite's highest peak, and deep Lyell Canyon. Leaving the bend, you now descend southwest 0.5 mile to the north end of a boulder-dotted tarn that occasionally reflects Lyell and its broad glacier—the largest one you'll see in the Sierra. Contour along the tarn's west shore, then briefly climb southwest to a gap in a low ridge. Next wind north and soon begin a steep northeast descent that ends at the north end of a small

meadow, where you cross Lyell Fork, usually via boulders (931.2–10,186'). Immediately above this crossing, the creek has widened almost to a narrow lake, and trekkers ascending in the opposite direction may assume (incorrectly) that they have reached the aforementioned tarn.

CAMPING There is no camping in the meadow area anymore, but large developed campsites soon appear on a forested bench by another Lyell Fork crossing (932.1–9,651'), via a bridge. In Yosemite National Park campfires are banned here and everywhere else above 9,600 feet. This is the last camping opportunity before you reach Tuolumne Meadows; camping is prohibited between here and 4 miles north of CA 120.

Now you'll stay on the west bank of the river all the way to Tuolumne Meadows. Beyond the bench you make your last major descent—a steep one—partly across rock-avalanche slopes down to the southern, upper end of Lyell Canyon. Your hike to CA 120 is now an easy, level, usually open stroll along meandering Lyell Fork.

Past the junction with a trail to Evelyn Lake and Vogelsang High Sierra Camp (936.1–8,888'), occasional backward glances at receding Potter Point mark your progress north along trout-inhabited Lyell Fork.

Shortly after Potter Point finally disappears from view, you curve northwest, descend between two bedrock outcrops, and then contour west. This area abounds in mosquitoes through late July, as does most of the Tuolumne Meadows area. Two-branched Rafferty Creek soon appears; its main branch can be crossed on a bridge. Just beyond it you meet the Vogelsang Trail (940.2–8,722'), which

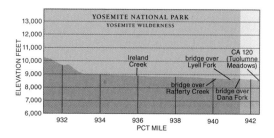

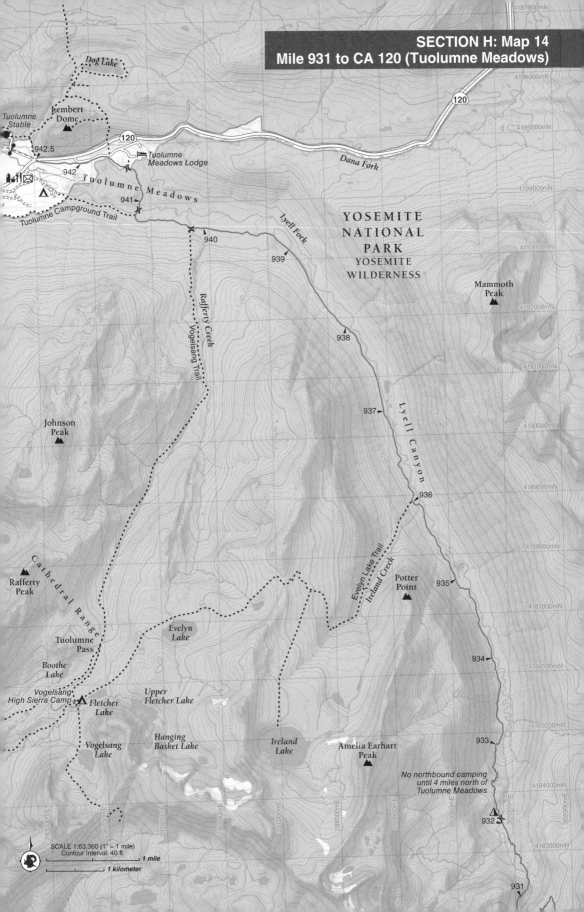

120

Dog Lake

Tuolumne Stable

Lembert Dome

942.5

120

Tuolumne Meadows Lodge

942

Tuolumne Meadows

941

Tuolumne Campground Trail

940

939

Lyell Fork

Dana Fork

YOSEMITE NATIONAL PARK
YOSEMITE WILDERNESS

Mammoth Peak

938

Rafferty Creek

Vogelsang Trail

937

Lyell Canyon

Johnson Peak

936

Cathedral Range

Rafferty Peak

Evelyn Lake Trail

Ireland Creek

Potter Point

935

Evelyn Lake

934

Tuolumne Pass

Boothe Lake

Vogelsang High Sierra Camp

Fletcher Lake

Upper Fletcher Lake

Ireland Lake

Amelia Earhart Peak

933

Vogelsang Lake

Hanging Basket Lake

No northbound camping until 4 miles north of Tuolumne Meadows

932

SCALE 1:63,360 (1" = 1 mile)
Contour Interval: 40 ft.

1 mile

1 kilometer

931

parallels Rafferty Creek and is part of the scenic and popular High Sierra Loop Trail. You continue west and soon meet another junction (940.8–8,669').

SIDE TRIP From here a trail goes 0.75 mile west to a junction immediately east of Tuolumne Meadows Campground, which has sites for backpackers and other nonmotorized walk-in visitors with overnight wilderness permits. It is generally open mid-July–September. From that junction the left branch skirts the campground's south perimeter, while the right branch quickly ends at the campground's main road. This road leads 0.5 mile west to CA 120, and just southwest on it, you'll find services.

Rather than head for the campground, you turn right (north) and soon come to bridges across the Lyell Fork. A photo pause here is well worth it, particularly when clouds are building over Mounts Dana and Gibbs in the northeast. A short, winding climb north followed by an equal descent brings you to a sturdy bridge across the Dana Fork (941.5–8,688') of the Tuolumne River, this bridging being only 130 yards past a junction with an east-climbing trail to the Gaylor Lakes. Immediately beyond the bridge you meet a short spur trail (signed) to the Tuolumne Meadows Lodge.

RESUPPLY ACCESS

The lodge, open seasonally from about late June until late September, offers showers, hot meals, and boxed lunches; reservations are required at dinner: 209-372-8413.

You parallel the Dana Fork downstream and soon hear the water making its small drop into a clear pool, almost cut in two by a protruding granite finger. At the base of this finger, about 8–10 feet down, there is a hole in it, essentially an underwater arch, which is an extremely rare feature in any kind of rock. Just beyond the pool you approach the lodge's road (941.7–8,671'), where a short path climbs a few yards up to it and takes you to the entrance of a large parking lot for backpackers. Now you parallel the paved road west, passing the Tuolumne Meadows Ranger Station and quickly reaching a junction. The main road curves north to the sometimes noisy highway, but you follow the spur road west, to where it curves into a second large parking lot for backpackers. In its east end you'll find an office where a summer ranger dispenses wilderness permits. The road past the lot diminishes to a wide trail before you arrive at this section's end, CA 120 (942.5–8,596'), across from the start of the Soda Springs road.

RESUPPLY ACCESS

A campground, store, and post office lie on CA 120 just southwest of the Tuolumne River bridge.

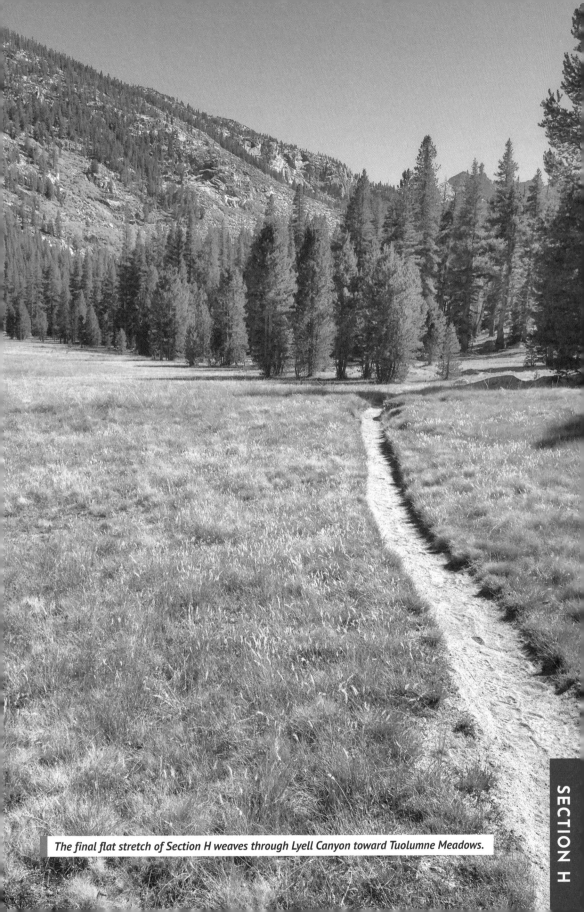

The final flat stretch of Section H weaves through Lyell Canyon toward Tuolumne Meadows.

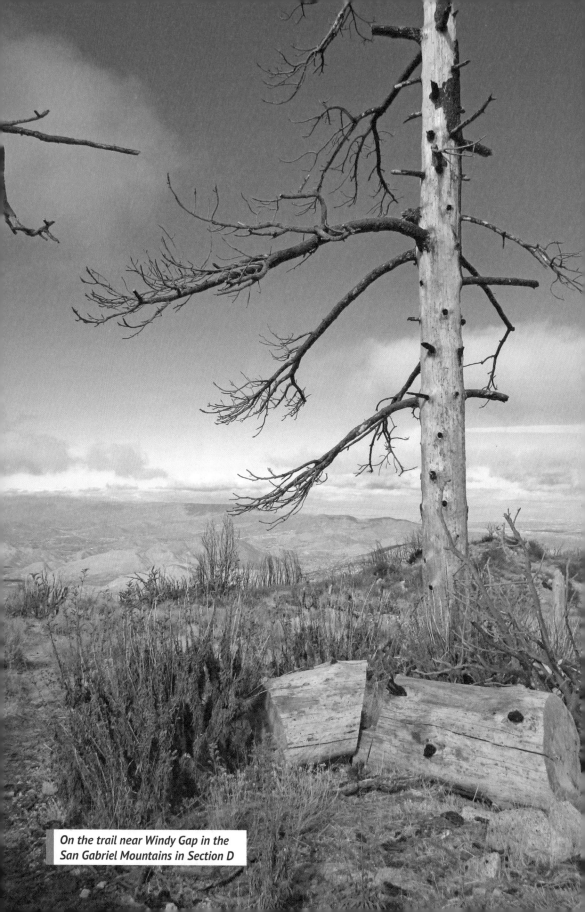

On the trail near Windy Gap in the
San Gabriel Mountains in Section D

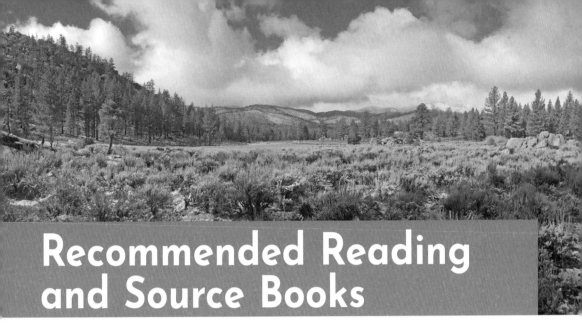

Recommended Reading and Source Books

Note: An asterisk (*) indicates an out-of-print book.

PACIFIC CREST TRAIL (PCT)

Berger, Karen, and Daniel R. Smith. *The Pacific Crest Trail: A Hiker's Companion.* 2nd ed. New York: The Countryman Press, 2014.

Bodnar, Paul. *Pocket PCT: Complete Data and Town Guide.* 4th ed. Scotts Valley, CA: CreateSpace Independent Publishing, 2016.

Clarke, Clinton C. *The Pacific Crest Trailway.* Pasadena, CA: The Pacific Crest Trail System Conference, 1945.*

Davis, Zach, and Carly Moree. *Pacific Crest Trials: A Psychological and Emotional Guide to Successfully Thru-Hiking the Pacific Crest Trail.* Golden, CO: Pacific Crest Trials, 2016.

Doherty, Kathleen Dodge, and Jordan Summers. *Day & Section Hikes: John Muir Trail.* Birmingham, AL: Menasha Ridge Press, 2017.

Egbert, Barbara. *Zero Days: The Real-Life Adventure of Captain Bligh, Nellie Bly, and 10-Year-Old Scrambler on the Pacific Crest Trail.* Berkeley: Wilderness Press, 2008.

Gerald, Paul. *Day & Section Hikes, Pacific Crest Trail: Oregon.* 3rd ed. Birmingham, AL: Wilderness Press, 2019.

Go, Benedict. *Pacific Crest Trail Data Book.* 6th ed. Birmingham, AL: Wilderness Press, 2020.

Green, David. *A Pacific Crest Odyssey: Walking the Trail from Mexico to Canada.* Berkeley: Wilderness Press, 1979.*

Harris, David. *Day & Section Hikes, Pacific Crest Trail: Southern California.* Birmingham, AL: Wilderness Press, 2012.

Above: A spacious view in Section G of Monache Meadow, the largest meadow in the Sierra (courtesy of the Pacific Crest Trail Association)

Hazard, Joseph T. *Pacific Crest Trails*. Seattle: Superior Publishing Co., 1946.*

Jardine, Ray. *The Pacific Crest Trail Hiker's Handbook*. 2nd ed. Arizona City, AZ: AdventureLore Books, 1996.*

Jenkins, J. C., and Ruby Johnson Jenkins. *Exploring the Southern Sierra: East Side*. 3rd ed. Berkeley: Wilderness Press, 1992.*

———. *Exploring the Southern Sierra: West Side*. 3rd ed. Berkeley: Wilderness Press, 1995.*

Larabee, Mark, and Barney Scout Mann. *The Pacific Crest Trail: Exploring America's Wilderness Trail*. New York: Rizzoli, 2016.

Lautner, Wendy. *Day & Section Hikes, Pacific Crest Trail: Northern California*. Berkeley: Wilderness Press, 2010.

McDonnell, Jackie. *Yogi's Pacific Crest Trail Handbook*. rev. ed. Inyokern, CA: Yogi's Books, 2019.

Ross, Cindy. *Journey on the Crest: Walking 2,600 Miles from Mexico to Canada*. Seattle: Mountaineers Books, 1987.

Ryback, Eric. *The High Adventure of Eric Ryback*. San Francisco: Chronicle Books, 1971.*

Schaefer, Adrienne. *Day & Section Hikes, Pacific Crest Trail: Washington*. 2nd ed. Birmingham, AL: Wilderness Press, 2017.

Strayed, Cheryl. *Wild: From Lost to Found on the Pacific Crest Trail*. New York: Vintage Books, 2013.

BACKPACKING, PACKING, AND MOUNTAINEERING

Back Country Horsemen of Montana. *Back Country Horsemen's Guidebook*. 5th ed. Columbia Falls, MT: Back Country Horsemen of Montana, 2019. bchmt.org/documents/Guide_Book_FINAL2019.pdf.

Back, Joe. *Horses, Hitches, and Rocky Trails*. 1987. Reprint, Denver: Johnson Books, 2018.

Beffort, Brian. *Joy of Backpacking*. Berkeley: Wilderness Press, 2007.

Brame, Rich, and David Cole. *NOLS Soft Paths: Enjoying the Wilderness Without Harming It*. 4th ed. Mechanicsburg, PA: Stackpole Books, 2011.

Brame, Susan C., and Chad Henderson. *NOLS Wilderness Ethics*. rev. ed. Mechanicsburg, PA: Stackpole Books, 2005.

Elser, Smoke, and Bill Brown. *Packin' In on Mules and Horses*. Missoula, MT: Mountain Press, 1980.

Gonzales, Laurence. *Deep Survival: Who Lives, Who Dies and Why*. 2003. Reprinted with a new introduction by the author. New York: W. W. Norton & Co., 2017.

Gookin, John, and Tom Reed. *NOLS Bear Essentials*. Mechanicsburg, PA: Stackpole Books, 2009.

Harvey, Mark. *The National Outdoor Leadership School's Wilderness Guide*. New York: Simon & Schuster, 1999.

Hinch, Stephen. *Outdoor Navigation with GPS*. 3rd ed. Berkeley: Wilderness Press, 2010.

Letham, Lawrence. *GPS Made Easy: Using Global Positioning Systems in the Outdoors*. 5th ed. Seattle: Mountaineers Books, 2008.

Light, Richard A. *Backpacking the Light Way*. Birmingham, AL: Menasha Ridge Press, 2015.

March, Laurie Ann. *A Fork in the Trail: Mouthwatering Meals and Tempting Treats for the Backcountry*. Berkeley: Wilderness Press, 2008.

The Mountaineers. *Mountaineering: The Freedom of the Hills*. 9th ed. Seattle: Mountaineers Books, 2017.

Powers, Phil. *NOLS Wilderness Mountaineering*. 3rd ed. Mechanicsburg, PA: Stackpole Books, 2008.

Schimelpfenig, Tod. *NOLS Wilderness Medicine*. 6th ed. Mechanicsburg, PA: Stackpole Books, 2016.

Tilton, Buck, and John Gookin. *NOLS Winter Camping*. Mechanicsburg, PA: Stackpole Books, 2005.

Trantham, Gene, and Darran Wells. *NOLS Wilderness Navigation*. 3rd ed. Mechanicsburg, PA: Stackpole Books, 2018.

Tremper, Bruce. *Avalanche Essentials: A Step-by-Step System for Safety and Survival*. Seattle: Mountaineers Books, 2013.

Wilkerson, James A., ed. *Hypothermia, Frostbite, and Other Cold Injuries*. 2nd ed. Seattle: Mountaineers Books, 2006.

———. *Medicine for Mountaineering & Other Wilderness Activities*. 6th ed. Seattle: Mountaineers Books, 2010.

HISTORY

Brewer, William H. *Up and Down California in 1860–1864: The Journal of William H. Brewer*. 4th ed. Berkeley: University of California Press, 2003. First published 1930 by Yale University Press (New Haven).

King, Clarence. *Mountaineering in the Sierra Nevada*. 1872. Reprint, Scotts Valley, CA: CreateSpace Independent Publishing, 2016.

Reid, Robert L., ed. *A Treasury of the Sierra Nevada*. Berkeley: Wilderness Press, 1983.*

GEOLOGY

Harden, Deborah R. *California Geology*. 2nd ed. Upper Saddle River, NJ: Prentice Hall, 2004.

Hill, Mary. *Geology of the Sierra Nevada*. 2nd ed. Berkeley: University of California Press, 2006.

Lynch, Dan R., and Bob Lynch. *Rocks & Minerals of California*. Cambridge, MN: Adventure Publications, 2017.

McPhee, John. *Annals of the Former World*. New York: Farrar, Straus and Giroux, 1998.

———. *Assembling California*. New York: Farrar, Straus and Giroux, 1994.

Sylvester, Arthur G., Robert P. Sharp, and Allen F. Glazner. *Geology Underfoot in Southern California*. 2nd ed. Missoula, MT: Mountain Press, 2020.

BIOLOGY

Alden, Peter, and Fred Heath. *National Audubon Society Field Guide to California*. New York: Alfred A. Knopf, 1998.

Jameson, E. W., Jr., and Hans J. Peeters. *Mammals of California*. rev. ed. Berkeley: University of California Press, 2004.

Laws, John Muir. *The Laws Field Guide to the Sierra Nevada*. Berkeley: Heyday Books, 2007.

Murie, Olaus J., and Mark Elbach. *Peterson Field Guide to Animal Tracks*. 3rd ed. Boston: Houghton Mifflin Harcourt, 2005.

Poppele, Jonathan. *Animal Tracks of California*. Cambridge, MN: Adventure Publications, 2017.

Schoenherr, Allan A. *A Natural History of California*. 2nd ed. Berkeley: University of California Press, 2017.

Sibley, David Allen. *The Sibley Guide to Birds*. 2nd ed. New York: Alfred A. Knopf, 2014.

Storer, Tracy I., Robert L. Usinger., and David Lukas. *Sierra Nevada Natural History*. Berkeley: University of California Press, 2004.

Tekiela, Stan. *Birds of California Field Guide*. Cambridge, MN: Adventure Publications, 2003.

BOTANY

Baldwin, Bruce G., Douglas Goldman, David J. Keil, Robert Patterson, Thomas J. Rosatti, and Dieter Wilken, eds. *The Jepson Manual: Higher Plants of California*. 2nd ed. Berkeley: University of California Press, 2012.

Barbour, Michael, Julie M. Evens, Todd Keeler-Wolf, and John O. Sawyer. *California's Botanical Landscapes: A Pictorial View of the State's Vegetation*. Sacramento: California Native Plant Society, 2016.

Blackwell, Laird R. *Wildflowers of California: A Month-by-Month Guide*. Berkeley: University of California Press, 2012.

———. *Wildflowers of the Tahoe Sierra*. Edmonton, AB: Lone Pine Publishing, 1996.

Johnston, Verna R., and Carla J. Simmons. *California Forests and Woodlands: A Natural History*. Berkeley: University of California Press, 1996.

Miller, George. *Wildflowers of Southern California*. Cambridge, MN: Adventure Publications, 2017.

Sawyer, John O., Todd Keeler-Wolf, and Julie Evens. *A Manual of California Vegetation*. 2nd ed. Sacramento: California Native Plant Society, 2009.

Stuart, John David, and John O. Sawyer. *Trees and Shrubs of California*. Berkeley: University of California Press, 2001.

Underhill, J. E. *Sagebrush Wildflowers*. Blaine, WA: Hancock House, 1986.

Watts, Tom. *Pacific Coast Tree Finder*. Rochester, NY: Nature Study Guild Publishers, 2004.

Wenk, Elizabeth. *Wildflowers of the High Sierra and John Muir Trail*. Birmingham, AL: Wilderness Press, 2015.

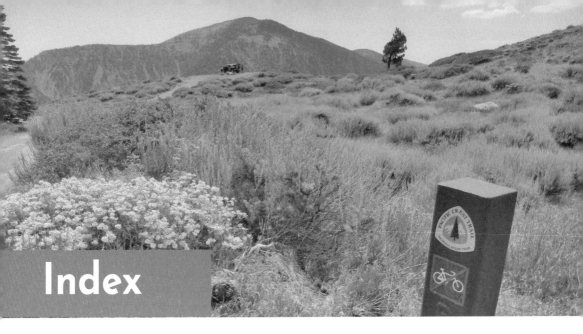

Index

Above: Wildflowers and Jeffrey pines flank the trail above Wrightwood in Section D.

N

O

Taking care of the Pacific Crest Trail is a full-time effort.

The Pacific Crest Trail Association's mission is to protect, preserve and promote the trail as a resource for hikers and equestrians and for the value that wild lands provide to all people.

Through a formal partnership with the U.S. Forest Service, our nonprofit membership organization is the primary caretaker of this 2,650-mile National Scenic Trail as it winds through the American West's most beautiful landscapes.

Each year, PCTA volunteers and paid staff members clear downed trees and repair washed out tread. We monitor threats to the trail and speak up on its behalf. We tell the trail's story in print and online. And we advocate for federal support by visiting our elected leaders in Washington, D.C.

All this effort safeguards the experiences and solitude people deserve when they venture into the wild.

Please help preserve this national treasure for future generations by joining the PCTA.

Your $35 annual membership will ensure that this trail will never end.

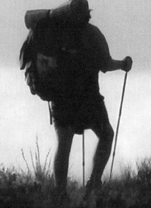

1331 Garden Highway, Suite 230
Sacramento, CA 95833

916-285-1846

www.pcta.org • info@pcta.org

**Pacific Crest Trail
Association**

Josh Meier

ABOUT THE AUTHORS

A journalist with more than 20 years of experience, Los Angeles resident **Laura Randall** has written about travel, film, education, and other topics for major newspapers and magazines, including *The New York Times, The Washington Post, Sunset,* and National Geographic News Service. She is the author of *60 Hikes Within 60 Miles: Los Angeles, Peaceful Places Los Angeles,* and *Day & Overnight Hikes: Palm Springs.*

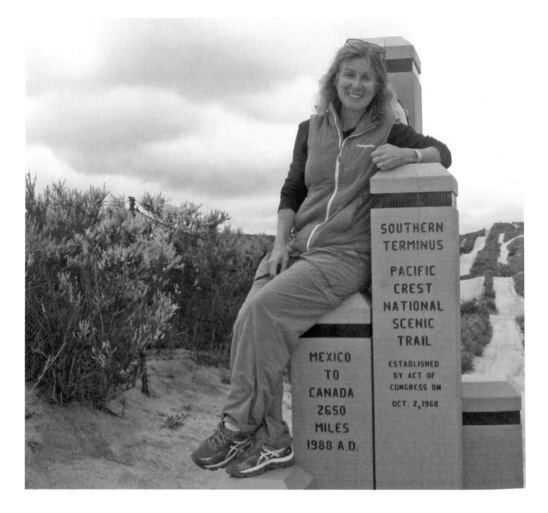

Wilderness Press would also like to acknowledge the contributions of **Ben Schifrin, Ruby Johnson Jenkins, Thomas Winnett,** and **Jeffrey P. Schaffer,** whose text from many prior editions was revised by Laura Randall for this edition.